Blood Transfusion Handbook

Blood Transfusion Handbook

Edited by **Martha Roper**

hayle
medical

New York

Published by Hayle Medical,
30 West, 37th Street, Suite 612,
New York, NY 10018, USA
www.haylemedical.com

Blood Transfusion Handbook
Edited by Martha Roper

International Standard Book Number: 978-1-63241-386-4 (Hardback)

The publisher's policy is to use permanent paper from mills that operate a sustainable forestry policy. Furthermore, the publisher ensures that the text paper and cover boards used have met acceptable environmental accreditation standards.

Trademark Notice: Registered trademark of products or corporate names are used only for explanation and identification without intent to infringe.

Printed in the United States of America.

Contents

Permissions

List of Contributors

Preface

This book was inspired by the evolution of our times; to answer the curiosity of inquisitive minds. Many developments have occurred across the globe in the recent past which has transformed the progress in the field.

Blood is the carrier of oxygen, which is essential for all life forms and for practically carrying out all the biological processes. Blood transfusion is the transfer of blood from one person to another in case of a medical emergency like accident, injury or a disease causing reduction in optimum levels of blood. It is a lifesaving technique. Blood transfusion techniques have seen some advancement over the years. Now only those components are required for transfusions that are present in lower concentration than required. While understanding the long term perspectives of the topics, this book makes an effort in highlighting their impact as a modern tool for the growth of the discipline. It aims to assist those with a goal of delving deeper into the field of blood transfusion. This book, with its detailed analyses and data, will prove immensely beneficial to professionals and students involved in this area at various levels.

This book was developed from a mere concept to drafts to chapters and finally compiled together as a complete text to benefit the readers across all nations. To ensure the quality of the content we instilled two significant steps in our procedure. The first was to appoint an editorial team that would verify the data and statistics provided in the book and also select the most appropriate and valuable contributions from the plentiful contributions we received from authors worldwide. The next step was to appoint an expert of the topic as the Editor-in-Chief, who would head the project and finally make the necessary amendments and modifications to make the text reader-friendly. I was then commissioned to examine all the material to present the topics in the most comprehensible and productive format.

I would like to take this opportunity to thank all the contributing authors who were supportive enough to contribute their time and knowledge to this project. I also wish to convey my regards to my family who have been extremely supportive during the entire project.

Editor

Quality of Red Blood Cells Isolated from Umbilical Cord Blood Stored at Room Temperature

Mariia Zhurova,[1] John Akabutu,[2] and Jason Acker[3]

[1] *Department of Laboratory Medicine and Pathology, University of Alberta, 8249-114 Street, Edmonton, AB, Canada T6G 2R8*
[2] *Alberta Cord Blood Bank, Suite 408 College Plaza, 8215-112 Street, Edmonton, AB, Canada T6G 2C8*
[3] *Research and Development, Canadian Blood Services, 8249-114 Street, Edmonton, AB, Canada T6G 2R8*

Correspondence should be addressed to Jason Acker, jacker@ualberta.ca

Academic Editor: Niranjan Bhattacharya

Red blood cells (RBCs) from cord blood contain fetal hemoglobin that is predominant in newborns and, therefore, may be more appropriate for neonatal transfusions than currently transfused adult RBCs. Post-collection, cord blood can be stored at room temperature for several days before it is processed for stem cells isolation, with little known about how these conditions affect currently discarded RBCs. The present study examined the effect of the duration cord blood spent at room temperature and other cord blood characteristics on cord RBC quality. RBCs were tested immediately after their isolation from cord blood using a broad panel of quality assays. No significant decrease in cord RBC quality was observed during the first 65 hours of storage at room temperature. The ratio of cord blood to anticoagulant was associated with RBC quality and needs to be optimized in future. This knowledge will assist in future development of cord RBC transfusion product.

1. Introduction

Fetal and neonatal anemias are among the most serious complications of pregnancy and postnatal development. The causes of fetal anemia include immune haemolytic disease [1], defects in hemoglobin structure and synthesis, fetomaternal or twin-to-twin hemorrhages, and parvovirus B19 infections [2]. Neonatal anemia, on the other hand, can either result from fetal anemia or develop after birth as a result of hemorrhage due to obstetric accidents, frequent drawing of blood for laboratory testing, or impaired red blood cell (RBC) production by bone marrow [2]. The most commonly used treatments for fetal and neonatal anemia are transfusions of red blood cells (RBCs), either intrauterine [1] or intravenous [3–6], to help replace the lost RBCs of the fetus or neonate.

RBCs used in intrauterine and neonatal (intravenous) transfusions are derived from adult donors [1, 3–7]. Adult RBCs are different from those present in the blood of a fetus or neonate [2, 8–12]. Neonatal RBCs obtained from umbilical cord blood (cord RBCs) are usually discarded during isolation of stem cells from cord blood [13–15]. This

waste product may offer a superior alternative for intrauterine and neonatal transfusions [16, 17].

Cord RBCs are unique cells that differ from adult RBCs in membrane composition and biophysical properties [2, 9], hemoglobin (Hb) structure [2, 8–12, 18], metabolism, and enzymatic profile [8, 10]. One of the most important physiological differences is the high concentration of fetal hemoglobin (HbF) in cord RBCs. This is practically absent in adult RBCs (normal adult HbF is <1%) [18]. HbF has a higher affinity for oxygen compared to adult hemoglobin (HbA). This allows HbF to bind oxygen more easily, with a left shift of the oxygen dissociation curve and the release of less oxygen to the tissues [18].

There are many problems associated with adult RBC transfusions to fetuses and neonates that can be resolved by replacing adult RBCs with cord RBCs. Due to the high concentration of HbF, fetal blood has higher affinity for oxygen than the mother's blood, which facilitates the uptake of oxygen from the placenta by the fetus [11]. The practice of administering adult RBC transfusions to premature infants has been associated with the increased incidence of retrolental fibroplasia—the abnormal growth of blood vessels in the retina that may lead to blindness [19–21]. Another possible complication of adult RBC transfusions to neonates is bronchopulmonary dysplasia, a chronic inflammatory lung disease that can lead to respiratory dysfunction [22]. Several researchers have demonstrated a direct correlation between the incidence of bronchopulmonary dysplasia and adult blood transfusions [23–25].

The practice of transfusions of RBCs derived from umbilical cord blood to treat neonatal anemia has recently gained a lot of interest [26–35]. A number of studies have demonstrated that transfusions of autologous cord RBCs are both safe and effective in the treatment of anemic neonates [26–32]. Some, however, have expressed concerns with cord blood transfusions, including the potential high risk of bacterial contamination, low hypothermic storage stability, and small volume of umbilical cord blood collections [28, 33]. At the same time, these can be overcome through use of novel or superior long-term storage techniques for cord RBCs.

Adult RBCs can be successfully stored at 1–6°C in an anticoagulant/preservative solution (e.g., citrate-phosphate-dextrose/saline-adenine-glucose-mannitol (CPD/SAGM)) for 42 days [36]. In contrast, cord RBCs deteriorate much faster under the same conditions and cannot be stored for more than 14 days without significant decrease in quality [28, 37]. Cryopreservation and subsequent storage at ultra-low temperatures may preserve cord RBCs and maintain a high quality of cord RBCs for use in intrauterine and neonatal transfusions. Despite many studies having documented the successful cryopreservation of adult RBCs, no protocol for cryopreservation of cord RBCs has been developed.

Since cord RBCs are currently treated as a waste product after processing of collected cord blood for stem cell extraction, there is no incentive to monitor or preserve their quality. After cord blood is collected, it can be stored ideally at room temperature for up to 48 hours before being processed for stem cell extraction [38]. Longer pre-processing room temperature storage for stem cell extraction is permissible when there is strict monitoring of cell viability, CD 34+ cell content and viability, and colony-forming assay potential. Presently, the effects of pre-processing storage on the quality of cord RBCs is unknown.

A number of conventional methods exist for assessing RBC quality. RBC hemolysis is used as an indicator of RBC membrane damage that results in the release of free Hb into extracellular space. A decrease in adenosine triphosphate (ATP), the energy substrate of RBCs, has been observed as one of the markers of RBC aging during hypothermic storage [39]. The concentration of 2,3-diphosphoglycerate (2,3-DPG) in RBCs is another important quality parameter, since 2,3-DPG regulates oxygen exchange between Hb and tissues by mediating the binding of oxygen to Hb, as well as the release of oxygen into tissues [8, 40]. Finally, the concentration of methemoglobin (metHb) acts as an indicator of RBC oxidative injury.

In addition, novel predictors of RBC *in vitro* quality, such as RBC deformability, microvesiculation, and extracellular expression of phosphatidylserine (PS) and CD47, have been recently incorporated into RBC quality assessments [41, 42]. The deformability of RBCs enables their passage through small blood capillaries and is therefore a critical property for maintaining normal blood flow [43]. Microvesiculation is the process of generating microparticles—phospholipid vesicles 0.04–1.5 μm in diameter—by eukaryotic cells as a result of different types of cell stimulation [44]. Notably, microvesiculation has been shown to increase during hypothermic storage of adult RBCs [45]. Glycophorin A (CD235a) is a glycoprotein abundantly present on the RBC membrane [46], and its expression on microparticles is used as a marker of RBC origin [44]. PS is a membrane phospholipid that is normally found within the inner leaflet of the plasma membrane, but during apoptosis, it is translocated to the outer leaflet. Annexin V is a phospholipid-binding protein with a high affinity for PS and is used to determine the percentage of cells within a population that are actively undergoing apoptosis. It has been shown that PS is exposed on the surface of RBCs during hypothermic storage [47]. CD47 is an erythrocyte surface antigen that has been shown to be a "marker of self." RBCs lacking this antigen on their surface are rapidly cleared from the circulation by macrophages in the spleen [48]. It has been demonstrated that the expression of CD47 on RBCs decreases during storage and may be an important determinant of posttransfusion *in vivo* survival [49].

If cord RBCs are to be cryopreserved for clinical use, it is critical to ensure that a high quality of cord RBC product remains, following isolation from cord blood. The objective of the present study was to examine if and how the quality of cord RBCs is affected by the duration of cord blood storage at room temperature and other cord blood characteristics.

2. Methods

2.1. Cord RBC Collection. Cord RBCs were obtained from the Alberta Cord Blood Bank, as a waste product, after stem cell isolation from umbilical cord blood. Women with healthy, full-term pregnancies who met the Alberta Cord Blood Bank criteria for inclusion and gave informed consent were eligible to donate cord blood. Cord blood collections were performed by a trained physician or midwife attending the delivery, from either the undelivered or delivered placenta. The umbilical vein was punctured, and cord blood was collected by gravity into a blood collection bag (Fenwal, Inc., Lake Zurich, IL, USA) containing 35 mL of citrate phosphate dextrose (CPD) anticoagulant. After collection, whole umbilical cord blood was stored at room temperature and processed at the Alberta Cord Blood Bank facility according to a previously described double collection procedure [50]. Ethics approval for the study was obtained from the University of Alberta Health Research Ethics Board (Biomedical Panel).

2.2. Cord Blood Characteristics. Upon receipt of a packed cord RBC unit, a number of cord blood characteristics were documented from the Alberta Cord Blood Bank Collection Form. The time between cord blood collection and the start of processing that cord blood spent at room temperature was calculated (age of cord blood). The baby's gender and weight, the cord blood collection method (*in utero* or delivered placenta), and cord blood hematocrit were recorded. The ratio of cord blood volume to anticoagulant volume (cord blood : CPD) was calculated by dividing the reported volume of cord blood in mL (w/o anticoagulant) by 35 mL (volume of CPD in blood bag). Additionally, the percentage of HbF in cord blood was determined using the standard Kleihauer-Betke kit (Sure Tech Diagnostic, Associates, Inc., St. Louis, MO, USA).

2.3. Assessment of Cord RBC Quality

2.3.1. Standard Indicators of RBC Quality. Cord RBCs were tested immediately after their isolation from cord blood for conventional indicators of RBC quality. RBC hemolysis was determined by spectrophotometric measurement of total and supernatant cyanmethemoglobin according to Drabkin's method [51]. Controls for total Hb were prepared from Stanbio Tri-Level Hemoglobin controls (Stanbio Laboratory, Boerne, TX, USA). Hematocrit of RBC sample was measured using the microhematocrit centrifuge (Hettich, Tuttlingen, Germany) as the ratio of the volume occupied by packed RBCs to the volume of a whole RBC sample [46]. ATP concentration in RBCs was determined using the commercial ATP Hexokinase FS kit (DiaSys Diagnostic Systems GmbH, Holzheim, Germany). A blank sample was prepared with distilled water, and a control sample was prepared using an ATP standard (DiaSys Diagnostic Systems GmbH, Holzheim, Germany). ATP concentration was subsequently converted from μmol/dL to μmol/g Hb using the following formula:

$$C(\mu\text{mol/gHb}) = C(\mu\text{mol/dL}) \times \frac{10}{\text{Hb(g/L)}} \quad (1)$$

2,3-DPG concentration in RBCs was determined using the commercially available 2,3-DPG assay kit (Roche Diagnostics GmbH, Mannheim, Germany). Concentration of metHb was measured spectrophotometrically on the SPECTRA max PLUS 384 microplate spectrophotometer (Molecular Devices Corporation, Sunnyvale, CA, USA). RBCs were diluted 1 : 500 in distilled water, and the concentration of each type of Hb (oxyhemoglobin, metHb, carboxyhemoglobin) was determined by measuring the absorption of lysed RBCs at four different wavelengths (560 nm, 576 nm, 630 nm, and 700 nm), since each type of Hb has a unique absorption peak. Concentrations of different types of Hb were calculated as the amount of heme monomer in mol/L using the following formulas [52]:

$$C_{\text{met}} = 501 \times [(-0.361416 \times (A_{560} - A_{700}))$$
$$+ (0.174064 \times (A_{576} - A_{700}))$$
$$+ (2.68255 \times (A_{630} - A_{700}))] \times 10^{-4},$$
$$C_{\text{oxy}} = 501 \times [(-0.741711 \times (A_{560} - A_{700}))$$
$$+ (1.01587 \times (A_{576} - A_{700}))$$

$$-(0.279425 \times (A_{630} - A_{700}))] \times 10^{-4},$$
$$C_{\text{deoxy}} = 501 \times [(1.35699 \times (A_{560} - A_{700}))$$
$$- (0.739456 \times (A_{576} - A_{700}))$$
$$-(0.671847 \times (A_{630} - A_{700}))] \times 10^{-4},$$

$$(2)$$

where C = concentration of each type of Hb (mol/L), and A = absorbance at each wavelength. Lastly, the percentage of metHb relative to total Hb was subsequently calculated.

2.3.2. Novel Indicators of RBC Quality. RBC deformability was analyzed via ektacytometry using the laser-assisted optical rotational cell analyzer (LORCA, Mechatronics, Zwaag, The Netherlands). In ektacytometry, the RBC suspension is subjected to different levels of shear stress during rotation at different speeds, which causes the RBCs to elongate to different extents. A laser beam, shone through the RBC suspension, is refracted by RBCs, and the shape of the diffraction pattern is used to determine EI_{max}, the maximum theoretical elongation index, and K_{EI}, the shear stress required to achieve half of the EI_{max} [43]. A high EI max suggests that RBCs are highly deformable, whereas a high KEI means that RBCs are very rigid and, hence, more force needs to be applied for RBCs to elongate. For ektacytometry experiments, RBCs were diluted 1 : 100 in polyvinylpyrrolidone (PVP, Mechatronics, Zwaag, The Netherlands). All measurements were performed at 37°C. Deformability data was analyzed using Eadie-Hofstee linearization as previously described by Stadnick et al. [53].

Flow cytometry was used to assess RBC microvesiculation, as well as expression of PS and CD47 by both RBCs and RBC microparticles. To prepare RBC samples, RBC concentrates were diluted 1 : 5650 in Annexin V binding buffer (prepared in-house and contained 140 mM sodium chloride, 2.5 mM calcium chloride, 10 mM 4-(2-hydroxyethyl)-1-piperazineethanesulfonic acid (HEPES)) in two steps. To eliminate any small particles originally present in the buffer, the buffer was sterile filtered through 0.2 μm Supor Membrane VacuCap 60 Bottle-top filters (Pall Life Sciences, Ann Arbor, MI, USA) before being used for any cell dilutions. Nine hundred eighty-five microliters of RBC suspension was then labelled with 5 μL each of FITC-conjugated anti-glycophorin A (Invitrogen Corporation, Camarillo, CA, USA), APC-conjugated Annexin V (BD Pharmingen, Frank- lin Lakes, NJ, USA), and PE-conjugated anti-CD47 (BD Pharmingen, Franklin Lakes, NJ, USA) and incubated for at least 15 minutes in the dark at room temperature.

A number of controls were used in this assay. Unstained RBCs served as a negative control. To determine the degree of nonspecific binding of antibodies, isotype controls were prepared by labeling 990 μL of RBCs with 5 μL each of PE-conjugated mouse IgG1, k (BD Pharmingen, Franklin Lakes, NJ, USA) and FITC-conjugated mouse IgG1, k (Invitrogen Corporation, Camarillo, CA,USA). The positive control for RBC microparticles and PS externalization was prepared by treating fresh RBCs with N-ethylmaleimide (NEM) (Sigma-Aldrich, St. Louis, MO, USA), as previously described by Stewart et al. [54], and subsequently labeling NEM-treated RBCs with fluorescent antibodies in the same way as a test sample. Annexin V binding buffer was run alone to check for the purity of the buffer and absence of microparticle artifacts, and the Annexin V binding buffer with added fluorescent antibodies was run as a blank control.

Prepared samples were then analyzed using an FACSCalibur flow cytometer (BD Biosciences, San Jose, CA, USA) with a low flow rate. Uniform Polystyrene Microspheres 1.01 μm in diameter (Bangs Laboratories, Inc., Fishers, IN, USA) were used as a size reference to set a gate around the desired population of microparticles, and only microparticles less than 1.01 μm in diameter were included in the analysis. Only microparticles positive for Glycophorin A were considered to be of RBC origin and, therefore, further quantified and analyzed for PS and CD47 expression. Data analysis was performed using CellQuest Pro software, Version 6.0 (BD Biosciences, San Jose, CA, USA). After analysis, flow cytometry output data was used to calculate the percentage of microparticle events in each RBC sample, the percentage of RBCs and RBC microparticles expressing PS and CD47, and the mean fluorescence intensity (MFI) of PS and CD47 on RBCs and RBC microparticles.

2.4. Statistical Analysis. Three types of statistical analysis were used in the present study: correlation, regression, and Student's *t*-test. Statistical analysis was conducted using statistical analysis system (SAS) software, version 9.1 (SAS institute Inc., Cary, NC, USA). To investigate the strength of the relationship between cord blood characteristics and cord RBC quality parameters, correlation analysis was performed. Spearman rank coefficients were calculated for the baby's gender and cord blood collection site, which are discrete variables, while Pearson's correlation coefficients were calculated for other cord blood characteristics. The use of regression analysis permitted the effects of multiple cord blood characteristics on RBC quality measures to be examined in a model simultaneously. In regression analysis, the backward selection approach was used to select the variable(s) for the final statistical model. First, all of the characteristic variables were entered into the model. Then, variables possessing the highest *P* values (indicating no effect) were removed one by one until all of the remaining variables comprising the model had a significance of a *P* value <0.1. Student's *t*-test was used for comparison of cord blood characteristics and cord RBC quality parameters between groups of cord blood units based on baby's gender and a method of cord blood collection. The significance level was set to 0.05.

3. Results

A total of 30 cord RBC samples were tested in this study. Most of the samples tested were between 17 and 48 hours old (Figure 1). The average age of cord blood samples was 30.6 ± 10.3 hours (mean ± SD). The ratio of cord blood volume to the volume of CPD anticoagulant in cord blood

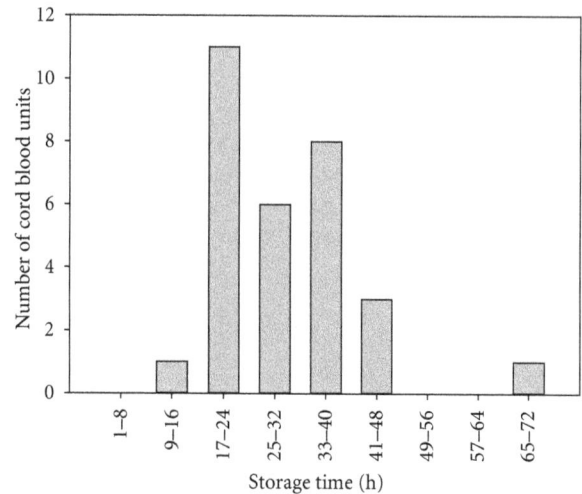

FIGURE 1: The duration cord blood samples spent at room temperature prior to testing.

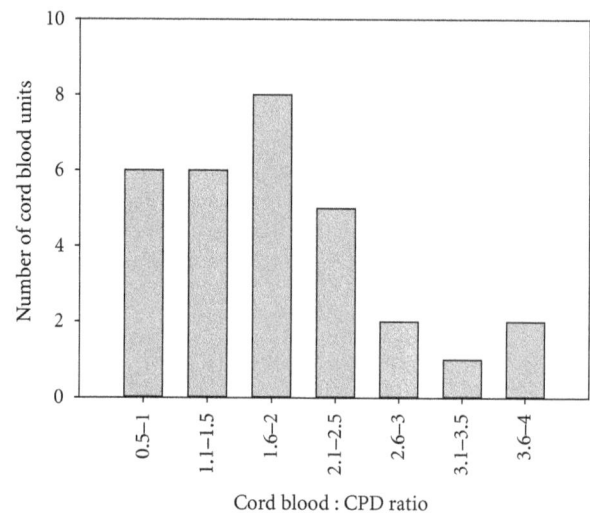

FIGURE 2: The distribution of the ratio of cord blood volume to CPD anticoagulant volume in collected cord blood samples.

collections ranged from 0.77 to 3.83 (Figure 2), the average ratio being 1.84 ± 0.80 (mean ± SD).

Table 1 shows correlations between cord blood characteristics and RBC quality measures. There was a fair, negative correlation between cord blood storage time and 2,3-DPG content of RBCs ($r = -0.431$, $P = 0.017$). A fair, positive correlation between cord blood hematocrit and deformability of RBCs was observed ($r = 0.392$, $P = 0.035$). Also, there was a moderately strong, positive relationship between the percentage of HbF in RBCs and their deformability ($r = 0.668$, $P = 0.002$). Other cord blood characteristics, such as baby's gender, baby's weight, cord blood volume, the ratio of cord blood volume to anticoagulant volume, and cord blood collection method, were not significantly correlated with any of the cord RBC quality measures.

TABLE 1: Correlation between cord blood characteristics and cord RBC quality measures.

Cord RBC quality measure	Cord blood characteristic							
	Age of cord blood (hours) 30.6 ± 10.3	Cord blood volume (mL) 64 ± 28	Cord blood Hct (L/L) 0.30 ± 0.04	Baby's gender	Baby's weight (g) 3468 ± 490	Cord blood collection site	HbF (%) 90.1 ± 5.8	Cord blood : CPD 1.84 ± 0.80
ATP (μmol/g Hb) **2.78 ± 0.69**	−0.229 (0.241)	0.337 (0.080)	0.316 (0.109)	−0.241 (0.216)	0.042 (0.841)	0.021 (0.914)	0.177 (0.497)	0.337 (0.080)
Hemolysis (%) **0.12 ± 0.04**	−0.127 (0.505)	−0.144 (0.448)	−0.104 (0.590)	0.055 (0.773)	−0.085 (0.672)	−0.013 (0.946)	−0.358 (0.145)	−0.144 (0.448)
MetHb (%) **4.60 ± 1.80**	0.098 (0.606)	−0.143 (0.451)	−0.236 (0.217)	0.019 (0.919)	−0.001 (0.995)	0.032 (0.866)	0.321 (0.194)	−0.143 (0.451)
2,3-DPG (mmol/L) **0.11 ± 0.20**	−0.431* (0.017)	−0.133 (0.484)	−0.181 (0.346)	−0.231 (0.220)	−0.072 (0.720)	0.019 (0.919)	−0.342 (0.165)	−0.133 (0.484)
Deformability **0.446 ± 0.030**	−0.119 (0.531)	0.323 (0.081)	0.392* (0.035)	0.012 (0.951)	0.254 (0.201)	0.160 (0.397)	0.668** (0.002)	0.323 (0.081)
Rigidity **1.47 ± 0.33**	−0.277 (0.138)	0.010 (0.960)	−0.093 (0.630)	0.144 (0.448)	−0.127 (0.529)	0.225 (0.233)	−0.375 (0.126)	0.010 (0.960)
Microparticle events (%) **0.3 ± 0.2**	−0.126 (0.540)	0.031 (0.882)	−0.240 (0.249)	−0.200 (0.327)	0.305 (0.156)	−0.088 (0.668)	0.145 (0.592)	0.031 (0.882)
PS-positive RBCs (%) **5.2 ± 0.9**	0.008 (0.969)	0.015 (0.938)	−0.023 (0.910)	−0.170 (0.388)	−0.080 (0.705)	0.193 (0.325)	−0.084 (0.741)	0.015 (0.938)
CD47-positive RBCs (%) **99.9 ± 0.1**	−0.144 (0.465)	−0.215 (0.271)	−0.371 (0.057)	−0.322 (0.095)	0.014 (0.947)	−0.236 (0.227)	−0.309 (0.212)	−0.215 (0.271)
PS-positive microparticles (%) **61.3 ± 18.2**	−0.151 (0.461)	−0.171 (0.404)	−0.292 (0.157)	0.084 (0.682)	−0.125 (0.569)	0.104 (0.612)	−0.056 (0.836)	−0.171 (0.404)
CD47-positive microparticles (%) **88.2 ± 24.2**	0.121 (0.557)	−0.076 (0.713)	−0.218 (0.295)	0.105 (0.608)	−0.209 (0.338)	0.265 (0.191)	0.137 (0.612)	−0.076 (0.713)
MFI of PS on RBCs **45 ± 10**	−0.086 (0.663)	0.102 (0.606)	−0.202 (0.313)	−0.152 (0.440)	0.093 (0.660)	−0.222 (0.257)	0.344 (0.163)	0.102 (0.606)
MFI of CD47 on RBCs **274 ± 83**	−0.129 (0.513)	−0.033 (0.869)	−0.105 (0.601)	−0.071 (0.718)	−0.070 (0.739)	−0.107 (0.587)	−0.070 (0.781)	−0.033 (0.869)
MFI of PS on microparticles **324 ± 55**	0.135 (0.494)	0.007 (0.972)	0.155 (0.439)	0.027 (0.892)	0.035 (0.868)	−0.164 (0.403)	−0.137 (0.588)	0.007 (0.972)
MFI of CD47 on microparticles **776 ± 370**	−0.168 (0.394)	−0.095 (0.632)	0.097 (0.629)	−0.080 (0.684)	−0.118 (0.574)	−0.136 (0.491)	−0.344 (0.163)	−0.095 (0.632)

The numbers in the table are correlation coefficients (P value in brackets), that show the strength of a relationship between two parameters. Coefficients between 0.3 and 0.5 represent a fair linear relationship, and coefficients between 0.6 and 0.8 represent moderately strong linear relationship. A +/− sign before the coefficient indicates the direction of the correlation (positive or negative). The numbers in bold are mean ± SD for each tested parameter. *Correlation is significant at 0.05 level, and **correlation is significant at 0.01 level. Hct—hematocrit, HbF—fetal hemoglobin, CPD—citrate-phosphate-dextrose (anticoagulant), ATP—adenosine triphosphate, MetHb—methemoglobin, 2,3-DPG—2,3-diphosphoglycerate, PS—phosphatidylserine, and MFI—mean fluorescence intensity.

Regression analysis revealed many significant effects of cord blood characteristics (predictor variables) on cord RBC quality measures (outcome variables). Regression coefficients show the nature of relationship between the predictor and the outcome. Absolute values of regression coefficients show how much the outcome changes when the predictor changes. A +/− sign before the coefficient shows the direction in which the change takes place (increase or decrease). There was a significant relationship between the age of cord blood and the 2,3-DPG concentration of RBCs, with a regression coefficient of −0.214 ($P = 0.012$). There was a significant relationship between the cord blood volume and the ATP content of RBCs, with a regression coefficient of 0.010 ($P = 0.030$). There was a significant negative relationship between the baby's weight and hemolysis, with a regression coefficient of −0.001 ($P = 0.018$). There were significant relationships between HbF content of RBCs and a number of cord RBC quality measures, such as hemolysis, with regression coefficient of −0.030 ($P = 0.009$), 2,3-DPG content, with a regression coefficient of −0.082 ($P = 0.007$), and deformability, with a regression coefficient of 0.004 ($P = 0.002$). The effect of HbF content on RBC rigidity was modified by baby's gender, so that no significant effect was observed for males; however, for females RBC rigidity decreased with the increase in HbF content (regression coefficient −0.068, $P = 0.002$). A positive relationship was

TABLE 2: Comparison of cord blood characteristics and cord RBC quality measures between cord blood groups based on baby's gender and a method of cord blood collection.

Cord blood characteristics and cord RBC quality parameters	Baby's gender			Method of cord blood collection		
	Male ($n = 17$)	Female ($n = 13$)	P value	Delivered placenta ($n = 3$)	Placenta *in utero* ($n = 27$)	P value
Age of cord blood	30.2 (11.8)	31.2 (8.3)	0.7908	24.5 (0.4)	31.3 (10.6)	0.0028*
Cord blood volume	60 (23)	70 (34)	0.3310	61 (25)	65 (29)	0.8113
Cord blood hematocrit	0.30 (0.05)	0.31 (0.04)	0.7943	0.31 (0.03)	0.30 (0.05)	0.8676
Baby's weight	3546 (557)	3336 (333)	0.2906	3230 (407)	3498 (499)	0.3821
HbF (%)	88.5 (5.6)	91.5 (6.0)	0.2891	· (·)	90.1 (5.8)	·
Cord blood : CPD	1.71 (0.66)	2.01 (0.96)	0.3310	1.73 (0.70)	1.85 (0.82)	0.8113
ATP (μmol/g Hb)	2.87 (0.58)	2.68 (0.83)	0.4811	2.68 (0.46)	2.80 (0.72)	0.7936
Hemolysis (%)	0.12 (0.05)	0.12 (0.05)	0.7987	0.11 (0.02)	0.12 (0.05)	0.6607
MetHb (%)	4.54 (1.62)	4.67 (2.07)	0.8531	4.46 (1.68)	4.61 (1.84)	0.8941
2,3-DPG (mmol/L)	0.11 (0.15)	0.11 (0.26)	0.9933	0.05 (0.03)	0.12 (0.21)	0.5923
Deformability	0.445 (0.029)	0.447 (0.032)	0.8972	0.437 (0.014)	0.447 (0.031)	0.5834
Rigidity	1.41 (0.21)	1.56 (0.43)	0.2025	1.27 (0.23)	1.49 (0.33)	0.2747
Microparticle events (%)	0.3 (0.2)	0.2 (0.1)	0.2483	0.9 (0.1)	0.3 (0.2)	0.8861
PS-positive RBCs (%)	5.4 (1.0)	5.1 (0.7)	0.3842	4.7 (1.4)	5.3 (0.8)	0.2113
CD47-positive RBCs (%)	99.9 (0.1)	99.8 (0.2)	0.0706	99.9 (0.1)	99.9 (0.1)	0.4089
PS-positive microparticles (%)	61.2 (21.8)	61.5 (11.2)	0.9770	57.2 (2.4)	61.9 (19.3)	0.6848
CD47-positive microparticles (%)	87.6 (30.1)	89.2 (10.2)	0.8674	76.3 (16.6)	89.8 (24.8)	0.3736
MFI of PS on RBCs	47 (7)	44 (13)	0.3924	51 (10)	45 (10)	0.2715
MFI of CD47 on RBCs	275 (73)	271 (99)	0.8983	299 (114)	271 (82)	0.5814
MFI of PS on microparticles	324 (62)	324 (46)	0.9946	366 (74)	319 (52)	0.1730
MFI of CD47 on microparticles	837 (434)	694 (258)	0.3209	899 (336)	761 (378)	0.5528

The numbers in the table are absolute values for each parameter (standard deviation in brackets), *P <0.05 (Student's t-test). HbF—fetal hemoglobin, CPD—citrate-phosphate-dextrose (anticoagulant), ATP—adenosine triphosphate, MetHb—methemoglobin, 2,3-DPG—2,3-diphosphoglycerate, PS—phosphatidylserine, and MFI—mean fluorescence intensity.

observed between the ratio of cord blood volume to anticoagulant volume and PS expression on RBCs with a regression coefficient of 3.836 ($P = 0.028$). Females had an increase in CD47 expression on RBCs of 0.742% compared to males ($P = 0.037$), which was modified by cord blood hematocrit. Cord blood RBCs collected from *in utero* placenta had an increase in PS expression on their surface of 4.106% compared to RBCs collected from delivered placenta ($P = 0.013$).

A number of interactions between predictor variables were observed, wherein the effect of one predictor on cord RBC quality measure was further enhanced by a similar direction change of another predictor. Interactions between the following parameters were found: baby's weight and HbF, age of cord blood and HbF, baby's gender and HbF, the ratio of cord blood volume to the volume of anticoagulant and the method of cord blood collection, and baby's gender and cord blood hematocrit. To illustrate some of the above interactions, there was an interaction between the effect of the age of cord blood and HbF content on 2,3-DPG concentration. Since both the age of cord blood and HbF content were negatively associated with 2,3-DPG, when the age of cord blood increased, for samples with higher HbF content, the decrease in 2,3-DPG content was stronger than for samples with lower HbF content. The effect of HbF on hemolysis was modified by the change in baby's weight; in

particular, cord blood samples with lower HbF content taken from smaller babies had higher hemolysis than those taken from larger babies. The effect of the ratio of cord blood volume to anticoagulant volume on RBC PS expression was modified by the method of cord blood collection, so that PS expression on RBCs collected from *in utero* placenta decreased with the increase in cord blood : CPD ratio.

The results of comparison of cord blood characteristics and cord RBC quality measures between cord blood groups based on baby's gender and a method of cord blood collection are presented in Table 2. There were no significant differences noted in the cord blood characteristics and cord RBC quality parameters between males and females, or between cord blood collected from delivered or *in utero* placentas (Table 2).

4. Discussion

The goal of this study was to examine if and how the quality of RBCs isolated from whole cord blood is affected during cord blood storage at room temperature and, secondly, whether or not any of several cord blood characteristics impact the quality of cord RBCs. The primary purpose of the cord blood units used in our study was for stem cell extraction according to well-established protocols. After collection, whole cord blood is stored at room temperature for a variable amount of time dictated by the time of birth, transportation to the processing facility, and laboratory processing hours. It is then processed for stem cell isolation. Little is known about the effect of such storage conditions on the quality of RBCs present in cord blood. If cord RBCs are potentially superior for intrauterine and neonatal transfusions and are to be cryopreserved for clinical use, there is an incentive to ensure their best quality upon isolation from umbilical cord blood.

During the first 65 hours of cord blood storage at room temperature, the only observed change was a decrease in the 2,3-DPG concentration of RBCs (Table 1). Other RBC quality measures were not affected. It has been reported that 2,3-DPG disappears very quickly from adult RBCs during hypothermic storage and is usually no longer detectable by the end of the first week [55], though it is easily replenished after RBCs are transfused into the patient [56]. Therefore, if cord RBCs are to be cryopreserved for clinical use within 65 hours after cord blood collection, the drop in 2,3-DPG may not pose a serious risk for maintaining an acceptable quality of cord RBCs after cryopreservation.

Evidence in the literature suggests that the ratio of adult blood volume to the volume of anticoagulant/preservative solution is important and affects RBC quality [57, 58]. For adult whole blood collections, the standard ratio of blood volume to CPD anticoagulant volume is 7 : 1 [59]. In our study, blood : CPD ratio for cord blood units ranged from 0.77 : 1 to 3.83 : 1, due to the variable volumes obtained at the time of collection. These volumes are not predictable, and hence, an optimal cord blood : CPD ratio cannot be specified. A number of scientific reports indicate that the quality of adult RBCs from under- [57, 58] or over-collected blood units is suboptimal as compared with defined standard collections [58]. Evidence from our study suggests that the same may be true for cord blood collections. Particularly, lower cord blood hematocrit was correlated with lower RBC deformability (Table 1). Since cord blood hematocrit was measured after cord blood was mixed with CPD, cord blood hematocrit was partly determined by the ratio of cord blood volume to the volume of anticoagulant. Anticoagulant is acidic; therefore, when this ratio is too low (in the case of small cord blood volumes), the pH of cord blood will be reduced. This eventually results in RBC damage early in storage. A positive association between cord blood volume and ATP content, observed in the present study, also supports the argument about the importance of ratio of volumes. Higher cord blood volumes result in higher blood : CPD ratio and, therefore, higher ATP concentration. Finally, our results show that a higher baby's weight was correlated with lower RBC hemolysis. This can be explained by the fact that in our study bigger babies on average had higher cord blood volumes, which in turn resulted in higher blood : CPD ratio. On the other hand, regression analysis showed that a lower ratio of cord blood to anticoagulant was associated with lower expression of the apoptotic marker PS on RBCs. Combined, these observations lead us to believe that cord RBC quality is governed by an optimal ratio of cord blood to anticoagulant

that will need to be maintained during cord blood collections for RBC transfusion *in utero* or for neonates.

We have observed the positive correlation between the content of HbF in RBCs and RBC deformability (Table 1). It is known that HbF decreases gradually during the last trimester of fetal development, and premature babies have higher percentage of HbF than full-term neonates [2]. Although the literature contains contradictory data on deformability of cord RBCs, Lindercamp et al. showed that RBCs of preterm babies have higher cellular deformability than RBCs of full-term babies [60]. Together, these two pieces of evidence are in agreement with our observation.

5. Conclusion

There was no significant decrease in quality measures of cord RBCs during the first 65 hours of whole cord blood storage at room temperature. The ratio of cord blood volume to anticoagulant volume in cord blood collection bag is important and needs to be optimized in order to ensure that a good quality cord RBCs are preserved. Knowledge of cord RBC quality upon isolation from cord blood is important to design procedures for cord RBC preservation. This, in turn, may result in the development of a novel blood product from a currently discarded byproduct of cord blood cell processing that may offer a superior alternative for treatment of fetal and neonatal anemias.

Acknowledgments

The authors would like to acknowledge Dr. Qi-long Yi (Canadian Blood Services) for performing statistical analysis for the present study. They also thank Ruqayyah Almizraq (Department of Laboratory Medicine and Pathology, University of Alberta), Jayme Tchir (Canadian Blood Services), and Ann Berg for help with developing flow cytometry method. Special thanks are due to Nanni Zhang and Sally Shahi from Alberta Cord Blood Bank for providing cord RBC samples and the Alberta Cord Blood Bank cord blood donors for providing cord blood samples. Funding for this study was provided by Canadian Blood Services Graduate Fellowship and Canadian Institutes of Health Research Operating Grant "Preservation of red cells from cord blood as a new blood product for intrauterine and neonatal transfusions."

References

[1] H. G. Liley, "Immune hemolytic disease," in *Hematology of Infancy and Childhood*, D. G. Nathan, S. H. Orkin, D. Ginsburg, and A. T. Look, Eds., pp. 56–85, Saunders, 6th edition, 2003.

[2] C. Brugnara and O. S. Platt, "The neonatal erythrocyte and its disorders," in *Hematology of Infancy and Childhood*, D. G. Nathan, S. H. Orkin, D. Ginsburg, and A. T. Look, Eds., pp. 19–55, Saunders, 6th edition, 2003.

[3] N. L. C. Luban, "Neonatal red blood cell transfusions," *Vox Sanguinis, Supplement*, vol. 87, no. 2, pp. S184–S188, 2004.

[4] H. Hume, "Red blood cell transfusions for preterm infants: the role of evidence- based medicine," *Seminars in Perinatology*, vol. 21, no. 1, pp. 8–19, 1997.

[5] W. H Tooley, "Neonatal anemia," in *Intensive Care Nursery House Staff Manual*, W. H. Tooley, Ed., pp. 108–110, UCSF Children's Hospital at UCSF Medical Center, 8th edition, 2004.

[6] S. R. Sloan, R. J. Benjamin, D. F. Friedman, I. J. Webb, and L. Silberstein, "Transfusion medicine," in *Hematology of Infancy and Childhood*, D. G. Nathan, S. H. Orkin, D. Ginsburg, and A. T. Look, Eds., pp. 1709–1756, Saunders, 6th edition, 2003.

[7] K. J. Moise Jr., "Intrauterine transfusion with red cells and platelets," *Western Journal of Medicine*, vol. 159, no. 3, pp. 318–324, 1993.

[8] F. A. Oski, "The unique fetal red cell and its function. E. Mead Johnson Award address," *Pediatrics*, vol. 51, no. 3, pp. 494–500, 1973.

[9] L. M. Matovcik and W. C. Mentzer, "The membrane of the human neonatal red cell," *Clinics in Haematology*, vol. 14, no. 1, pp. 203–221, 1985.

[10] S. K. Jain, "The neonatal erythrocyte and its oxidative susceptibility," *Seminars in Hematology*, vol. 26, no. 4, pp. 286–300, 1989.

[11] F. A. Oski, "Fetal hemoglobin, the neonatal red cell, and 2,3-diphosphoglycerate," *Pediatric Clinics of North America*, vol. 19, no. 4, pp. 907–917, 1972.

[12] R. L. Nagel, "Hemoglobins: normal and abnormal," in *Hematology of Infancy and Childhood*, D. G. Nathan, S. H. Orkin, D. Ginsburg, and A. T. Look, Eds., pp. 745–789, Saunders, 6th edition, 2003.

[13] F. Bertolini, M. Battaglia, C. Zibera et al., "A new method for placental/cord blood processing in the collection bag. I. Analysis of factors involved in red blood cell removal," *Bone Marrow Transplantation*, vol. 18, no. 4, pp. 783–786, 1996.

[14] P. Perutelli, S. Catellani, L. Scarso, P. Cornaglia-Ferraris, and G. Dini, "Processing of human cord blood by three different procedures for red blood cell depletion and mononuclear cell recovery," *Vox Sanguinis*, vol. 76, no. 4, pp. 237–240, 1999.

[15] T. Sousa, M. E. De Sousa, M. I. Godinho, C. Mendes, A. Carvalhais, and I. L. Barbosa, "Umbilical cord blood processing: volume reduction and recovery of CD34+ cells," *Bone Marrow Transplantation*, vol. 19, no. 4, pp. 311–313, 1997.

[16] F. C. Battaglia, W. Bowes, H. R. McGaughey, E. L. Makowski, and G. Meschia, "The effect of fetal exchange transfusions with adult blood upon fetal oxygenation," *Pediatric Research*, vol. 3, no. 1, pp. 60–65, 1969.

[17] J. C. Fouron, H. Bard, J. C. Le Guennec, and M. R. Van Amerigen, "Effect of fetal or adult red cells on tissue oxygenation and myocardial function in normoxemic newborn lambs," *Pediatric Research*, vol. 15, no. 6, pp. 967–970, 1981.

[18] B. F. Ludvigsen, "Hemoglobin synthesis and function," in *Clinical Hematology: Principles, Procedures, Correlations*, E. A. Stiene-Martin, C. A. Lotspeich-Steininger, and J. A. Koepke, Eds., pp. 73–86, Lippincott, 2nd edition, 1997.

[19] C. Clark, J. A.H. Gibbs, and R. Maniello, "Blood transfusion: a possible risk factor in retrolental fibroplasia," *Acta Paediatrica Scandinavica*, vol. 70, no. 4, pp. 535–539, 1981.

[20] W. R. Hepner and A. C. Krause, "Retrolental fibroplasia: clinical observations," *Pediatrics*, vol. 10, no. 4, pp. 433–443, 1952.

[21] H. Mallek and P. Spohn, "Retrolental fibroplasia," *Canadian Medical Association journal*, vol. 63, no. 6, pp. 586–588, 1950.

[22] J. P. Kinsella, A. Greenough, and S. H. Abman, "Bronchopulmonary dysplasia," *Lancet*, vol. 367, no. 9520, pp. 1421–1431, 2006.

[23] K. J. Collard, S. Godeck, and J. E. Holley, "Blood transfusion and pulmonary lipid peroxidation in ventilated premature babies," *Pediatric Pulmonology*, vol. 39, no. 3, pp. 257–261, 2005.

[24] R. W. I. Cooke, J. A. Drury, C. W. Yoxall, and C. James, "Blood transfusion and chronic lung disease in preterm infants," *European Journal of Pediatrics*, vol. 156, no. 1, pp. 47–50, 1997.

[25] P. Korhonen, O. Tammela, A. M. Koivisto, P. Laippala, and S. Ikonen, "Frequency and risk factors in bronchopulmonary dysplasia in a cohort of very low birth weight infants," *Early Human Development*, vol. 54, no. 3, pp. 245–258, 1999.

[26] T. Brune, H. Garritsen, R. Hentschel, F. Louwen, E. Harms, and G. Jorch, "Efficacy, recovery, and safety of RBCs from autologous placental blood: clinical experience in 52 newborns," *Transfusion*, vol. 43, no. 9, pp. 1210–1215, 2003.

[27] T. Brune, H. Garritsen, R. Witteler et al., "Autologous placental blood transfusion for the therapy of anaemic neonates," *Biology of the Neonate*, vol. 81, no. 4, pp. 236–243, 2002.

[28] H. Eichler, T. Schaible, E. Richter et al., "Cord blood as a source of autologous RBCs transfusion to preterm infants," *Transfusion*, vol. 40, no. 9, pp. 1111–1117, 2000.

[29] K. Imura, H. Kawahara, Y. Kitayama, A. Yoneda, M. Yagi and N. Suehara, "Usefulness of cord-blood harvesting for autologous transfusion in surgical newborns with antenatal diagnosis of congenital anomalies," *Journal of Pediatric Surgery*, vol. 36, no. 6, pp. 851–854, 2001.

[30] A. Ballin, E. Arbel, G. Kenet et al., "Autologous umbilical cord blood transfusion," *Archives of Disease in Childhood*, vol. 73, no. 5, pp. F181–F183, 1995.

[31] D. V. Surbek, R. Glanzmann, H. P. Senn, I. Hoesli, and W. Holzgreve, "Can cord blood be used for autologous transfusion in preterm neonates?" *European Journal of Pediatrics*, vol. 159, no. 10, pp. 790–791, 2000.

[32] M. V. Appalup and T. A. Fedorova, "The effectiveness and safety of autologous umbilical blood derived red blood cells in a treatment of postoperative anaemia in newborns with a surgical pathology," *Vox Sanguinis*, vol. 99, supplement 1, p. 408, 2010.

[33] R. G. Strauss, "Autologous transfusions for neonates using placental blood: a cautionary note," *American Journal of Diseases of Children*, vol. 146, no. 1, pp. 21–22, 1992.

[34] C. M. Khodabux and A. Brand, "The use of cord blood for transfusion purposes: current status," *Vox Sanguinis*, vol. 97, no. 4, pp. 281–293, 2009.

[35] C. M. Khodabux, J. S. Von Lindern, J. A. Van Hilten, S. Scherjon, F. J. Walther, and A. Brand, "A clinical study on the feasibility of autologous cord blood transfusion for anemia of prematurity," *Transfusion*, vol. 48, no. 8, pp. 1634–1643, 2008.

[36] K. L. Scott, J. Lecak, and J. P. Acker, "Biopreservation of red blood cells: past, present, and future," *Transfusion Medicine Reviews*, vol. 19, no. 2, pp. 127–142, 2005.

[37] C. M. Khodabux, J. M. van Beckhoven, J. G. M. Scharenberg, F. El Barjiji, M. C. Slot, and A. Brand, "Processing cord blood from premature infants into autologous red-blood-cell products for transfusion," *Vox Sanguinis*, vol. 100, no. 4, pp. 367–373, 2011.

[38] "Processing of Cord Blood-Double Collection Procedure. Alberta Cord Blood Bank Standard Operating Procedure Manual," CP004.LS04DCv2.5. Effective 01 November 2010.

[39] G. J. C. G. M. Bosman, J. M. Werre, F. L. A. Willekens, and V. M. J. Novotný, "Erythrocyte ageing in vivo and in vitro: Structural aspects and implications for transfusion," *Transfusion Medicine*, vol. 18, no. 6, pp. 335–347, 2008.

[40] J. F. Dailey, Ed., *Dailey's Notes on Blood*, Medical Consulting Group, Arlington, Mass, USA, 3rd edition, 1996.

[41] J. L. Holovati, K. A. Wong, J. M. Webster, and J. P. Acker, "The effects of cryopreservation on red blood cell microvesiculation, phosphatidylserine externalization, and CD47 expression," *Transfusion*, vol. 48, no. 8, pp. 1658–1668, 2008.

[42] H. Stadnick, J. P. Acker, and J. L. Holovati, "Eadie-Hofstee analysis of ektacytometric deformability data from hypothermically stored red blood cells," *Cryobiology*, vol. 61, no. 3, p. 390, 2010.

[43] J. G. G. Dobbe, *LORCA Laser-Assisted Optical Rotational Cell Analyzer Version 2.1 User's Manual*, Academic Medical Centre, University of Amsterdam, Amsterdam, The Netherlands, 2004.

[44] J. Simak and M. P. Gelderman, "Cell membrane microparticles in blood and blood products: potentially pathogenic agents and diagnostic markers," *Transfusion Medicine Reviews*, vol. 20, no. 1, pp. 1–26, 2006.

[45] T. J. Greenwalt, "The how and why of exocytic vesicles," *Transfusion*, vol. 46, no. 1, pp. 143–152, 2006.

[46] D. M. Harmening, Ed., *Clinical Hematology and Fundamentals of Hemostasis*, F. A. Davis Company, Philadelphia, Pa, USA, 4th edition, 2002.

[47] I. Chin-Yee, N. Arya, and M. S. D'Almeida, "The red cell storage lesion and its implication for transfusion," *Transfusion Science*, vol. 18, no. 3, pp. 447–458, 1997.

[48] P.-A. Oldenborg, A. Zheleznyak, Y.-F. Fang, C. F. Lagenaur, H. D. Gresham, and F. P. Lindberg, "Role of CD47 as a marker of self on red blood cells," *Science*, vol. 288, no. 5473, pp. 2051–2054, 2000.

[49] A. M. Anniss and R. L. Sparrow, "Expression of CD47 (integrin-associated protein) decreases on red blood cells during storage," *Transfusion and Apheresis Science*, vol. 27, no. 3, pp. 233–238, 2002.

[50] H. Yang, J. P. Acker, D. Abley, L. E. McGann, and J. Akabutu, "High-efficiency volume reduction of cord blood using pentastarch," *Bone Marrow Transplantation*, vol. 27, no. 4, pp. 457–461, 2001.

[51] A. Zwart, O. W. Van Assendelft, B. S. Bull, J. M. England, S. M. Lewis, and W. G. Zijlstra, "Recommendations for reference method for haemoglobinometry in human blood (ICSH standard 1995) and specifications for international haemiglobincyanide standard (4th edition)," *Journal of Clinical Pathology*, vol. 49, no. 4, pp. 271–274, 1996.

[52] R. E. Benesch, R. Benesch, and S. Yung, "Equations for the spectrophotometric analysis of hemoglobin mixtures," *Analytical Biochemistry*, vol. 55, no. 1, pp. 245–248, 1973.

[53] H. Stadnick, R. Onell, J. P. Acker, and J. L. Holovati, "Eadie-Hofstee analysis of red blood cell deformability," *Clinical Hemorheology and Microcirculation*, vol. 47, no. 3, pp. 229–239, 2011.

[54] A. Stewart, S. Urbaniak, M. Turner, and H. Bessos, "The application of a new quantitative assay for the monitoring of integrin-associated protein CD47 on red blood cells during storage and comparison with the expression of CD47 and phosphatidylserine with flow cytometry," *Transfusion*, vol. 45, no. 9, pp. 1496–1503, 2005.

[55] D. De Korte, M. Kleine, H. G. H. Korsten, and A. J. Verhoeven, "Prolonged maintenance of 2,3-diphosphoglycerate acid and adenosine triphosphate in red blood cells during storage," *Transfusion*, vol. 48, no. 6, pp. 1081–1089, 2008.

[56] A. Heaton, T. Keegan, and S. Holme, "In vivo regeneration of red cell 2,3-diphosphoglycerate following transfusion of DPG-depleted AS-1, AS-3 and CPDA-1 red cells," *British Journal of Haematology*, vol. 71, no. 1, pp. 131–136, 1989.

[57] J. Joseph, J. Pink, A. Ribeiro, and I. M. Stewart, "In vitro characteristics of "undercollected" units of whole blood in CP2D-A," *Vox Sanguinis*, vol. 67, no. 3, pp. 275–279, 1994.

[58] V. Weisbach, I. Hunold, R. Zimmermann et al., "In vitro characteristics of red blood cell concentrates prepared from under- and overcollected units of whole blood and from a paediatric blood bag system," *Transfusion Medicine*, vol. 10, no. 1, pp. 23–30, 2000.

[59] R. Kakaiya, C. A. Aronson, and J. Julleis, "Whole blood collection and component processing," in *AABB Technical Manual*, J. D. Roback, M. R. Combs, B. J. Grossman, and C. D. Hillyer, Eds., pp. 189–228, AABB, 16th edition, 2008.

[60] O. Linderkamp, "Cellular and membrane deformability of red blood cells in preterm infants with and without growth retardation," *Clinical Hemorheology and Microcirculation*, vol. 17, no. 4, pp. 279–283, 1997.

Testing for Partial RhD with a D-Screen Diagast Kit in Moroccan Blood Donors with Weak D Expression

Z. Kabiri,[1,2] M. Benajiba,[1] K. Hajjout,[3] N. Dakka,[2] and H. Bellaoui[2]

[1] Centre National de Transfusion Sanguine, rue Lamfadel Cherkaoui, Madinat Al Irfane, P.O. Box 180, 10000 Rabat, Morocco
[2] Departement de Biologie, Faculté des Sciences, University MDV Rabat Agdal, 1014 Rabat, Morocco
[3] Centre Regional de Transfusion Sanguine, rue Lamfadel Cherkaoui, Madinat Al Irfane, P.O. Box 180, 10000 Rabat, Morocco

Correspondence should be addressed to Z. Kabiri; kabiri_zh@yahoo.com

Academic Editor: Maria Rios

The aim of this study was to search for the partial D phenotype in Moroccan blood donors with weak D expression. The study included 32 samples with weak D phenotype, and partial D category red blood cells were detected with the D-Screen Diagast kit, which consists in 9 monoclonal anti-D antibodies specific for the most common categories of partial D. Among the 32 samples studied, we identified 13 specific reactions to a partial D antigen (3 DVI, 2 DVa, 2 DIII$^{(a,b,c)}$, and 6 DVII), with 8 reactions suggesting a weak D and 11 reactions providing no formal argument in favor of a partial D antigen. This work can be used to validate the performance of the anti-D reagent and to improve the safety of transfusion of red blood cells from donors expressing the partial D antigen by integrating the finding into the recipient file with a recommendation concerning the appropriate care.

1. Introduction

Rhesus is one of the most important and clinically significant blood group systems. D antigen (ISBT 004.001; RH1) is the most immunogenic and clinically important of this system because of the ability of anti-D to cause transfusion reactions and hemolytic disease of the foetus and newborn. The Rh system was described for the first time in 1939 and is now considered to be a mosaic of epitopes (antigenic determinants). Partial D variants lack one or more epitopes of D antigen while weak D variants have all epitopes present but express a significantly reduced amount of D antigen per red blood cell and are usually identified by the indirect antiglobulin test (IAT). Partial D and weak D are the most commonly found D variants. Individuals whose red blood cells do not carry all the parts of the D mosaic can, when exposed to the full D antigen, produce anti-D alloantibodies directed against one or more of the missing epitopes, thus defining the phenotype "partial D." Loss of D epitopes is associated with either gene rearrangements or point mutations affecting extracellular portions of the RhD protein [1, 2]. The great diversity of D variants (weak D and partial D) explains the discrepancies noted between two serological determinations and the lack of reactivity of certain variants by serology [3]. It is very important to identify a donor having a D variant (weak D or D partial D) since in some instances these red blood cells can trigger an immune response if transfused to a recipient who is D negative.

The study of D variants in blood donors for immunohematological qualification was little studied in Morocco and thus in order to provide elements of information on the prevalence of weak D and the identification and the frequency of certain D variants, our earlier study [4], conducted among Moroccan blood donors in which we tested 23098 samples of Moroccan blood donors to determine the incidence of weak D phenotype, showed that 9.5% (2204) of the donors were RhD negative and the weak D phenotype was detected in about 0.4%. Therefore, the purpose of this present study was to identify the partial D phenotype among 32 Moroccan blood donors with weak D expression collected in total of 59693 samples using the D-Screen Diagast kit of nine anti-D monoclonal antibodies and to guide immunohematologist in the resolution of serological difficulties (discrepancies) in order that the correct D antigen status can be assigned and in choosing the right strategy adapted to the Moroccan population in terms of prevention of alloimmunization and fetal-maternal transfusion.

2. Subjects and Methods

2.1. Subjects. This study is concerned with 32 samples of Moroccan blood donors with D variant phenotype, collected in total of 59693 blood donors at the National Blood Transfusion Centre of Rabat, for over one year.

2.2. Methods

2.2.1. Determination of the RhD Phenotype and Weak D Phenotype. The RhD phenotype was performed with an Olympus pk7300 analyzer. We used the anti-D IgM Diagast (clone P3 × 61) for the first determination and the anti-D IgG Diagast TOTEME (clones P3 × P3 × 61 + 21223B10 + P3 + P3 × 290 × 35) for the second determination. Weak D expression of the D antigen was performed systematically for all RhD negative blood donors using the indirect Coombs test. Red blood cells of blood donors with the weak D phenotype were subsequently studied, using the hemagglutinin tube technique, with a panel of nine monoclonal antibodies anti-D IgM and IgG of the D-Screen Diagast kit. These reagents were selected for their ability to define specific reaction profiles of the most frequent partial D following the classifications DII, DIIIa, DIIIb, DIIIc, DIVa, DIVb, DVa, DVI, DVII, DFR, DBT, DHAR, and DHMi.

(i) For the anti-D antibody of IgM type, the reaction used a direct hemagglutinin test tube, while for the D-type anti IgG antibody, the reaction consisted in the indirect Coombs test tube of antiglobulin human (AHG) Mestria IGG or IGG + C3D.

3. Results

(i) In total of 59693 samples analyzed by Olympus pk7300, 6612 of the donors were RhD negative and the weak D phenotype was detected in about 0.5% ($n = 32$).

(ii) Screening for Rh partial D with the D-Screen Diagast kit of nine anti-D monoclonal antibodies allowed us to identify in the 32 samples the following phenotypes: (Table 1)

(a) 13 (40.7%) specific reactions to the partial D antigen defined as follows: 3 (9.37%) DVI, 2 (6.25%) DV^a, 2 (6.25%) DIII$^{(a,b,c)}$, and 6 (18.75%) DVII.

(b) 8 (25%) reactions positive only with IgM anti-D and with most performed IgG anti-D, suggesting a weak D antigen.

(c) 11 (34.37%) positive reactions with all the kit reagents, which does not provide formal arguments in favor of a partial D antigen.

4. Discussion

The distinction between D positive and D negative red blood cells is not always obvious in the case of D variants [5]. The partial D and weak D phenotypes give discrepant results when using different marketed monoclonal anti-RhD reagents [6, 7]. Depending on the presence or absence of D epitopes on red blood cells, those with partial D may be typed as D positive or negative with commercial anti-D reagents [8].

In our study, which consisted of a population of 32 weak D phenotype donors, we identify, 13 samples with a partial D phenotype (3 DVI, 2 DVa, 2 (DIIIa, DIIIb, DIIIc), and 6 DVII), identified with the D-Screen Diagas kit. However, we cannot provide any conclusions regarding the frequency of these variants in the Moroccan population due to the limited number of samples obtained in our study (32 weak D), because the weak D phenotype is infrequent in Morocco (0.4%) [4].

The frequency of partial D varies from one ethnic group to another, and in the Caucasian population the frequency of variants DVI is 1 : 6.200 [9] and among black individuals the frequency of certain partial D variants (DIIIa, DIIIb, and DIVa) is relatively high [10, 11]. In addition, it is very important to identify and assess the frequency of partial D variants, in particular the partial DVI variant, because this category is characterized by a reduced number of antigenic sites per cell. These variants can be typed by serology as false negatives (DVI type I: 300 antigens/cell) [12, 13]. On other hand the absence of detection of certain variants by serological techniques has been reported by several authors. Engelfriet et al. [14] calculated that in Southern California alone each year the red cells from at least 120 weak D or DEL donors, typed D negative serologically, are transfused to D negative recipients. Yet, no cases of unexpected anti-D immunization have been recorded, because very weak D or Del cells, with a very small number of D sites, only very rarely induce a primary anti-D immune response in D negative recipients and are only found to be D positive by RHD genotyping.

In our study using D-Screen Diagast kit containing a panel of nine monoclonal anti-D, we identified 13 (40.7%) reactions of partial D phenotype, 8 (25%) reactions of weak D phenotype, and 11 (34.37%) indeterminate reactions. However, based on our findings in this study, this kit was not very useful for the identification of most D variants. Therefore it is very important to identify these samples of weak D and the 11 indeterminate phenotypes in the further work, by using another kit of D partial or by analyzing the samples with PCR and sequencing, because they could not exclude the possibility for partial D.

Although it is difficult in blood banks to differentiate between partial D and weak D, it is important to identify a donor as having a D variant as the red cells of such a donor could elicit an immune response if transfused to a D negative recipient.

In Europe, DVI is most frequently associated with alloimmunization. Therefore, an unexpected feature of DVI type III was its almost normal number of RhD proteins per cell [15]. Furthermore to limit anti-D immunization for DVI recipient,

TABLE 1: Reaction profile of the D-Screen Diagast kit.

(a)

Number	Clone	Type	Two reactions DIIIa DIIIb DIIIc	Two reactions (Dva)	Three reactions (DVI)	Six reactions (DVII)	Eight reactions (weak D)							
1	HM10	IgM	+	+	−	+	+	+	+	+	+	+	+	+
2	HM16	IgG	+	+	−	+	−	−	+	−	+	+	−	−
3	P3 × 61	IgM	+	+	−	+	+	+	+	+	+	+	+	+
4	P3 × 35	IgG	+	−	−	+	+	+	+	−	−	+	−	+
5	P3 × 21211F1	IgM	+	+	−	−	+	+	+	+	+	+	+	+
6	P3 × 21223B10	IgM	+	+	+	+	+	+	+	+	+	+	+	+
7	P3 × 241	IgG	+	−	−	+	−	−	−	+	+	−	+	+
8	P3 × 249	IgG	+	+	−	+	−	+	+	−	−	−	−	−
9	P3 × 290	IgG	+	+	+−	+	+	−	+	−	+	−	−	+
Frequency			6.25%	6.25%	9.37%	18.75%	25%							

(b)

Number	Clone	Type	11 indeterminate reactions (34.37%)										
1	HM10	IgM	+	+	+	+	+	+	+	+	+	+	+
2	HM16	IgG	+	++	+	+−	++	++	++	++	++	+	++
3	P3 × 61	IgM	−	+	+	+	+	+	+	+	+−	+	+
4	P3 × 35	IgG	+	+	+	+	+−	+	+−	+	+	+	+
5	P3 × 21211F1	IgM	+	+	++	+	+	+	+	+	+	+	+
6	P3 × 21223B10	IgM	++	+	+	+	+	+	+	+	+	+	+
7	P3 × 241	IgG	+	+	+	+	+	+	++	+	+	+	−
8	P3 × 249	IgG	+	+−	+	+	+	+−	+	−	+	+−	+
9	P3 × 290	IgG	+	+	−	+	+	+	+	+	+	+	+

+: positive reaction.

−: negative reaction.

+−: positive or negative reaction.

the strategy of screening was essentially RhD antigen density-based transfusion strategy that is today considered wasteful, as it became apparent that most weak D (types 1 and 2) may be safely transfused RhD positive such that the goal of Wanger et al. [16]. The wastage might be reduced by lowering of the weak D threshold for RhD negative transfusion. However, this measure would trigger RhD positive transfusion in partial D like DVI type III, while still many RhD negative units would be transfused to weak D patients not requiring RhD negative transfusion. In this context, a strategy based on two monoclonal anti-D that do not react with DVI is advantageous [9]. This RhD epitope-based transfusion strategy abandons RhD antigen density as the trigger for RhD negative transfusions and became mandatory in Germany in 1996 [17]. For donor typing, weak D is considered Rhesus positive [18]. DVI type III proved that DVI erythrocytes may carry rather high RhD antigen densities. The threshold of RhD antigen density and RhD epitopes that most likely cause anti-D immunization is not fully established [15].

Based on our findings in this study, it seems appropriate to use molecular test in the next study which will identify the majority of D variants in our population and also resolve serological discrepancies. On the other hand, it is important to follow a strategy that consists firstly in selecting a monoclonal anti-D antibody that does not recognize DVI category for potential recipients of blood products. This should lead to better prevention of alloimmunization and to optimization of fetal-maternal transfusion [1]. Secondly, we need to increase the number of samples in order to better study the frequency of the most frequent partial D phenotypes in our population to guide immunohematologist in resolving serological discrepancies and in choosing the right strategy adapted to our population in terms of prevention of anti-D alloimmunization.

5. Conclusion

In conclusion, our study identified D variants (weak D and partial D categories) of the antigen D. This work can be used to validate the performance of the anti-D reagent and to improve the safety of transfusion of red blood cells from donors expressing the partial D antigen by integrating the finding into the recipient file with a recommendation concerning the appropriate care.

Conflict of Interests

The authors declare that there is no conflict of interests regarding the publication of this paper.

Authors' Contribution

Z. Kabiri collected the data and performed the research. M. Benajiba and K. Hajjout provided the reagents and materials. N. Dakka and H. Bellaoui analyzed the data and validated the paper.

Acknowledgments

The authors are grateful to all blood donors who contributed their blood samples to the study. The authors thank Dr. MC Brahimi-Horn for editorial assistance. Z. Kabiri, M. Benajiba, and K. Hajjout were supported by the CNTS, Ministry of Health. N. Dakka and H. Bellaoui were supported by MV University, Rabat.

References

[1] J. Chiaroni, V. Ferrera, I. Dettori, and F. Roubinet, "Groupes sanguins érythrocytaires: red-cell blood groups," *EMC: Hématologie*, vol. 2, no. 2, pp. 53–112, 2005.

[2] W. A. Flegel and F. F. Wagner, "Molecular biology of partial D and weak D: implications for blood bank practice," *Clinical Laboratory*, vol. 48, no. 1-2, pp. 53–59, 2002.

[3] J. Chiaroni, M. Touinssi, S. Chapel-Fernandes, T. Granier, A. Bokilo, and P. Bailly, "Molecular analysis of inactive and active RHD alleles in native Congolese cohorts," *Transfusion*, vol. 49, no. 7, pp. 1353–1360, 2009.

[4] Z. Kabiri, M. Benajiba, K. Hajjout, N. Dakka, and H. Bellaoui, "Weak D prevalence among Rh D negative blood donors in Morocco," *Immuno-Analyse et Biologie Specialisee*, vol. 28, no. 1, pp. 36–38, 2013.

[5] K. F. K. Fung, E. Eason, J. Crane et al., "Maternal fetal medicinal committee, genetics committee prevention of Rh alloimmunisation," *Journal of Obstetrics & Gynaecology*, vol. 25, pp. 765–773, 2003.

[6] S. S. Kulkarni, K. Vasantha, S. C. Gupte, D. Mohanty, and K. Ghosh, "Potential of commercial anti-D reagents in the identification of partial D variants in Indian population," *Indian Journal of Medical Research*, vol. 125, no. 5, pp. 641–644, 2007.

[7] J. Jones, M. L. Scott, and D. Voak, "Monoclonal anti-D specificity and Rh D structure: criteria for selection of monoclonal anti-D reagents for routine typing of patients and donors," *Transfusion Medicine*, vol. 5, no. 3, pp. 171–184, 1995.

[8] J. W. Jones, D. Voak, M. L. Scott, and H. H. Sonneborn, "Policies for the selection of monoclonal RHD typing reagents," *Biotest Bulletin*, vol. 5, pp. 485–494, 1997.

[9] F. F. Wagner, D. Kasulke, M. Kerowgan, and W. A. Flegel, "Frequencies of the blood groups ABO, Rhesus, D category VI, Kell, and of clinical relevant high-frequency antigens in South-Western Germany," *Infusionstherapie und Transfusionsmedizin*, vol. 22, no. 5, pp. 285–290, 1995.

[10] P. Tippett, C. Lomas-Francis, and M. Wallace, "The Rh antigen D: partial D antigens and associated low incidence antigens," *Vox Sanguinis*, vol. 70, no. 3, pp. 123–131, 1996.

[11] N. D. Avent, J. Poole, B. K. Singleton et al., "Studies of two partial Ds: DMH and DOL," *Transfusion Medicine*, vol. 9, supplement 1, p. 33, 1999.

[12] C. Loma, P. Tippett, K. M. Thompson, M. D. Melamed, and N. C. Hughes-Jones, "Demonstration of seven epitopes on the Rh antigen D using human monoclonal anti-D antibodies and red cells from D categories," *Vox Sanguinis*, vol. 57, no. 4, pp. 261–264, 1989.

[13] N. D. Avent, W. Liu, J. W. Jones et al., "Molecular analysis of Rh transcripts and polypeptides from individuals of Rh transcripts and polypeptides from individuals expressing the DVI variant phenotype and RHD gene deletion event does not generate all DVI phenotype and RHD gene deletion event does not generate all DVI ccEe phenotypes," *Blood*, vol. 83, pp. 1129–1135, 1994.

[14] C. P. Engelfriet, H. W. Reesink, G. F. Körmöczi et al., "Testing for weak D," *Vox Sanguinis*, vol. 90, no. 2, pp. 140–153, 2006.

[15] B.-N. Pham, M. Roussel, T. Peyrard et al., "Anti-D investigations in individuals expressing weak D Type 1 or weak D Type 2: allo- or autoantibodies?" *Transfusion*, vol. 51, no. 12, pp. 2679–2685, 2011.

[16] F. F. Wagner, C. Gassner, T. H. Müller, D. Schönitzer, F. Schunter, and W. A. Flegel, "Three molecular structures cause rhesus D category VI phenotypes with distinct immunohematologic features," *Blood*, vol. 91, no. 6, pp. 2157–2168, 1998.

[17] Wissenschaftlicher Beirat der Bundesärztekammer Paul-Ehrlich-Institut, *Richtlinien zur Blutgruppenbestimmung und Bluttransfusion (Hämotherapie)*, Deutscher Ärzte, Köln, Germany, 1996.

[18] H. G. Klein, *Standards for Blood Banks and Transfusion Services*, American Association of Blood Banks, 1996.

Anti-A and Anti-B Haemolysins amongst Group "O" Voluntary Blood Donors in Northeastern Nigeria

M. B. Kagu,[1,2] Sagir G. Ahmed,[2] Aisha A. Mohammed,[3] Waheed K. Moshood,[1] Mohammed B. Malah,[2] and Jimoh M. Kehinde[2]

[1] North-East Zonal Centre, National Blood Transfusion Service, Maiduguri, Nigeria
[2] Department of Haematology & Blood Transfusion, University of Maiduguri Teaching Hospital, P.M.B.1414 Maiduguri, Borno State, Nigeria
[3] Department of Haematology & Blood Transfusion, Aminu Kano Teaching Hospital, P.M.Bc 3452 Kano, Nigeria

Correspondence should be addressed to M. B. Kagu, bmk449@yahoo.com

Academic Editor: Mike Murphy

Background and Objective. The aim of this study was to determine the prevalence and haemolytic significance of alpha- and beta-haemolysins in our voluntary group "O" donor population. *Methods.* This was a prospective study carried out at North-East Zonal Centre, the National Blood Transfusion Service, Maiduguri, Nigeria from April 2007 to April 2009. One thousand nine hundred and twenty nine voluntary group "O" blood donors (1609 males and 320 females, median age 26 years $\pm$ 7.6 SD) were screened for alpha- (anti-A) and beta- (anti-B) haemolysins using the standard tube technique at 37 degrees C for 1 hour. All samples showing haemolysis were titrated for anti-A and anti-B haemolysins. *Results.* The overall prevalence of haemolysins in group O donors was 55.4%. Prevalence of alpha- and beta-haemolysins only was 10.3% and 12.6%, respectively, while that of donors having both alpha- and beta-haemolysins in their sera was 32.5%. Visual titre of 8 was seen in 0.4% of lytic alpha-haemolysin and 0.2% of lytic beta-haemolysin whereas donors with both alpha- and beta-haemolysins had a titre of 1.8%. Lytic titre of 16 and 32 was very low in our donor population. *Conclusion.* This study has shown that although the prevalence of haemolysins is high in our voluntary group "O" donor population, the strength of the lytic antibodies is low. Therefore, despite the labour intensiveness of our haemolysis titration technique and the frequent transfusion of group O blood to certain recipients of blood group A, B, and AB in our environments, there is the need to routinely screen our donors for haemolysins in order to identify those posing the greatest risk to recipients. Further studies to determine episodes of clinically significant haemolysis in recipients of blood group O may be necessary.

1. Introduction

The importance of a blood group system in clinical blood transfusion practice lies in the frequency of its antibodies and in the possibility that such antibodies will destroy incompatible cells in vivo [1]. Almost everybody over the age of 6 months has clinically significant anti-A and/or anti-B in their serum if they lack the corresponding antigens on their red cells [1]. Blood group "O" red cells can be given to A, B, or AB recipients and were formerly inappropriately called "Universal donor red cells". Early studies from Nigeria have shown high frequency of potentially lytic anti-A and lytic anti-B in blood group "O" persons [2, 3]. These high

frequency of alpha- and beta-haemolysins has been suggested to be responsible for the high frequency of ABO-haemolytic disease of the newborn seen in Africans [4, 5]. Blood group "O" is the commonest and most prescribed blood group type in our environment [6]. The fractionation of blood into its various components is still a nightmare in Nigerian blood transfusion service centres and the hospital blood banks. Apathy to blood donation coupled with poor funding is mostly responsible for these difficulties. As such most clinicians often transfused group compatible whole blood to recipients who ordinarily need packed red cells and/or fresh plasma. The occurrence of anti-A (alpha-haemolysin) and anti-B (beta-haemolysin) in group "O" donors was reported

TABLE 1: Distribution pattern of haemolysins among the group "O" donors.

Gender	Anti-A	Anti-B	Anti-A+B	Negative for haemolysins	Total (%)
Male	159 (8.2)	220 (11.4)	528 (27.4)	702 (36.4)	1609 (83.4)
Female	40 (2.1)	24 (1.2)	98 (5.1)	158 (8.2)	320 (16.6)
Total	199 (10.3)	244 (12.6)	626 (32.5)	860 (44.6)	1929 (100)

TABLE 2: Visual titres of anti-A, anti-B, and anti-A+B among the group "O" donors.

Titre	Anti-A	Anti-B	Anti- A+B	Total (%)
1	33 (3.0)	34 (3.2)	87 (8.1)	154 (14.3)
2	106 (9.9)	127 (11.9)	336 (31.4)	569 (53.2)
4	53 (5.0)	78 (7.3)	179 (16.7)	310 (29.0)
8	4 (0.4)	2 (0.2)	19 (1.8)	25 (2.4)
16	2 (0.2)	1 (0.1)	4 (0.4)	7 (0.7)
32	1 (0.1)	2 (0.2)	1 (0.1)	4 (0.4)
Total	199	244	626	1069 (100.0)

to be high in African population [7–9], and as such, some laboratories still spend a great deal of time screening for these lytic haemolysins using the labour-intensive technique due to the nonavailability of automated technique. The prevalence of these haemolysins also varies with age and gender [8, 9].

No similar study was carried out in this part of the country to investigate the prevalence and the strength of alpha- and beta-haemolysins in our voluntary group "O" donor population, hence the necessity of this study.

2. Materials and Methods

2.1. Materials. Blood samples for the study were obtained from voluntary group "O" donors, who had been screened, found fit, and accepted as donors. About 4 mls of haemoglobin-free serum was obtained from clotted samples, and these were stored at minus 18–20°C until they were analyzed (all samples were tested within 12 hours of separation after addition of absorbed fresh O serum as a source of complement). Although the lytic property of serum deteriorates rapidly on storage due to decay of complements, storage is to avoid the effect of high temperature in our environment that would also affect the potency of antibodies [10].

2.2. Methods. One volume of donor serum and one volume of absorbed fresh O serum (as a source of complement because the lytic property of serum deteriorates rapidly on storage due to decay of complements) were placed into each of 3 test tubes. To each tube was added 1 volume of 5% suspension in saline solution of red cells of group A, B, and 0, respectively. The O cells were used as negative control. The tubes were then incubated at 37°C for 1 hour, after which all tubes were centrifuged. They were then held before a source of light, and with minimal disturbances, the supernatant was examined for haemolysis microscopically. Haemolysis

was graded as follows: 3+: complete haemolysis, 2+: partial (more than 50% but not complete) haemolysis, 1+: trace haemolysis, and negative, no visual visible haemolysis. All samples showing haemolysis were titrated for anti-A and anti-B haemolysins as follows: 2 mls of each serum was double diluted serially in saline up to 256 and 0.5 mls of each serum dilution and 0.5 mls of absorbed fresh group O serum were placed in each of 3 tubes. To each tube was than added 0.5 mls of 5% A-cells, B-cells, and O-cells, respectively and the mixture was incubated at 37°C. At 1 hour, the samples were examined for haemolysis microscopically, and the titres were recorded. Titres were recorded as the dilution showing the weakest haemolysis microscopically. All data were analysed by standard statistical software (SPSS, Chicago, IL, USA). A P value of <.05 was considered significant.

3. Results

One thousand nine hundred and twenty nine sera from voluntary group "O" donors (1855-Rhesus D Positive and 74 Rhesus D Negative) were examined by the method described for anti-A and anti-B haemolysins. The median age of the donors was 26 years +7.6 SD. These included 1609 males and 320 females. The overall prevalence of haemolysins in group O donors was 55.4%. Alpha- and beta-haemolysins only was seen in 10.3% and 12.6% of the donors, respectively, while that of donors having both alpha- and beta-haemolysins in their sera was 32.5% (Table 1). Visual titre of 8 was seen in 0.4% of lytic alpha-haemolysin and 0.2% of lytic beta-haemolysin whereas donors with both alpha- and beta-haemolysins had a titre of 1.8% (Table 2). Lytic titre of 16 and 32 was very low (Table 2). There was no statistically significant difference between male and female donors in the frequency of haemolysins. Age also has no significant impact on the frequency of haemolysins in this study.

4. Discussion

This study has confirmed the high frequency of haemolysins in Nigerian group "O" donors. The prevalence of 55.4% observed in this study is higher than those reported by Olawumi and Olatunji in Ilorin (Southwestern Nigeria) [8] in 2001, Worlledge et al. (Southsouthern Nigeria) [3] in 1974, and Kulkarni et al. in Zaria (Northwestern Nigeria) [2] in 1985 as well as the work reported by Onwukeme and Nanna in Jos (North-central Nigeria) [11] in 1990. The higher prevalence rate observed in this study could be due to the methods and the fact that large population of group "O" donors were screened. Another possible reason could be the geographical location of Maiduguri bordering the Republic of Cameroun to the south, the Republic of Niger to the North, and the Republic of Tchad to the east. Admixture of blood of immigrants as a result of intermarriages could also be responsible for the higher prevalence. This geographical variation in the prevalence has been described in the literature [2, 11]. There was no statistically significant difference between male and female donors in the frequency of haemolysins. This is in conformity with the work reported by other workers [8, 10]. There was also no significant age difference in the prevalence of haemolysins. This is consistent with the findings of other workers [8, 12]. Although episodes of haemolysis in the recipients were not determined in this study so as to justify the clinical significance of such antibodies, it will be an overstatement to state that the frequency of strongly lytic anti-A and anti-B is low in this study. Taking a visual titre of 8 and above as being able to cause significant in vivo haemolysis [13], only 0.4% of the sera positive for alpha-haemolysin and 0.2% of those positive for beta-haemolysin had significant visual titre of 8. Similarly, a titre of 16 was seen in only 0.2% for haemolytic anti-A and 0.1% for haemolytic anti-B. This finding is lower than that reported by Olawumi and Olatunji [8] who found a significant prevalence titre of 2.0% for anti-A and 2.8% for anti-B. The difference could be due to the methods and the large sample size used in this study. In a study of the distribution of anti-A haemolysins in group "O" donors, David-West [14] found most titres to be not more than 16. In this study, most titres are between 2 and 4. This study has shown that although the prevalence of haemolysins is high in our voluntary group "O" donor population, the strength of the lytic antibodies is low. Therefore, despite the labour intensiveness of our haemolysis titration technique and the frequent transfusion of group O blood to certain recipients of blood group A, B, and AB in our environments, there is the need to routinely screen our donors for haemolysins in order to identify those posing the greatest risk to recipients. A further study to determine the episodes of haemolysis in the recipients of blood group O is needed so as to justify the clinical significance of such antibodies.

Acknowledgment

The authors would like to acknowledge the contributions of all the staff of the National Blood Transfusion Service, Northeast Zonal Centre, Maiduguri, Nigeria.

References

[1] C. Marcela and L. Antole, "Antigens in human blood," in *Postgraduate Haematology*, chapter 10, pp. 186–189, Butterworth-Heinemann, Boston, Mass, USA, 4th edition, 1999.

[2] A. G. Kulkarni, R. Ibazebe, and A. F. Fleming, "High frequency of anti-A and anti-B haemolysins in certain ethnic groups of Nigeria," *Vox Sanguinis*, vol. 48, no. 1, pp. 39–41, 1985.

[3] S. Worlledge, S. E. Ogiemudia, and C. O. Thomas, "Blood group antigens and antibodies in Nigeria," *Annals of Tropical Medicine and Parasitology*, vol. 68, no. 3, pp. 249–264, 1974.

[4] C. Chintu, A. Zipursky, and M. Blajchman, "ABO haemolytic disease of the newborn," *East African Medical Journal*, vol. 56, no. 7, pp. 314–319, 1979.

[5] H. N. Kirkman Jr., "Further evidence for a racial difference in frequency of ABO hemolytic disease," *Journal of Pediatrics*, vol. 90, no. 5, pp. 717–721, 1977.

[6] M. B. Kagu, S. G. Ahmed, and B. H. Askira, "Utilization of blood transfusion service in north eastern Nigeria," *Highland Medical Research Journal*, vol. 5, no. 2, pp. 27–30, 2007.

[7] L. A. Okafor and S. Enebe, "Anti-A and anti-B haemolysins, dangerous universal blood donors and the risk of ABO antagonism in a Nigerian community," *Tropical and Geographical Medicine*, vol. 37, no. 3, pp. 270–272, 1985.

[8] H. O. Olawumi and P. O. Olatunji, "Prevalence and titre of alpha and beta haemolysins in blood group 'O' donors in Ilorin," *African Journal of Medicine and Medical Sciences*, vol. 30, no. 4, pp. 319–321, 2001.

[9] A. O. Emeribe, "The status of alpha and beta haemolysins in Nigerian blood donors," *East African Medical Journal*, vol. 67, no. 3, pp. 205–208, 1990.

[10] H. G. Klein and D. J. Anstee, "Blood grouping techniques," in *Mollison's Blood Transfusion in Clinical Medicine*, pp. 302–310, Blackwell Scientific Publications, Oxford, UK, 11th edition, 2005.

[11] K. E. Onwukeme and O. U. Nanna, "Frequency of anti-A and anti-B haemolysins in Nigerians living in Jos," *The Nigerian Medical Practitioner*, vol. 20, p. 29, 1990.

[12] J. O. Adewuyi, C. Gwanzura, and D. Mvere, "Characteristics of anti-A and anti-B in black Zimbabweans," *Vox Sanguinis*, vol. 67, no. 3, pp. 307–309, 1994.

[13] D. G. Saphire, N. S. Rudolph, S. M. Hackleman, and W. H. Stone, "The effect of age on the level of human ABO blood group antibodies," *Aging*, vol. 5, no. 3, pp. 177–184, 1993.

[14] A. S. David-West, "Blood transfusion and blood bank management in a tropical country," *Clinics in Haematology*, vol. 10, no. 3, pp. 1013–1028, 1981.

Process Improvement by Eliminating Mixing of Whole Blood Units after an Overnight Hold Prior to Component Production Using the Buffy Coat Method

Cherie Mastronardi,[1] Peter Schubert,[2] Elena Levin,[2] Varsha Bhakta,[3] Qi-Long Yi,[1] Adele Hansen,[4] Tamiko Stewart,[5] Craig Jenkins,[1] Wanda Lefresne,[1] William Sheffield,[3] and Jason P. Acker[4,5]

[1] Canadian Blood Services, 1800 Alta Vista Drive, Ottawa, ON, K1G 4J5, Canada K1G 4J5

[2] Canadian Blood Services, Centre for Blood Research, 2350 Health Sciences Mall, University of British Columbia, Vancouver, BC, Canada V6T 1Z3

[3] Canadian Blood Services Research and Development, McMaster University, HSC 4N66, 1200 Main Street West, Hamilton, ON, Canada L8N 3Z5

[4] Canadian Blood Services Research and Development, 8249 114th Street, Edmonton, AB, Canada T6G 2R8

[5] Canadian Blood Services, Network Centre for Applied Development, Suite 207, 2150 Western Parkway, Vancouver, BC, Canada V6T 1V6

Correspondence should be addressed to Jason P. Acker; jacker@ualberta.ca

Academic Editor: Erwin Strasser

The elimination of a thorough manual mixing of whole blood (WB) which takes place following the overnight hold, but before the first centrifugation step, during buffy coat component production at Canadian Blood Services (CBS) was investigated. WB was pooled after donation and split. Pairs of platelet, red blood cell (RBC), and plasma components were produced, with half using the standard method and half using a method in which the mixing step was eliminated. Quality assessments included yield, pH, CD62P expression and morphology for platelets, hemoglobin, hematocrit, hemolysis, and supernatant K^+ for RBCs, and volume and factor VIII activity levels for plasma. All components, produced using either method, met CBS quality control criteria. There were no significant differences in platelet yield between components produced with and without mixing. A significant difference was seen for RBC hemolysis at expiry ($P = 0.03$), but for both groups, levels met quality control requirements. Noninferiority of components produced without mixing was confirmed for all parameters. Manual mixing is laborious and has a risk of repetitive strain for production staff and its significance is unclear. Elimination of this step will improve process efficiencies without compromising quality.

1. Introduction

Whole blood (WB) collection and storage and processing conditions can have critical consequences not only for the immediate quality of the resulting components but also for their long-term quality during storage. At Canadian Blood Services (CBS), production of pooled platelet components (PCs) is a semiautomated process in which WB is held overnight and then separated by a hard centrifugation step into RBCs, plasma, and buffy coats (BCs), from which PCs are

subsequently produced [1, 2]. CBS current practice includes a thorough, manual mixing of WB units following the overnight hold immediately prior to the first centrifugation step. In consultation with the bag vendors, this step was introduced during the implementation of semiautomated component production at CBS [1] and was thought to improve the separation of platelets from the other components in blood and hence results in a higher platelet yield.

In contrast with other mixing steps, such as the proper mixing of WB with anticoagulant at donation [3, 4], there is no evidence regarding the benefits of mixing WB immediately prior to centrifugation. Mixing of WB units does not appear to have been investigated previously nor does it appear in most descriptions of component production methods found in the literature, yet desired platelet yields are still reported [5–8]. The aim of this study was to examine the impact of eliminating this nonevidence based step in our component production process, as it is labour intensive, time consuming, and has the additional disadvantage of creating a risk of repetitive strain injury for production staff.

2. Materials and Methods

2.1. Whole Blood Collection, Pooling, and Splitting. Ethical approval for this study was granted by CBS Research Ethics Board. The study was designed as a noninferiority study which used a pool and split design to generate homogenous starting samples. WB donations were collected from consenting healthy blood donors into 70 mL citrate-phosphate-dextrose anticoagulant. Following a minimum 3-hour rest period on cooling trays at room temperature (18–24°C), eight or nine ABO-matched units were docked together using sterile tubing with multiple connectors (MacoPharma) and an automated Compodock (Fresenius-Kabi, Bad Homburg, Germany) and drained into a 5 L pooling bag (waste bag from RBC Cell Wash Set, Haemonetics, Braintree, MA). Following gentle but thorough mixing, the pool was split back into the original blood bags in random order, with volumes based on the net weight of the WB pool (minus 3% for losses incurred during pooling and splitting) divided by the number of units in the pool. WB units were prelabeled either mixed (M) or nonmixed (NM) and were stored for approximately 8 h at room temperature prior to component production the following day.

2.2. Component Production. WB units from each pool were processed into leukoreduced pooled PCs in plasma, leukoreduced RBCs in saline-adenine-glucose-mannitol preservative, and frozen plasma following the standard semiautomated BC production method currently in place at CBS, as described previously [1, 2]. The 4 WB units labeled M were manually and thoroughly mixed prior to the first centrifugation step, while those labeled NM were not. A total of 12 WB pools were used for the study, each of which generated 2 pooled PCs (1 M, 1 NM), 8 RBC components (4 M, 4 NM), and 6 plasma components (3 M, 3 NM).

2.3. Sampling and Testing of PCs. PCs were sampled on Day 1 and Day 5 and were tested on Day 1 (all tests), Day 5 (for CD62P, extent of shape change (ESC) and morphology), and after expiry (Days 7-8 of storage for pH and platelet yield). Unit weight was used to calculate volume based on a specific gravity of 1.03 g/mL. Calculations for platelet yield on Day 1 and after expiry were made using this calculated volume. A total of 24 PCs was tested (12 M, 12 NM).

2.3.1. CBS QC Requirements for PCs. Platelet yield (platelet count/unit) was calculated using the component volume and the platelet count, measured on an ADVIA 120 Hematology Analyzer (Siemens, Mississauga, ON, Canada), as described previously [1]. pH was measured using a GEM premier 3000 blood gas analyzer (Instrumentation Laboratory, Orangeburg, NY) and corrected to 22°C or a Thermo Orion 3-Star pH Meter (ThermoFisher Scientific, Nepean, Ontario, Canada). Residual leukocyte count was measured on the day of production using a flow cytometric assay as described previously [9], and sterility was tested on the day of production and at expiry using the BacT/ALERT system (automated BacT/ALERT 3D system, bioMérieux Canada Inc., St Laurent, Quebec, Canada) as described previously [10].

2.3.2. Platelet Quality Assays. Assessment of platelet degranulation, a marker of platelet activation, was conducted using CD62P expression by flow cytometry on a FACS Canto II (BD, Mississauga, Ontario, Canada), as described previously [1, 11]. Platelet morphology was assessed by modified Kunicki scoring, as described previously [1, 11, 12]. ESC was measured using a SPA-2000 (Chronolog Corp., Havertown, PA) according to Holme et al. [13] and described in detail previously [1].

2.4. Sampling and Testing of RBC Components. RBCs were tested at Day 3 and Day 43 after collection. Unit volume was determined based on the net RBC unit weight and a specific gravity of 1.06 g/mL. Components were sampled and prepared for residual leukocyte count within 24 hours of production. In total, forty (20 M/20NM) RBCs were tested.

2.4.1. CBS QC Requirements for RBCs. Total hemoglobin (g/L) was measured on an ADVIA 120 automated hematology analyzer and g/unit determined using the calculated volume of the RBC unit. RBCs were tested for rWBC levels using a flow cytometric approach as described previously [9] and were tested after expiry for sterility using the BacT/ALERT system. RBCs were tested for hemolysis levels using two methods. For the manual Drabkin's method, hematocrit (Hct) was determined visually following centrifugation in a Hettich 2010 microhematocrit centrifuge (Hettich Lab Technology, Tuttlingen, Germany) at 12,800 RPM. Supernatant and total hemoglobin were measured using the Drabkin's method as described previously [14], with trilevel commercial hemoglobin controls (Stanbio Laboratories, Boerne, TX) used for quality control. For automated hemolysis determination, Hb_T and Hct were determined using the ADVIA 120 automated hematology analyzer. Hb_S levels were measured using a HemoCue Plasma/Low automated hemoglobin analyzer (HemoCue AB, Ängelholm, Sweden). For both methods, percentage hemolysis was calculated using the following equation:

$$\% \text{ hemolysis} = [(100 - \text{Hct}) \times Hb_S]/Hb_T. \tag{1}$$

2.4.2. Additional RBC Quality Testing. Extracellular K^+ concentrations were determined by indirect potentiometry using ion selective electrodes on a Beckman Coulter DXC 800 (Beckman Coulter Inc., Fullerton, CA).

TABLE 1: Quality control acceptance criteria, noninferiority margins, and testing time points for platelet, RBC, and plasma components.

Parameter (unit)	Testing point	QC acceptance criteria	Noninferiority margin[*]	Sample size (pairs)[†]	Number of pairs tested[‡]
Platelets					
Platelet yield/unit ($\times 10^9$/unit)	Day 1 and at expiry	>240 in 75% of units at expiry	50	12	
pH	Day 1 and at expiry	6.4–7.8 in 100% of units at expiry	0.2	4	
rWBC ($\times 10^6$/unit)	Day 1	<5 in 100% of units	0.05	4	12
Sterility (growth/no growth)	Day 1 and at expiry	No growth in 100% of units	N/A	N/A	
Platelet CD62P (%)	Day 1 and Day 5	N/A	7	10	
RBC					
Hematocrit (L/L)	Day 3 and Day 43	0.5–0.7 in 90% of units	0.03	11	
Hemoglobin (g/unit)	Day 3 and Day 43	≥35 g/unit (in 100%) & ≥40 g/unit (in 90% of units)	5	11	
rWBC ($\times 10^6$/unit)	Day 1	<5 in 100% of units	1	20	20
Hemolysis %	Day 3 and Day 43	<0.8 in 100% of units at expiry	0.06	11	
Sterility (growth/no growth)	At expiry	No growth in 100% of units	N/A	N/A	
Supernatant potassium (mmol/L)	Day 3 and Day 43	N/A	1.3/4[§]	9	
Plasma					
Factor VIII (IU/mL)	<8 weeks after production	>0.52 in 75% of units	0.3	7	7
Volume (mL)	<8 weeks after production	≥100	10	18	20
Sterility (growth/no growth)	<8 weeks after production	No growth in 100% of units	N/A	N/A	

[*]Noninferiority margins were determined using previous CBS quality control and quality monitoring program data.
[†]Sample size calculations assumed a significance level of 5% and a power of 80%.
[‡]The number of paired samples (mixed/not mixed) tested for each component type equals the largest sample size required for each component type, except for plasma, for which 7 pairs were tested for FVIII activity and 20 pairs were used to assess volume.
[§]As supernatant potassium levels increase during storage, noninferiority margins were determined based on levels early in storage (Day 3—1.3 mM) and after expiry (Day 43—4 mM).
N/A: not applicable and rWBC: residual white blood cells.

2.5. Sampling and Testing of Plasma Components. The volume of 36 (18 M/18 NM) plasma components was measured. Plasma was placed into storage at ≤ −20°C and 14 randomly selected components (7 M/7 NM) were shipped frozen for FVIII activity testing within 8 weeks of production, as described previously [15, 16].

2.6. Data Analysis. Two approaches were applied. Firstly, it was determined whether all components met acceptable QC criteria based on the CBS standard panel of QC tests (Table 1). Some tests were conducted both early and late in storage to determine whether quality was affected immediately after processing. Secondly, all QC parameters were assessed to determine whether components produced without mixing were noninferior to those produced using the standard protocol, based on noninferiority/equivalence margins, determined by reviewing one year of CBS QC data and data from an on-going internal Quality Monitoring Program (QMP) [11, 15]. Additional quality parameters were also measured, and if there were sufficient prior QMP data (CD62P expression for platelets and supernatant K^+ for RBCs), noninferiority margins were determined and applied (Table 1). Sample size

calculations assumed a significance level of 5% and a power of 80% (Table 1).

The data are clustered for each WB pool from which multiple components of the same type and group (i.e., M or NM) were produced. A paired t-test was used to confirm whether the difference between the two groups was statistically significant. To confirm noninferiority of the nonmixing process, the difference between the two groups and the 95% confidence interval was calculated. If the upper and/or lower bounds of the 95% confidence interval were within the specified noninferiority margin, then noninferiority was confirmed. A two-sided P value of <0.05 was considered significant.

3. Results

3.1. PCs

3.1.1. Quality Control of PCs.
There was no significant difference in volume between pooled PCs produced with or without mixing (334 ± 10.6 mL versus 334 ± 10.1 mL, resp.), indicating that pooling and splitting produced uniform components. Both the M and NM components produced from

TABLE 2: Quality of pooled platelets produced with and without mixing. Sample size was 12 pairs (mixed/not mixed) for all parameters on Day 1 and after expiry. On Day 5, sample size was 10 pairs for CD62P and 11 pairs for morphology. In keeping with current QC processes at CBS, rWBC/unit was assessed at the beginning of storage, and platelet yield/unit and pH were tested after expiry. All QC criteria (parameters in bold) were met and noninferiority of platelets produced without being mixed was confirmed.

Testing time	Parameter	Study arm	Mean ± SD	Passed QC? (pass rate)	Difference (95% CI)
Day 1	**rWBC/unit**	NM	$3.40 \times 10^4 \pm 1.78 \times 10^3$	Yes (100%)	−0.000 (−0.001, 0.001)
		M	$3.37 \times 10^4 \pm 1.32 \times 10^3$	Yes (100%)	
	Platelet yield/unit ($\times 10^9$/unit)	NM	256 ± 36.4	N/A	−0.08 (−8.87, 8.70)
		M	256 ± 28.3	N/A	
	pH (corrected to 22°C)	NM	6.93 ± 0.03	N/A	0.02 (−0.01, 0.06)
		M	6.95 ± 0.05	N/A	
	CD62P (% of population)	NM	15.71 ± 4.06	N/A	−0.19 (−2.28, 1.90)
		M	15.53 ± 3.78	N/A	
	Morphology	NM	358 ± 8.78	N/A	−0.29 (−7.89, 7.31)
		M	358 ± 12.39	N/A	
	Extent of shape change (%)	NM	37.7 ± 3.07	N/A	2.85 (1.22, 4.47)
		M	40.5 ± 3.78	N/A	
Day 5	CD62P (% of population)	NM	26.00 ± 3.53	N/A	1.169 (−0.021, 2.358)
		M	27.17 ± 4.28	N/A	
	Morphology	NM	327 ± 7.0	N/A	−4.864 (−11.150, 1.423)
		M	322 ± 8.9	N/A	
	Extent of shape change (%)	NM	36.2 ± 5.52	N/A	0.588 (−1.757, 2.932)
		M	36.8 ± 5.25	N/A	
After expiry	**Platelet yield/unit ($\times 10^9$/unit)**	NM	279 ± 29.3	Yes (91.6%)	−0.667 (−10.920, 9.587)
		M	278 ± 27.4	Yes (91.6%)	
	pH (corrected to 22°C)	NM	7.38 ± 0.058	Yes (100%)	0.033 (−0.006, 0.073)
		M	7.42 ± 0.058	Yes (100%)	

SD: standard deviation, QC: quality control, CI: confidence interval, NI: noninferiority, rWBC: residual white blood cells, M: mixed, NM: not mixed, and N/A: not applicable.

one pool did not meet QC criteria for platelet yield after expiry, possibly due to low donor platelet counts in that specific WB pool (Table 2). Otherwise, all PCs produced from M or NM blood met current QC acceptance criteria, and no bacteria were found in any unit.

3.1.2. Comparison of PC Quality. Significant differences between M and NM groups were not observed, and noninferiority of the NM samples was confirmed for rWBC count on Day 1 and platelet yield and pH both on Day 1 and after expiry (Table 2). Using previous QMP data [11], a noninferiority margin of 7% was determined for CD62P expression (Table 1). Both on Day 1 and at expiry, no significant difference in CD62P expression between M and NM platelets was observed (Table 2). Similar to CD62P expression, ESC and morphology are not part of the routine QC panel but are often used as a means to assess platelet quality [11, 13], although there was insufficient QMP data to determine noninferiority margins (Table 2). No significant differences in morphology between NM and M platelets at Day 1 or Day 6 were seen. A significant difference in ESC between the 2 arms was observed at Day 1 ($P < 0.01$) with NM pooled platelets displaying lower ESC compared to M pooled

platelet products. No difference between M and NM groups was seen at expiry (Table 2).

3.2. RBCs

3.2.1. Quality Control of RBC Components. For RBCs, there was also no significant difference in volume between components produced from whole blood units with or without mixing (277 ± 3.6 mL versus 277 ± 3.8 mL, resp.). Bacterial growth was not detected in any unit, and all QC criteria were met with 100% pass rates for all parameters for both M and NM samples (Table 3).

3.2.2. Comparison of RBC Component Quality. No significant difference was observed for rWBCs/unit between M and NM groups (Table 3). Total hemoglobin levels on Day 3 and Day 43 were similar between the two arms, and no significant differences in Hct were seen. Based on the predetermined margins for rWBCs/unit, hemoglobin, and Hct, noninferiority of RBCs produced from WB that was not mixed was confirmed (Table 3). Hemolysis was measured using the CBS standard QC HemoCue/ADVIA method, and no significant

TABLE 3: Quality of red cell concentrates produced with and without mixing. Sample size was 20 pairs (mixed/not mixed) for all parameters. All QC criteria (parameters in bold) were met and noninferiority of RBCs produced without mixing was confirmed for all parameters.

Testing time	Parameter	Study arm	Mean ± SD	Passed QC? (pass rate)	Difference (95% CI)
Day 3	**rWBC/unit**	NM	$1.18\times10^5\pm7.11\times10^4$	Yes (100%)	$0.89\,(-3.62, 5.41)\times10^4$
		M	$1.27\times10^5\pm9.96\times10^4$	Yes (100%)	
	Hemoglobin (g/unit)	NM	52.5 ± 1.53	Yes (100%)	$-0.061\,(-0.499, 0.376)$
		M	52.4 ± 1.40	Yes (100%)	
	Hematocrit (L/L)	NM	0.626 ± 0.009	Yes (100%)	$-0.002\,(-0.006, 0.002)$
		M	0.624 ± 0.008	Yes (100%)	
	Hemolysis (%): hemoCue/ADVIA	NM	0.045 ± 0.042	N/A	$-0.011\,(-0.029, 0.006)$
		M	0.033 ± 0.023	N/A	
	Hemolysis (%): Drabkin's	NM	0.084 ± 0.019	N/A	$0.001\,(-0.007, 0.008)$
		M	0.084 ± 0.021	N/A	
	Supernatant potassium (mM)	NM	5.830 ± 0.207	N/A	$-0.095\,(-0.175, -0.015)$
		M	5.735 ± 0.220	N/A	
Day 43	**Hemoglobin (g/unit)**	NM	52.3 ± 1.47	Yes (100%)	$-0.128\,(-0.575, 0.318)$
		M	52.2 ± 1.64	Yes (100%)	
	Hematocrit (L/L)	NM	0.649 ± 0.011	Yes (100%)	$-0.004\,(-0.006, 0.002)$
		M	0.646 ± 0.009	Yes (100%)	
	Hemolysis (%): hemoCue/ADVIA	NM	0.162 ± 0.044	Yes (100%)	$0.016\,(0.002, 0.029)$
		M	0.178 ± 0.039	Yes (100%)	
	Hemolysis (%): Drabkin's	NM	0.198 ± 0.034	N/A	$0.012\,(-0.008, 0.032)$
		M	0.210 ± 0.036	N/A	
	Supernatant potassium (mM)	NM	40.460 ± 1.898	N/A	$-0.615\,(-1.259, 0.029)$
		M	39.845 ± 1.484	N/A	

SD: standard deviation, QC: quality control, CI: confidence interval, NI: noninferiority, rWBC: residual white blood cells, M: mixed, NM: not mixed, and N/A: not applicable.

differences were observed between M and NM groups at Day 3. A significant difference was seen at expiry ($P = 0.03$), with the NM units showing greater hemolysis. Despite this, noninferiority was confirmed, as the upper bound of 95% confidence interval of 0.029% was less than the margin (0.06%).

Measurement of hemolysis using the Drabkin method showed no significant differences between the M and NM arms and noninferiority was again confirmed (Table 3). There was a significant difference in supernatant K^+ between the 2 arms at Day 3 ($P = 0.02$) with higher supernatant K^+ observed in the NM units, but no difference at Day 43. Early in storage, levels of supernatant K^+ are low (~5 mM), and they rise steadily during hypothermic storage [17]. Therefore, two noninferiority margins were determined and applied, one based on levels early in storage and one based on levels after expiry. Noninferiority of the NM units was confirmed at both time points (Table 3).

3.3. Plasma Components. Volumes were not significantly different between plasma produced from M or NM WB (294 ± 5.8 mL versus 295 ± 6.0 mL, resp., $P = 0.08$), and all units passed QC requirements for sterility. FVIII activity was examined as this is one of the most labile of the coagulation factors, is often used as an indicator of plasma quality [16],

and is a regulated QC requirement in Canada (Table 1). FVIII activity levels were 0.79 ± 0.10 IU/mL and 0.78 ± 0.12 IU/mL for M and NM components, respectively, with no significant difference found ($P = 0.41$). Noninferiority of the NM units was confirmed.

4. Discussion

Many aspects of the processes used to produce components from WB have been intensively investigated, including collection and storage bags [18], the anticoagulant used for WB collection, the importance of adequate mixing of the WB and anticoagulant at donation [19, 20], and the optimal time and temperature of WB storage prior to component production [21, 22]. However, there are elements of the process that are nonevidence based, and this study assessed one such step to determine whether it is value added or has any effect on product quality. Elimination of the mixing step produced acceptable products as all QC criteria were met. For all parameters tested, noninferiority criteria were met, indicating that components produced without WB mixing prior to centrifugation are not inferior to those produced with mixing. For some *in vitro* quality tests, differences were found between the M and NM groups. Early in storage, there were differences between the two arms for platelet ESC, with lower ESC, indicating less responsive platelets [13, 23], seen in the NM platelets; however, these differences disappeared when platelets were tested at expiry. Although lower ESC was seen in the NM group, both M and NM groups displayed responsiveness of greater than 30%, indicating overall good quality.

Similarly for RBCs, supernatant potassium levels were found to be significantly different between the M and NM groups at Day 3 of storage, a difference also not seen at expiry. The levels seen between the groups early in storage differ by just 0.1 mmol/L, and although statistically significant, this difference should not affect product quality. A significant difference between M and NM RBCs was also observed for hemolysis measured using the standard HemoCue/ADVIA method used for QC at CBS but not using the Drabkin's method. Levels of hemolysis measured early in storage and at expiry using the Drabkin's method were higher than those measured using the HemoCue/ADVIA method. This underestimation of hemolysis by the HemoCue/ADVIA method has been observed before [24], and the differences in measurement of hemolysis using different methods are well documented [14, 25].

Communication with a number of blood centres in Europe and Australia which use a similar component production method to CBS reveals that some mix and some do not, but all achieve their desired platelet yields (personal communication with Dr. Denese Marks, Australian Red Cross, Australia; Gordon Nicholson, National Health Service Blood and Transplant England; Dr. Pieter van der Meer, Sanquin, The Netherlands and Dr. Alex Morrison, Scottish National Blood Transfusion Service, Scotland). Among the centres we contacted, none have transitioned from a process that mixed WB prior to centrifugation to one that did not, and so we are not aware of any validation or investigation of the effect of this process change. The results of the current study demonstrate that elimination of the mixing step is not detrimental to product quality, and components produced without mixing of the WB will meet all necessary QC criteria. In terms of process efficiency, and also for the health and safety of the production staff processing the blood, removal of this step may indeed be beneficial, and at CBS we are currently planning to implement this change.

Abbreviations

BC: Buffy coat
CBS: Canadian blood services
ESC: Extent of shape change
Hct: Hematocrit
Hb_S: Supernatant haemoglobin
Hb_T: Total haemoglobin
M: Mixed
NM: Not mixed
PC: Platelet component
QC: Quality control
QMP: Quality monitoring program
RBC: Red blood cell
WB: Whole blood.

Conflict of Interests

The authors declare that they have no conflict of interests.

Acknowledgments

The authors would like to thank the following for technical assistance with this study: Riki Roberts and Nobu Nakane, CBS NetCAD, Vancouver, BC; Helen Yu, Shadi Sarshad, and Janice Fujisawa, CBS BC & Yukon, Vancouver, BC, Jayme D. R. Tchir and Tracey R. Turner, CBS NetCAD, Edmonton, AB; Brankica Culibrk, CBS Research and Development, Centre for Blood Research, University of British Columbia, Vancouver, BC; Heather Perkins and Yuntong Kou, CBS NetCAD, Ottawa, ON and the CBS National Testing Laboratory, Ottawa, ON. The authors would also like to thank Dr. Sandra Ramirez, CBS NetCAD, Ottawa, ON, for scientific input and Dr. Geraldine Walsh, CBS Scientific Writer, for assistance with the paper preparation and editing. The generous donation of all CBS blood donors is gratefully acknowledged. Funding for this study was provided by CBS.

References

[1] E. Levin, B. Culibrk, M. I. C. Gyöngyössy-Issa et al., "Implementation of buffy coat platelet component production: comparison to platelet-rich plasma platelet production," *Transfusion*, vol. 48, no. 11, pp. 2331–2337, 2008.

[2] E. Semple, A. Bowes-Schmidt, Q. L. Yi, S. Shimla, and D. V. Devine, "Transfusion reactions: a comparative observational study of blood components produced before and after implementation of semiautomated production from whole blood," *Transfusion*, vol. 52, no. 12, pp. 2683–2691, 2012.

[3] P. F. Van Der Meer and R. N. Pietersz, "An evaluation of automated blood collection mixers," *Vox Sanguinis*, vol. 91, no. 3, pp. 275–277, 2006.

[4] M. A. Blajchman, J. Cid, and M. Lozano, Eds., *Blood Component Preparation: From Benchtop to Bedside*, AABB Press, Bethesda, Md, USA, 1st edition edition, 2010.

[5] J. Cid, M. Claparols, A. Pinacho et al., "Comparison of blood component preparation methods from whole blood bags based on buffy coat extraction," *Transfusion and Apheresis Science*, vol. 36, no. 3, pp. 243–247, 2007.

[6] C. H. Mondéjar, S. Bonanad, M. A. Soler et al., "Quality analysis of blood components obtained by automated buffy-coat layer removal with a top and bottom system," *Haematologica*, vol. 85, no. 4, pp. 390–395, 2000.

[7] F. Q. Lu, W. Kang, Y. Peng, and W. M. Wang, "Characterization of blood components separated from donated whole blood after an overnight holding at room temperature with the buffy coat method," *Transfusion*, vol. 51, no. 10, pp. 2199–2207, 2011.

[8] S. Thomas, M. Beard, M. Garwood, M. Callaert, and R. Cardigan, "Platelet concentrates produced from whole blood using the Atreus processing system," *Vox Sanguinis*, vol. 97, no. 2, pp. 93–101, 2009.

[9] D. S. Palmer, P. Birch, J. O'Toole, D. Henderson, and V. Scalia, "Flow cytometric determination of residual white blood cell levels in preserved samples from leukoreduced blood products," *Transfusion*, vol. 48, no. 1, pp. 118–128, 2008.

[10] C. Jenkins, S. Ramirez-Arcos, M. Goldman, and D. V. Devine, "Bacterial contamination in platelets: incremental improvements drive down but do not eliminate risk," *Transfusion*, vol. 51, no. 12, pp. 2555–2565, 2011.

[11] E. Levin, C. Jenkins, B. Culibrk, M. I. Gyongyossy-Issa, K. Serrano, and D. V. Devine, "Development of a quality monitoring program for platelet components: a report of the first four years' experience at Canadian Blood Services," *Transfusion*, vol. 52, no. 4, pp. 810–818, 2012.

[12] T. J. Kunicki, M. Tuccelli, G. A. Becker, and R. H. Aster, "A study of variables affecting the quality of platelets stored at 'room temperature'," *Transfusion*, vol. 15, no. 5, pp. 414–421, 1975.

[13] S. Holme, G. Moroff, and S. Murphy, "A multi-laboratory evaluation of in vitro platelet assays: the tests for extent of shape change and response to hypotonic shock," *Transfusion*, vol. 38, no. 1, pp. 31–40, 1998.

[14] J. P. Acker, I. Croteau, and Q. L. Yi, "An analysis of the bias in red blood cell hemolysis measurement using several analytical approaches," *Clinica Chimica Acta*, vol. 413, no. 21-22, pp. 1746–1752, 2012.

[15] W. P. Sheffield, V. Bhakta, C. Jenkins, and D. V. Devine, "Conversion to the buffy coat method and quality of frozen plasma derived from whole blood donations in Canada," *Transfusion*, vol. 50, no. 5, pp. 1043–1049, 2010.

[16] W. P. Sheffield, V. Bhakta, C. Mastronardi, S. Ramirez-Arcos, D. Howe, and C. Jenkins, "Changes in coagulation factor activity and content of di(2-ethylhexyl)phthalate in frozen plasma units during refrigerated storage for up to five days after thawing," *Transfusion*, vol. 52, no. 3, pp. 493–502, 2012.

[17] L. Van De Watering, "Red cell storage and prognosis," *Vox Sanguinis*, vol. 100, no. 1, pp. 36–45, 2011.

[18] L. Eriksson, G. Eriksson, and C. F. Högman, "Storage of buffy coat preparations at 22°C in plastic containers with different gas permeability," *Vox Sanguinis*, vol. 73, no. 2, pp. 74–80, 1997.

[19] P. Burger, H. Korsten, A. J. Verhoeven, D. de Korte, and R. van Bruggen, "Collection and storage of red blood cells with anticoagulant and additive solution with a physiologic pH," *Transfusion*, vol. 52, no. 6, pp. 1245–1252, 2012.

[20] D. De Korte and H. A. Veldman, "Automated blood-mixing devices still fail to mix at low bleeding rates," *Vox Sanguinis*, vol. 80, no. 1, pp. 34–39, 2002.

[21] S. Thomas, "Ambient overnight hold of whole blood prior to the manufacture of blood components," *Transfusion Medicine*, vol. 20, no. 6, pp. 361–368, 2010.

[22] P. F. Van Der Meer, J. A. Cancelas, R. Cardigan et al., "Evaluation of overnight hold of whole blood at room temperature before component processing: effect of red blood cell (RBC) additive solutions on in vitro RBC measures," *Transfusion*, vol. 51, supplement 1, pp. 15S–24S, 2011.

[23] S. Holme and S. Murphy, "Quantitative measurements of platelet shape by light transmission studies; application to storage of platelets for transfusion," *Journal of Laboratory and Clinical Medicine*, vol. 92, no. 1, pp. 53–64, 1978.

[24] J. P. Acker, A. L. Hansen, S. Payant, and C. DiFranco, "Evaluation of percent hemolysis measurement methods for use in the Canadian Blood Services quality control program," *Vox Sanguinis*, vol. 99, supplement 1, p. 212, 2010.

[25] V. Han, K. Serrano, and D. V. Devine, "A comparative study of common techniques used to measure haemolysis in stored red cell concentrates," *Vox Sanguinis*, vol. 98, no. 2, pp. 116–123, 2010.

Comparative Efficacy of Three Forms of Parenteral Iron

Richard Dillon,[1] Ibrahim Momoh,[2] Yvonne Francis,[1] Laura Cameron,[1] Claire N. Harrison,[1] and Deepti Radia[1]

[1] Department of Haematology, Guy's and St Thomas' NHS Foundation Trust, London SE1 9RT, UK
[2] Department of Haematology, Kings College Hospital, London SE5 9RS, UK

Correspondence should be addressed to Richard Dillon, richard.dillon@gstt.nhs.uk

Academic Editor: P. M. Kopko

Intravenous iron therapy is a useful treatment for the rapid correction of iron deficiency anaemia and can be used to avoid or reduce the requirement for allogeneic blood transfusion. Several intravenous iron preparations are available commercially which differ in cost, mode of administration and side effect profile. There are few data directly comparing the efficacy of these preparations. In this retrospective single-centre study, we present the results from two hundred and eight patients treated using three different iron preparations (iron dextran, iron sucrose and ferric carboxymaltose) and compare the effect on haemoglobin levels and other measures of iron deficiency six weeks after treatment. Within the limitations of our study design, we show a statistically and clinically significant difference in efficacy between these preparations.

1. Introduction

Intravenous iron can be a useful treatment for iron-deficiency anaemia in several clinical situations, including in patients who are intolerant to or unresponsive to oral iron [1], patients undergoing elective surgery [2], and in patients in whom the severity of the anaemia requires rapid correction [3]. Intravenous iron therapy may reduce the requirement for allogeneic blood transfusion [4]. Iron deficiency is the most common cause of anaemia worldwide and in the United Kingdom; "Better Blood Transfusion" guidelines require hospitals to provide alternatives to allogeneic blood transfusion where possible, and the use of intravenous iron may be an effective way to achieve this.

At the time of writing, there were three commercially available forms of intravenous iron in use in the United Kingdom. Iron sucrose (IS, Venofer, Vifor Pharma) is administered as an intravenous infusion containing 200 mg of iron over two hours, and subsequent doses may be given at 48-hour intervals until the desired dose of iron has been achieved. Iron dextran (ID, CosmoFer, Vitaline Pharma) is given as an intravenous infusion containing any dose up to 2000 mg of iron depending upon the patients' calculated iron deficit; the rate of infusion is titrated according to patient tolerance, and, for example, a 1000 mg dose would usually be infused over a total of 5 hours. Ferric carboxymaltose (FCM, Ferinject, Vifor Pharma) has become available recently and is administered as an intravenous bolus (containing 500 mg elemental iron) or intravenous infusion over 30 minutes (containing 1 g of elemental iron) (source: British National Formulary).

Although FCM has been shown to be safe and effective in the treatment of iron-deficiency anaemia [5], at present there are no data comparing it to existing preparations. Furthermore, although the costs of ID and IS are comparable, FCM is significantly more expensive (basic NHS prices for 1 g of iron: iron sucrose £70.80, iron dextran £79.70, of ferric carboxymaltose £217.50) (British National Formulary).

In addition to the drug cost, factors that need to be taken into account when selecting an intravenous iron preparation include the number of hospital visits required, the administration costs (e.g., staff time, bed occupancy time), and whether any benefits will be achieved by reducing pressure on ambulatory care facilities (e.g., ability to increase other treatments).

Comparative efficacy data would therefore be useful in deciding which preparation to use in a given clinical setting. Although this should be in the form of a randomised trial, we have been able to study a large number of patients treated with these preparations through our haematology service.

2. Patients and Methods

We performed a retrospective analysis of all patients who had been treated in our service for iron-deficiency anaemia over a two-year period. During that period, all three preparations had been in use at different times because the supply of both ID and IS had been interrupted at times due to manufacturing problems, and FCM was introduced onto our local formulary part of the way through the period of our study.

Patients were referred to our service by their general practitioners or by other medical or surgical teams within the same hospital for assessment and management of anaemia. After clinical assessment by a haematology doctor or clinical nurse specialist, patients underwent intravenous iron treatment if they had proven iron-deficiency anaemia and were either intolerant to or unresponsive to oral iron treatment, severely anaemic to the extent that it was felt by a consultant haematologist that oral iron treatment alone would be insufficient treatment, or if they had elective surgery scheduled and required a rapid correction of their anaemia. Treatment was delivered by a nurse-led service initiative. Patients were not treated in our service if they were under the age of 16 years or if they had chronic kidney disease stage 4 or worse (eGFR < 29 mL/min—these patients were managed in a separate renal anaemia service). The mean age of the patients was 39 years with a range of 22–75 years.

In parallel to iron therapy, patients also underwent investigations for the cause of iron deficiency as was clinically appropriate in each case. All patients were stable with no active bleeding. The choice of iron therapy was based on which iron preparation was available in our unit at the time patients presented for treatment, and where more than one preparation was available, choice was by clinician's preference.

Eighty-four patients (72 female) were given iron sucrose. After a 25 mg test dose on the first infusion only, this was given at a dose of 200 mg by intravenous infusion over two hours diluted in 100 mL of normal saline, repeated a variable number of times over the following 7–14 days depending on the severity of the anaemia (although there was no set formula for this). The median number of infusions was 4, and the range was 3–6.

Forty-two patients (35 female) were given iron dextran at a dose of 20 mg/kg by intravenous infusion. After an initial test dose of 25 mg, the remainder of the dose was given in 500 mL of normal saline over 4–6 hours.

Eighty-two patients (seventy female) were treated with ferric carboxymaltose at a dose of either 500 mg by slow intravenous bolus injection (patients below 60 kg body weight) or 1 g diluted in 500 mL of normal saline and infused over 30 minutes (patients above 60 kg).

Six weeks after intravenous iron treatment, patients were reviewed and had a blood sample taken for measurement of the full blood count and serum ferritin.

3. Results

The three groups of patients were similar with respect to age, gender, baseline haemoglobin level, baseline red cell

TABLE 1: Baseline characteristics.

Preparation	Iron dextran	Iron sucrose	Ferric carboxymaltose
Number of patients	44	84	82
% Female	84	85	85
Mean haemoglobin	9.7	9.3	9.0
Median (SD) haemoglobin	9.6 (1.37)	9.5 (1.8)	9.0 (1.75)
Mean MCV	79	78	76
Median (SD) MCV	79 (9.51)	79 (14.4)	75 (10.8)
Mean ferritin	23	14	27
Median (SD) ferritin	9 (36.9)	11 (42.4)	27 (52.9)

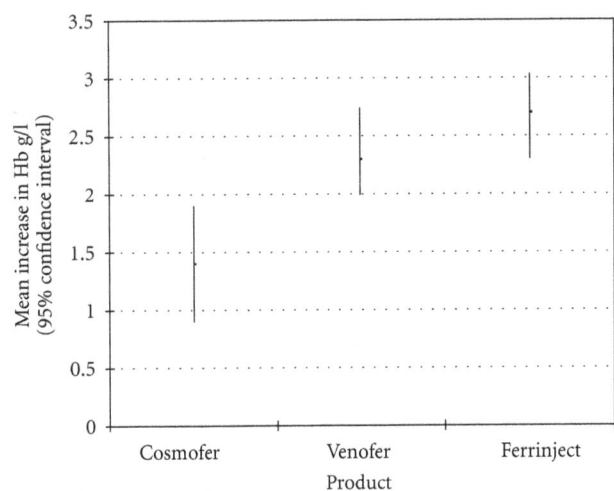

FIGURE 1: Mean increase in Hb six weeks after intravenous iron treatment with each product.

indices, and serum ferritin (see Table 1). At six weeks after infusion (or six weeks after the last infusion in patients who received IS), the mean haemoglobin had risen from baseline significantly in all three groups. The mean (± standard deviation) increase in haemoglobin level from baseline was 1.4 g/dL (0.9–1.9) with ID, 2.4 g/dL (1.99–2.74) with IS, and 2.7 g/dL (2.30–3.03) with FCM (see Figure 1).

When we compared these three groups using Student's t-test, we found that the increase in haemoglobin concentration was significantly greater in both IS and FCM compared with ID ($P = 0.04$ and <0.01, resp.). However, there was no statistically significant difference between the groups treated with IS and FCM.

There was a significant increase in both mean serum ferritin concentration and mean MCV after treatment in all groups (see Table 2); however, we were unable to show a statistically significant difference in these variables between the groups.

Two patients experienced an adverse event attributable to intravenous iron therapy. One patient in the ID group experienced hypotension and a rash during infusion, and one patient in the FCM group noticed an urticarial rash shortly after the infusion.

TABLE 2: Increase from baseline in Hb, Ferritin, and MCV in each group.

Preparation	Iron dextran	Iron sucrose	Ferric carboxymaltose
Mean ($\pm$ SD) haemoglobin increase g/dL	1.4 (0.9–1.9)	2.4 (1.99–2.74)	2.7 (2.30–3.03)
Mean ($\pm$ SD) MCV increase (fl)	5.8 (4.0–7.6)	5.6 (2.9–8.3)	7.0 (4.6–9.7)
Mean ($\pm$ SD) ferritin increase (mcg/dL)	149 (93–205)	109 (84–133)	149 (99–200)

4. Discussion

There are several limitations to our study. First, the doses of elemental iron received by the three treatment groups were different. However, the dosing system we used and therefore our results reflect the way in which these preparations are typically used in clinical practice. Furthermore, this factor would have biased our results in favour of iron dextran because patients usually received a higher dose of elemental iron if they were given ID (any patient who weighed over 50 kg would have received more than 1 g of iron in the ID group), and yet our results still show a significantly greater increase in Hb with FCM and IS compared with ID. Second, as we took our followup sample for full blood count six weeks after the last infusion, and patients treated with IS typically received 4–6 infusions over a two-week period, theoretically our results would have been biased in favour of IS because the patients in this treatment group would have had a slightly longer time for the earlier doses of iron to take effect.

In spite of these two major limitations, both of which would have biased our results against FCM, we saw increases in haemoglobin level that were significantly greater than in patients treated with ID and equivalent to those treated with IS. The results of cost versus benefit analysis will vary in different settings, but in many cases, we suggest that the higher cost of FCM may well be offset by savings in staff time and bed space (especially compared with IS: one infusion compared with 4–6) and with greater efficacy (especially compared with ID).

Our study was much too small to assess differences in adverse effects; however, ID has been reported previously to have a higher rate of anaphylaxis compared with newer preparations [6].

As this is a retrospective study with several limitations, our observations will require verification, preferably with a randomised controlled trial.

References

[1] O. Schröder, O. Mickisch, U. Seidler et al., "Intravenous iron sucrose versus oral iron supplementation for the treatment of iron deficiency anemia in patients with inflammatory bowel disease—a randomized, controlled, open-label, multicenter study," *American Journal of Gastroenterology*, vol. 100, no. 11, pp. 2503–2509, 2005.

[2] O. M. Theusinger, P. F. Leyvraz, U. Schanz, B. Seifert, and D. R. Spahn, "Treatment of iron deficiency anemia in orthopedic surgery with intravenous iron: efficacy and limits," *Anesthesiology*, vol. 107, no. 6, pp. 923–927, 2007.

[3] S. B. Silverstein and G. M. Rodgers, "Parenteral iron therapy options," *American Journal of Hematology*, vol. 76, no. 1, pp. 74–78, 2004.

[4] J. A. Serrano-Trenas, P. F. Ugalde, L. M. Cabello, L. C. Chofles, P. S. Lázaro, and P. C. Benítez, "Role of perioperative intravenous iron therapy in elderly hip fracture patients: a single-center randomized controlled trial," *Transfusion*, vol. 51, no. 1, pp. 97–104, 2011.

[5] S. Kulnigg, S. Stoinov, V. Simanenkov et al., "A novel intravenous iron formulation for treatment of anemia in inflammatory bowel disease: the ferric carboxymaltose (FERINJECT) randomized controlled trial," *American Journal of Gastroenterology*, vol. 103, no. 5, pp. 1182–1192, 2008.

[6] S. Fishbone and E. A. Kowalski, "The comparative safety of intravenous iron dextran, iron saccharate, and sodium ferric gluconate," *Seminars in Dialysis*, vol. 13, no. 6, pp. 381–384, 2000.

6

Screening Donated Blood for Transfusion Transmitted Infections by Serology along with NAT and Response Rate to Notification of Reactive Results: An Indian Experience

Rahul Chaurasia, Shamsuz Zaman, Bankim Das, and Kabita Chatterjee

Department of Transfusion Medicine, All India Institute of Medical Sciences, New Delhi 110029, India

Correspondence should be addressed to Shamsuz Zaman; rxhope@gmail.com

Academic Editor: Silvano Wendel

Background. Transfusion safety begins with healthy donors. A fundamental part of preventing transfusion transmitted infections (TTIs) is to notify and counsel reactive donors. Donor notification and counselling protect the health of the donor and prevent secondary transmission of infectious diseases. *Methods.* 113,014 donations were screened for TTIs, namely, HIV, HBV, HCV, and syphilis, by serology and nucleic acid testing. All reactive donors were retested (wherever possible) and notified of their status by telephone or letter. All initial reactive screens were followed over six months. *Results.* We evaluated 2,838 (2.51%) cases with reactive screening test results (1.38% HBV, 0.54% HCV, 0.27% HIV, and 0.32% syphilis). Only 23.3% of donors (662) responded to notification. The response among voluntary donors was better as compared to the replacement donors (43.6% versus 21.2%). Only 373 (56.3%) responsive donors followed their first attendance at referral specialties. Over six months, only 176 of 662 (26.6%) reactive donors received treatment. *Conclusion.* Our study shed light on the importance of proper donor counselling and notification of TTI status to all reactive donors who opt to receive this information. There is also an urgent need to formulate the nationally acceptable guidelines for notification and follow-up of reactive donors.

1. Introduction

Blood transfusion is safer than ever before through continuous improvements in donor recruitment, screening, testing of donated blood with increasingly sensitive assays, and appropriate clinical use of blood [1]. Serologic testing for transfusion transmitted diseases had historically been the foundation of blood screening, while newer strategies like nucleic acid testing (NAT) have helped further shorten the "window period" [2]. Currently, no technology exists to completely detect all window period donations. No matter how sensitive NAT becomes, we will never be able to completely close the exposure-to-seroconversion window period. The general public and media might believe that with the advancement in testing technologies zero risk blood products are currently available. This generalization is far from reality as judged by our current experience with new testing

methodologies. Breakthrough transmissions of viruses (HIV-1 and HCV) had occurred as late as 2009 due to NAT failures because of low level of viraemia and/or suboptimal amplification efficiency [3]. Moreover, threat of infectious agents entering the blood supply is not static and may evolve as new pathogens emerge or as old ones change their epidemiological pattern [4]. Therefore, regardless of testing modality chosen, a nonzero risk of disease transmission still exists in all its seriousness [5]. Under current practice in India, potential blood donors, after registration, filling of donor-health questionnaire, and brief medical examination, are sent for predonation counseling. During counseling process of blood donation, postdonation care and the outcomes of donation are explained. After blood donation, samples are collected for screening for anti-HIV-1/2, anti-HCV, and HBsAg, RPR for syphilis, and slide/card test for malaria. In addition to ELISA, NAT is being increasingly used in many centers to further improve blood safety although it is not mandated by national authorities.

In 2002, the Government of India adopted the National Blood Policy *"An action plan for blood safety"* to ensure safe blood supply. This policy advocates notification to all reactive blood donors. Blood banks are thus now required to obtain written consent from donors at time of donation for screening blood for TTI (Transfusion-transmitted Infections) and whether they wish to be informed about their abnormal tests results [6]. If any of the screening tests are abnormal, before notification to the donors the tests are repeated either using two assays of differing principles or in duplicate with the same assay so as to avoid notification of false-positive results. Donors who report back to the transfusion facility are retested and if found repeat reactive are referred to integrated counseling and testing centers (ICTC) for HIV and gastroenterology and STD clinic for HBV/HCV and syphilis, respectively, for counseling, confirmatory testing, and management.

Currently in India, most of the blood banks including ours do not have the facility to perform confirmatory tests for TTI. The donors are informed only on the basis of their screening tests available in blood bank. As most of the donors do not expect to hear that they have reactive results they may become extremely distressed to hear this news. These donors may be highly motivated to donate, having desire to help others, or simply want some time off work or may have other motives. This, unfortunately, may leave the donor with a negative feeling towards blood donation or diminish his/her own self-worth [7, 8]. On the other hand, a small minority of individuals appear to ignore notification and continue to donate blood elsewhere. Some of the donors even use blood donations as a means for free testing because of their high risk behavior *(test seekers)* [9].

Donor notification can therefore be a challenging task demanding special skills from the staff involved who should always be prepared to meet new challenges and help donors come to terms with their newly discovered status. Although the blood policy advocates disclosure of TTI status, donors are not, in practice, informed about their results. The onus lies with the donor to contact the blood bank [10]. There is very little information available about donor behavior on receipt of reactive TTI results. We undertook this study to determine the response rate following notification of reactive status to the donors. We also assessed the prevalence of TTI using serology as well as NAT among blood donors attending our center.

2. Material and Methods

Between January 2011 and December 2013, 113,014 donations at Main Blood Bank, All India Institute of Medical Sciences, New Delhi, were screened by ELISA using 4th generation ELISA test kits for HIV-1/2, 3rd generation ELISA test for HBsAg and HCV infections, and rapid immunochromatographic test for syphilis. All donations were also screened individually using the Procleix Ultrio assay (Novartis, Emeryville, CA), a multiplex NAT assay

for the detection of hepatitis B virus (HBV) DNA, hepatitis C virus (HCV) RNA, and human immunodeficiency virus-1 (HIV-1) RNA. If initial NAT result was positive, sample was retested again in triplicate. If any of these three tests were positive, sample was drawn from plasma bag and tested in triplicate. Discriminatory NAT was run if any test from plasma bag came positive. The analytical sensitivities of the Procleix Ultrio assay for HBV DNA, HCV RNA, and HIV-1 RNA are 10.4 (9.2–12.2) IU/mL, 3.0 (2.7–3.4) IU/mL, and 47.9 (43.3–54.5) IU/mL, respectively. The analytical sensitivities for the Procleix dHBV (d = discriminatory), dHCV, and dHIV assays are 8.5 (7.6–9.8) IU/mL, 3.2 (2.8–3.6) IU/mL, and 53.6 (47.9–61.2) IU/mL, respectively.

If the results of either serology and/or NAT were found to be positive, blood unit was discarded as per hospital SOPs and donor was notified of his/her status either by telephone or by letter. The first follow-up call was made on the 10th day of notification. If the donor did not respond to this first call, second and third follow-up calls were made every 10 days. The case was closed only if the donor did not respond to any of the three telephone calls/letters and the case was labeled as nonresponder. Donors who responded to the call/letters and came back to transfusion facility were counseled and retested by ELISA with fresh blood sample. Donors whose results from fresh sample were concordant with earlier tests were referred to concerned clinical specialty and donors who tested nonreactive were asked to remain in follow-up (Figure 1).

3. Results

A total of 113,014 donors were evaluated comprising 85.4% replacement and 14.6% voluntary donors. The majority of the donors (97%) donated blood for the first time. The demographic details of donors are given in Table 1. Total of 2838 (2.51%) donors tested reactive for TTI. Prevalence of TTI was 1.38% for HBV, 0.54% for HCV, 0.27% for HIV, and 0.32% for syphilis (Table 2). For HIV, HBV, and HCV testing, concordant serological and NAT reactive results were found in 1643/2480 (66.25%) positive donations. NAT yield in our study was 1 in 628 donations (180 NAT+ELISA– cases) (Table 2). Of all the donors who were notified of their reactive status only 662 (23.3%) donors reported back to transfusion facility. The response among voluntary donors was better as compared to the replacement donors (43.6% versus 21.2%) (Table 3). Donors residing in the urban nearby areas responded better than those who lived in rural or far-off areas. Donor notification using telephone was more beneficial as more donors turned up to transfusion facility. Only 373 (56.3%) responsive donors followed their first attendance at referral specialties. Over six months, 176 of 662 (26.6%) responsive donors were undergoing treatment.

4. Discussion

With over 93 million donations made every year worldwide, blood transfusion continues to save millions of lives each year and improve the life expectancy and quality of life of patients

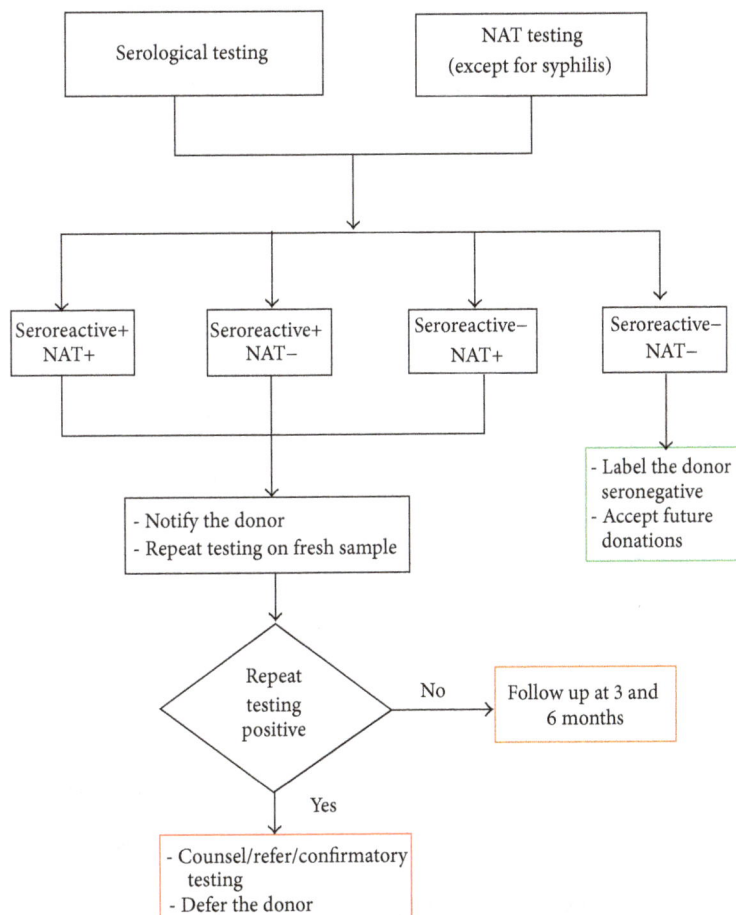

FIGURE 1: Algorithm for donor testing and recall.

TABLE 1: Demographic details of donations.

Donor demographics ($n = 113,014$)		
	Number	%
Gender		
Male	108,042	95.6
Female	4,972	4.4
Age group		
18–25	36,390	32.2
26–40	61,367	54.3
41–65	15,257	13.5
Residence		
Urban	78,206	69.2
Rural	34,808	30.8
Donation type		
Voluntary	16,516	14.6
Replacement	96,498	85.4
Donor repeatability		
First time donors	109,669	97
Repeat donor	3,345	3

suffering from life-threatening conditions [11]. At the same time, blood transfusion is an important mode of transmission of infection to the recipients. Prevalence of TTI in India is 1.8–4%, 0.4–1.09%, 0.2–1%, and 0.05–0.9% for HBV, HCV, HIV, and syphilis, respectively [12–17]. Prevalence of TTI in the present study was in agreement with other seroprevalence studies carried out in various parts of India. NAT yield in our study was 1 in 628 donations which was comparable to a previous study performed at the same institution [18]. There was high proportion of ELISA positive/NAT negative for HIV (50%) and HBV (15%) in our study (Table 2). This could be either due to low viral load below detection limits of the NAT assay or due to false-positive results in ELISA. The differences in the proportion of ELISA positive/NAT negative for HIV (50%) and HBV (15%) in our study can be explained by the fact that we performed fourth generation ELISA testing for HIV which has a high potential risk for nonspecific reactivity [19].

Transfusion safety begins with healthy donors. A fundamental part of preventing TTI is to notify and counsel reactive donors. Donor notification and counseling protect the health of the donor, prevent secondary transmission of infectious diseases to sexual partners, reduces risk of vertical transmission and provide feedback about the effectiveness of donor selection procedures such as predonation education and medical history [20]. We attempted to contact all

TABLE 2: Prevalence of TTI markers and comparison of ELISA versus NAT.

Marker	Reactive donors	ELISA+/NAT− (%)	ELISA+/NAT+ (%)	ELISA−/NAT+ (%)	Prevalence (%)
HBV	1557	232 (0.21)	1218 (1.08)	107 (0.09)	1.38
HCV	612	269 (0.24)	272 (0.24)	71 (0.06)	0.54
HIV	311	156 (0.14)	153 (0.13)	2 (0.002)	0.27
Syphilis (RPR)	358	NA	NA	NA	0.32
Total	**2838**	**657**	**1643**	**180**	**2.51**

*NA: not applicable.

TABLE 3: Donor response rate.

Marker	Reactive donors	Voluntary donors			Replacement donors		
		Notified	Response	%	Notified	Response	%
HBV	1557	143	69	48.2	1414	244	17.3
HCV	612	75	42	56	537	140	26.1
HIV	311	39	5	12.8	272	91	33.5
Syphilis	358	18	4	22.2	340	67	19.7
Total	**2838**	**275**	**120**	**43.6**	**2563**	**542**	**21.2**

2838 (2.51%) reactive donors about their TTI status either telephonically or by letter. Only 662 (23.3%) reactive donors responded to the notification. In an Indian study by Patel et al. 236 (60.36%) donors showed a positive response following donor notification [6]. In another study by Agarwal et al. involving 416 reactive donors, only 249 (59.8%) donors turned to transfusion facility and attended counseling after receipt of their reactive status [21]. The counseling success rate at large blood center in southern India was 41.18%, 11.11%, and 14.63% for HBV, HIV, and HCV, respectively [22]. Donor response rate in our study was low as compared to other studies from the country. This may be due to poor health care knowledge, social stigma associated with TTIs (especially HIV), and inadequate understanding of implications of screening tests among the general population [21, 23]. Also, as our center is a large volume referral center in India, most of the donors belonged to far-off places; thus distance could be a reason for the donors not reporting back to transfusion facility. Given the large volume of daily donations coupled with limited resources (only one counselor), it is difficult to ensure that every donor had understood the meaning and intent of counseling to the best of his/her intelligence. Another explanation which we think of for low response rate was nonreceipt of postal letters as donors tend to write inadequate postal address in donor registration forms. The study by Kleinman et al. reports that following notification 27% of donors contacted the blood center for further information [24].

One more finding of this study that should be a serious concern for blood transfusion authorities is that only 373 (56.3%) of 662 responsive donors responded to the first call and followed up their attendance at the ICTC or with the physicians they were asked to meet. Rest of the 289 donors (43.7%) was lost to follow up at this very first stage. This raises questions about the way donors are counseled and made aware of the consequences of not taking proper

treatment. It is also alarming that only 176 donors (6.2%) of all the reactive donors either were taking treatment or had completed it 6 months after having received notification of their infectious status. We could not find any studies from India to compare this data. The donors who did not turn up to transfusion facility (nonresponders) may continue to donate blood at other centers especially those centers which do not use biometric donor identification, hence posing serious threat to safety of blood supply. This threat is amplified by the fact that though ELISA is the recommended and preferred screening technique, many blood centers still do not have this facility and rely on "rapid kits" which may have high false-negative rate. Donors who are ELISA/NAT reactive elsewhere may escape TTI screening [25].

As per objective 4.16 of the Indian action plan for blood safety, the blood donors are counseled about TTIs prior to donation and are offered the option of knowing their seroreactive status provided they give their consent. Low donor response rate suggest that we are not able to meet this goal with reasonable satisfaction. Another important problem which we encounter in our daily transfusion practice is about donors who are notified because of NAT reactive/ELISA nonreactive status. These donors have their tests repeated by their personal physicians and return with discrepant results as most of the laboratories again screen samples by ELISA. These donors usually demonstrate an angry behaviour in blood bank and question the accuracy of screening performed in blood bank. More often than not despite our best attempts we are not able to explain the meaning of sensitivity and specificity of testing methods to the donors up to their level of understanding. We need to follow up such cases over 6 months as 95% of infected persons will seroconvert in this timeframe [26].

Our study has two limitations. First, we did not perform confirmatory testing of TTIs prior to notification. Second, repeat NAT was not done on the returning reactive donors (although a quantitative viral load is being performed at the referral center, unfortunately the results of which are not available to us). Our study was a small endeavor in determining donor behavior when informed about their reactive status according to results based on screening assays including NAT. Transfusion safety rests heavily on the health of blood donors. To improve donor response rate, we have switched to exclusive telephonic notification to all donors who test reactive in screening tests. Donors should undergo optimal predonation counseling so as to educate them about the risk of infections and the window period. It is the collective duty of transfusion community to inform these donors and do as much as possible to allay their anxiety about reactive result and to advise them about available treatment options. There is an urgent need to formulate the nationally acceptable guidelines for notification of all reactive donors. We have tried to formulate such schema (Figure 1). We expect that other blood centers will carry out such studies and further refine the algorithm.

Conflict of Interests

The authors declare that there is no conflict of interests regarding the publication of this paper.

References

[1] Z. S. Bharucha, "Safe blood transfusion practices," *Indian Journal of Pediatrics*, vol. 68, no. 2, pp. 127–131, 2001.

[2] R. Hans and N. Marwaha, "Nucleic acid testing-benefits and constraints," *Asian Journal of Transfusion Science*, vol. 8, no. 1, pp. 2–3, 2014.

[3] C. M. Nübling, M. Heiden, M. Chudy et al., "Experience of mandatory nucleic acid test (NAT) screening across all blood organizations in Germany: NAT yield versus breakthrough transmissions," *Transfusion*, vol. 49, no. 9, pp. 1850–1858, 2009.

[4] F. Bihl, D. Castelli, F. Marincola, R. Y. Dodd, and C. Brander, "Transfusion-transmitted infections," *Journal of Translational Medicine*, vol. 5, article 25, 2007.

[5] L. M. Kucirka, H. Sarathy, P. Govindan et al., "Risk of window period HIV infection in high infectious risk donors: systematic review and meta-analysis," *The American Journal of Transplantation*, vol. 11, no. 6, pp. 1176–1187, 2011.

[6] D. P. Patel, D. S. Patel, D. J. Bhatt, D. N. Bhatnagar, and D. M. G. Shah, "Evaluation of response to donor notification of reactive transfusion transmitted infections (ttis) result," *National Journal of Integrated Research in Medicine*, vol. 3, no. 2, pp. 20–25, 2012.

[7] L. A. Bashawri, "A review of predonation blood donor deferrals in a university hospital," *Journal of Family and Community Medicine*, vol. 12, no. 2, pp. 79–84, 2005.

[8] K. A. Munsterman, A. J. Grindon, M. T. Sullivan et al., "Assessment of motivations for return donation among deferred blood donors," *Transfusion*, vol. 38, no. 1, pp. 45–50, 1998.

[9] T. M. Roshan, H. Rosline, S. A. Ahmed, M. Rapiaah, and M. N. Khattak, "Response rate of malaysian blood donors with reactive screening test to transfusion medicine unit calls," *The Southeast Asian Journal of Tropical Medicine and Public Health*, vol. 40, no. 6, pp. 1315–1321, 2009.

[10] L. P. Choudhury and S. Tetali, "Ethical challenges in voluntary blood donation in Kerala, India," *Journal of Medical Ethics*, vol. 33, no. 3, pp. 140–142, 2007.

[11] Global blood safety and availability. Key facts and figures, 2010.

[12] P. Kaur and S. Basu, "Transfusion-transmitted infections: existing and emerging pathogens," *Journal of Postgraduate Medicine*, vol. 51, no. 2, pp. 146–151, 2005.

[13] D. Arora, B. Arora, and A. Khetarpal, "Seroprevalence of HIV, HBV, HCV and syphilis in blood donors in Southern Haryana," *Indian Journal of Pathology and Microbiology*, vol. 53, no. 2, pp. 308–309, 2010.

[14] P. Pallavi, C. K. Ganesh, K. Jayashree, and G. V. Manjunath, "Seroprevalence and trends in transfusion transmitted infections among blood donors in a University Hospital blood bank: a 5 year study," *Indian Journal of Hematology and Blood Transfusion*, vol. 27, no. 1, pp. 1–6, 2011.

[15] K. Chatterjee, P. Coshic, M. Borgohain, R. M. Thapliyal, S. Chakroborty, and S. Sunder, "Individual donor nucleic acid testing for blood safety against HIV-1 and hepatitis b and c viruses in a tertiary care hospital," *National Medical Journal of India*, vol. 25, no. 4, pp. 207–209, 2012.

[16] T. Chandra, S. N. F. Rizvi, and D. Agarwal, "Decreasing prevalence of transfusion transmitted infection in Indian scenario," *The Scientific World Journal*, vol. 2014, Article ID 173939, 4 pages, 2014.

[17] M. Meena, T. Jindal, and A. Hazarika, "Prevalence of hepatitis B virus and hepatitis C virus among blood donors at a tertiary care hospital in India: a five-year study," *Transfusion*, vol. 51, no. 1, pp. 198–202, 2011.

[18] N. Agarwal, K. Chatterjee, P. Coshic, and M. Borgohain, "Nucleic acid testing for blood banks: an experience from a tertiary care centre in New Delhi, India," *Transfusion and Apheresis Science*, vol. 49, no. 3, pp. 482–484, 2013.

[19] L. Gürtler, A. Mühlbacher, U. Michl et al., "Reduction of the diagnostic window with a new combined p24 antigen and human immunodeficiency virus antibody screening assay," *Journal of Virological Methods*, vol. 75, no. 1, pp. 27–38, 1998.

[20] C. Bianco and D. Kessler, "Donor notification and counseling management of blood donors with positive test results," *Vox Sanguinis*, vol. 67, no. 3, pp. 255–259, 1994.

[21] N. Agarwal, "Response rate of blood donors in the uttarakhand region of india after notification of reactive test results on their blood samples," *Blood Transfusion*, vol. 12, no. 1, pp. s51–s53, 2014.

[22] S. Dontula, A. Mathur, T. Kamaladoss, S. Adimurthy, and L. Jagannathan, "Donor disclosure—a donor's right and blood bank's responsibility," *Transfusion Alternatives in Transfusion Medicine*, vol. 12, no. 3-4, pp. 44–50, 2012.

[23] N. Choudhury, P. Singh, and H. Chandra, "AIDS awareness in blood donors in north India," *Transfusion Medicine*, vol. 5, no. 4, pp. 267–271, 1995.

[24] S. Kleinman, B. Wang, Y. Wu et al., "The donor notification process from the donor's perspective," *Transfusion*, vol. 44, no. 5, pp. 658–666, 2004.

[25] V. P. Torane and J. S. Shastri, "Comparison of ELISA and rapid screening tests for the diagnosis of HIV, hepatitis B and hepatitis C among healthy blood donors in a tertiary care hospital in Mumbai," *Indian Journal of Medical Microbiology*, vol. 26, no. 3, pp. 284–285, 2008.

[26] C. A. Ciesielski and R. P. Metler, "Duration of time between exposure and seroconversion in healthcare workers with occupationally acquired infection with human immunodeficiency virus," *The American Journal of Medicine*, vol. 102, no. 5, pp. 115–116, 1997.

7

Massive Transfusion Protocol Activation Does Not Result in Preferential Use of Older Red Blood Cells

Lauren M. McDaniel,[1] Darrell J. Triulzi,[2,3] James Cramer,[3] Brian S. Zuckerbraun,[4] Jason L. Sperry,[4] Andrew B. Peitzman,[4] Jay S. Raval,[5] and Matthew D. Neal[4]

[1] University of Pittsburgh School of Medicine, Pittsburgh, PA 15261, USA

[2] Department of Pathology, University of Pittsburgh, Pittsburgh, PA 15213, USA

[3] The Institute for Transfusion Medicine, Pittsburgh, PA 15213, USA

[4] Division of Trauma and General Surgery, Department of Surgery, University of Pittsburgh, Pittsburgh, PA 15213, USA

[5] Department of Pathology and Laboratory Medicine, University of North Carolina, Chapel Hill, NC 27599, USA

Correspondence should be addressed to Matthew D. Neal; nealm2@upmc.edu

Academic Editor: Donald M. Arnold

Widespread, anecdotal belief exists that patients receiving massive transfusion, particularly those for whom a massive transfusion protocol (MTP) is activated, are more likely to receive older red blood cells (RBCs). Retrospective review of blood bank records from calendar year 2011 identified 131 patients emergently issued ≥10 RBC units (emergency release (ER)) prior to obtaining a type and screen. This cohort was subclassified based on whether there was MTP activation. For comparison, 176 identified patients transfused with ≥10 RBC units in a routine fashion over 24 hours represented the nonemergency release (nER) cohort. Though the median age of ER RBCs was 5 days older than nER RBCs (ER 20, nER 15 days, $P < 0.001$), both fell within the third week of storage. Regardless of MTP activation, transfused ER RBCs had the same median age (MTP 20, no-MTP 20 days, $P = 0.069$). In the ER cohort, transition to type-specific blood components increased the median age of transfused RBC units from 17 to 36 days ($P < 0.001$). These data refute the anecdotal belief that MTP activation results in transfusion of older RBCs. However, upon transition to type-specific blood components, the age of RBCs enters a range in which it is hypothesized that there may be a significant effect of storage age on clinical outcomes.

1. Background

The influence of duration of storage of red blood cells (RBCs) on clinical outcomes is currently unknown. Multiple retrospective and observational studies suggest that transfusion of older RBCs, particularly in trauma patients, is associated with increased morbidity including multiple organ failure and nosocomial infection [1–6]. However, the inherent limitations of the study designs of these analyses weaken the conclusions. Furthermore, other authors contend that there is no increase in complication rates attributable to RBC duration of storage [7–10].

The age of stored RBCs in massive transfusion has received particular interest. Most blood banks in the United States practice a "first-in-first-out" inventory policy, which could potentially result in the delivery of large volumes of older RBCs to massively hemorrhaging patients [11–13]. Some have hypothesized that patients receiving massive transfusion, particularly trauma patients, are more likely to receive older RBCs than other patients requiring transfusion [4]. Despite the concern regarding the age of RBCs transfused to patients with massive hemorrhage, there are no studies specifically designed to address whether the use of a massive transfusion protocol (MTP) results in the delivery of older RBCs. Furthermore, although studies exist to suggest that certain ABO blood types may be stored for longer duration due to infrequent use [11, 13], there is no data to suggest how ABO blood type impacts the age of RBCs given in massive transfusion. Our goal was to characterize the age and ABO type of RBCs utilized during massive transfusion at a large, tertiary referral academic medical center. We hypothesized that MTP activation would not result in the transfusion of older RBCs.

2. Materials and Methods

A retrospective analysis was performed using blood bank emergency release (ER) and massive transfusion records at the University of Pittsburgh Medical Center and the Institute for Transfusion Medicine from January 1, 2011, through December 31, 2011. This research was conducted after approval by the University of Pittsburgh Medical Center Quality Assurance Committee (QIRB878).

An ER was defined as a request for the immediate release of RBCs in any quantity. This included the issuing of type O units (and not type-specific units) in situations in which there was insufficient time to obtain a patient sample for performance of a type and screen and to release type-specific units. At our institution, at the time of this study, a physician in any location of the hospital had the option to emergently order a massive transfusion of RBCs, defined as ≥10 units in a 24-hour period, with or without activation of the massive transfusion protocol (MTP) described previously [14]. Patients who had ≥10 RBC units issued to them in a single release were identified from the ER records and represented the ER cohort of this study. Using information from the electronic medical records, patients with an issuance of ≥10 RBC units were further categorized based on whether the MTP was or was not activated during their care (MTP or no-MTP subgroups, resp.). Both the ER cohort and the MTP subgroup included patients with traumatic and nontraumatic sources of massive hemorrhage.

Additional data were collected from University of Pittsburgh Medical Center records to identify all patients in 2011 who received massive transfusion. In addition to the ER cohort of patients, this dataset included those who had met massive transfusion criteria but instead received exclusively type-specific products since they had valid type and screens at the time of RBC requests. The majority of these patients were individuals with postsurgical complications and medically bleeding patients who met the criteria for massive transfusion through the serial transfusion of ≥10 RBCs over 24 hours as opposed to an up-front single request. This group represented the nonemergency release (nER) cohort. Importantly, the physicians caring for patients in this group had not requested an ER or activated the MTP at any point, suggesting that they may not have anticipated that the patient would require massive transfusion at the time of initial assessment and RBC infusion. This nER cohort of patients was chosen as a comparison group to the ER patient cohort since patients in both groups had similar RBC transfusion needs.

After identification of the patients within the ER and nER cohorts, an Institute for Transfusion Medicine blood bank database was queried to determine the age of each RBC unit transfused into each patient during the 24-hour period of massive transfusion. The age of each unit was defined as the difference in time between the collection and transfusion date. Additionally, the ABO type of each unit and of each patient was recorded. The vast majority (>95%) of RBCs at

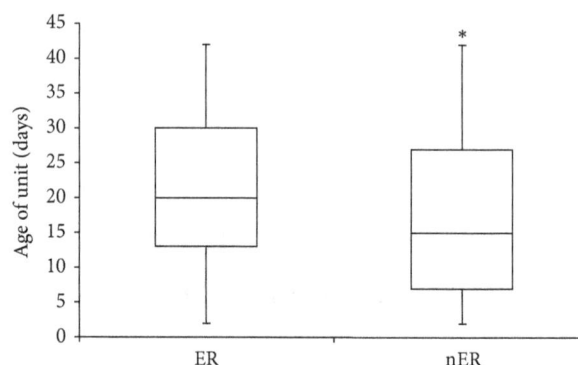

FIGURE 1: Difference in unit age between ER and nER cohorts. ER, emergency release; nER, nonemergency release; *P < 0.001.

our institution have a 42-day shelf life. Of note, universal leukoreduction is not employed at our institution, but rather patients are selectively given leukoreduced RBCs for either prevention of febrile nonhemolytic transfusion reactions, need for CMV risk reduction, or decreasing likelihood of HLA sensitization.

Patients in the ER cohort initially received type O RBCs during their resuscitation. Once the results of their type and screens were known, ABO type-specific units were transfused. However, the point at which the patients began to receive type-specific RBCs could only be determined for non-type O patients due to limitations in the dataset.

Lastly, to estimate the distribution and availability of the different ABO type RBCs available to the patients at our medical center, the regional blood donor center records were analyzed over a 30-year period. Between 1980 and 2010, deidentified records of unique individuals making a donation were analyzed and the ABO type of each donor was recorded.

Statistical analyses were performed using SPSS software, versions 22 (SPSS, Inc.). Mann-Whitney U or ANOVA tests were used to compare continuous variables and chi-square tests were used for categorical variables. Statistical significance was defined as P < 0.05.

3. Results

3.1. ER Cohort. In the ER cohort, 1500 units of RBCs were transfused into 131 patients. The median RBC age at time of transfusion of these emergently released units was 20 days [IQR 13, 30] (Figure 1). A total of 779 of these ER units were used in MTP activations. Regardless of whether RBCs were requested with or without MTP activation, the median ages of transfused units between the two subgroups were identical with similar interquartile ranges (MTP 20 [IQR 12, 29], nMTP 20 [IQR 13, 31], P = 0.069) (Figure 2).

The number of transfused units that were >28 and 35 days was calculated for each patient. In the ER cohort, the median number of units >28 days and 35 days was 2 (IQR 0, 1) and 0 (IQR 0, 0) units, respectively. In the MTP subgroup, the median number of units of each age transfused per patient was 3 (IQR 0, 6) and 0 (IQR 0, 3.5). In the nMTP subgroup, the median number of units >28 days and 35 days was 1

TABLE 1: Difference in number of transfused units of older ages between cohorts.

	ER	nER	P value	MTP	nMTP	P value
Total # of pts	**131**	**176**		**51**	**80**	
# (%) of pts who received ≥1 unit ≥28 days old	82 (62.6%)	120 (68.2%)	0.31	37 (72.5%)	45 (56.2%)	0.06
# (%) of pts who received ≥5 units ≥28 days old	32 (24.4%)	50 (28.4%)	0.44	18 (35.3%)	14 (17.5%)	0.02
# (%) of pts who received ≥1 unit ≥35 days old	54 (41.2%)	79 (44.9%)	0.52	24 (47.0%)	30 (37.5%)	0.28
# (%) of pts who received ≥5 units ≥35 days old	14 (10.7%)	25 (14.2%)	0.36	4 (13.7%)	7 (8.8%)	0.37

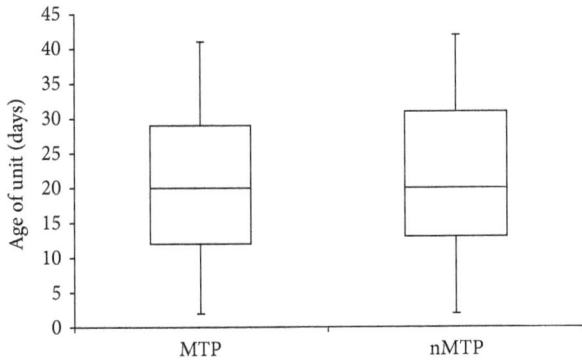

FIGURE 2: Difference in unit age between MTP and nMTP cohorts. MTP, massive transfusion protocol; nMTP, no massive transfusion protocol; $P = 0.069$.

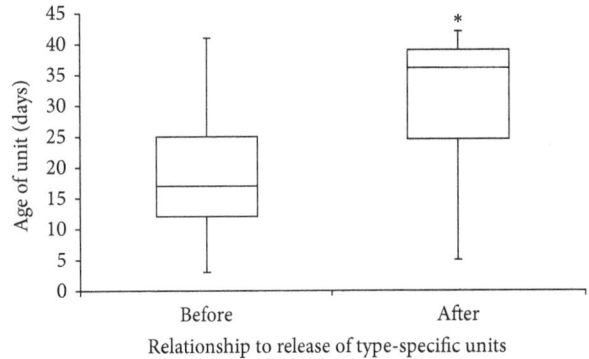

FIGURE 4: Difference in unit age before and after receiving type-specific units in non-type O patients. $^{*}P < 0.001$.

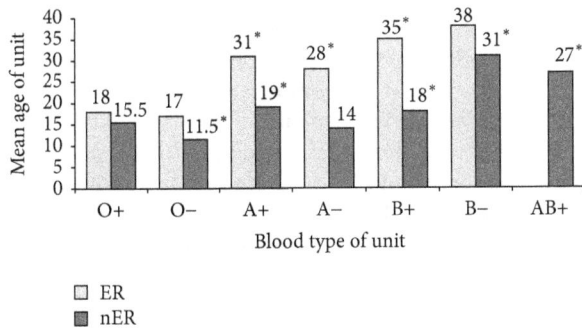

FIGURE 3: Median age of RBC units categorized by ABO type of unit. Storage ages of RBCs were computed for all transfused units as divided by ABO type. ER, emergency release; nER, nonemergency release; O+, O-positive; O−, O-negative, A+, A-positive; A−, A-negative; B+, B-positive; B−, B-negative; AB+, AB-positive; $^{*}P < 0.05$ when compared to O+ group.

(IQR 0, 3) and 0 (IQR 0, 3) units, respectively. The number of patients who received ≥1 and 5 units ≥28 and 35 days old was calculated (Table 1). There were no statistically significant differences between groups except for the percentage of patients receiving ≥1 unit older than 28 days, which was higher in the MTP group ($P = 0.02$) (Table 1).

When the 1500 transfused RBC units were stratified by ABO type, there were 1180 O-positive, 41 O-negative, 233 A-positive, 7 A-negative, 38 B-positive units, and 1 B-negative unit. Patients in the ER cohort who received type O RBCs received younger units than those who received non-type O blood (Figure 3), as the median age of an O-positive unit

was 18 days and the median age of an O-negative unit was 17 days. The median ages of each of the other non-type O units were ≥28 days. Additionally, when the 81 patients in the ER cohort with non-type O blood groups were switched from type O RBCs to type-specific RBCs, the median ages of the transfused units significantly increased by over 2 weeks (17 [IQR 12, 25] days to 36 [IQR 24.5, 39] days; $P < 0.001$) (Figure 4). The average number of type O units transfused in these patients (with blood types other than O) prior to the switch to type-specific units was 8.5 units.

3.2. nER Cohort. In the nER cohort, 2849 units were transfused into 176 patients. The median RBC age at time of transfusion of these nonemergently released units was 15 [IQR 7, 27] days. The median number of units older than 28 and 35 days transfused per patient was 2 (IQR 0, 5) and 0 (IQR 0, 3) units, respectively. Importantly, there were no statistically significant differences in the percentage of patients receiving ≥1 or 5 units ≥28 or 35 days between the ER and nER cohorts (Table 1).

When the RBC units transfused to patients in the nER cohort were stratified by ABO type, there were 1415 O-positive, 115 O-negative, 928 A-positive, 83 A-negative, 272 B-positive, 29 B-negative, and 7 AB-positive units. Similar to the ER cohort, differences in RBC unit age were also observed when the nER cohort was stratified by ABO type (Figure 3). The median age of an O-positive unit was 15 days and the median age of an O-negative unit was 11.5 days. A-positive, A-negative, and B-positive units had median ages between 14 and 19 days of age, while B-negative and AB-positive units had median ages of 31 and 27 days, respectively.

TABLE 2: Distribution of ABO type blood products from the regional donor population compared to ER and nER cohort RBCs. Data is presented as number (% of total).

	Donors	ER	nER
O	313276 (44.1%)	49 (37.4%)	79 (44.9%)
A	277461 (39.1%)	61 (46.6%)	71 (40.3%)
B	86009 (12.1%)	18 (13.7%)	23 (13.1%)
AB	33148 (4.7%)	0 (0.0%)	3 (1.7%)
Unknown*	0 (0.0%)	3 (2.3%)	0 (0%)
Total	709,894 (100.0%)	131 (100.0%)	176 (100.0%)

*The blood type of 3 patients in the ER cohort was unable to be obtained in the available dataset.

3.3. ER Cohort versus nER Cohort Comparisons. The median RBC unit age in the ER cohort was significantly greater compared to the median unit age in the nER cohort (20 [IQR 13, 30] versus 15 [IQR 7, 27] days, resp.; $P < 0.001$). However, it is important to note that both cohorts were within the same week of storage with an absolute difference of 5 days. A recent national survey reported that the mean storage age of a RBC unit transfused in the United States is 17.9 days [15]; this is consistent with the internal quality data at our institution (data not shown) as well as the current findings. Lastly, the majority of RBC units issued in both cohorts were type O (ER 81.4%, nER 53.7%) and the mean ages of these type O units from both cohorts fell within the third week of storage (ER 19.1 days, nER 15.7 days; $P < 0.001$). For non-type O RBCs, the mean ages of these units were significantly different between the two cohorts (ER 31.0 days, nER 20.1 days, $P < 0.001$).

3.4. Distribution of ABO Type Blood Products from the Regional Donor Population. Over the 30-year analysis period, 709,894 unique blood donors were identified. The distribution of ABO types of these donors and their respective products is shown in Table 2. As the data demonstrates, while type O donors represented the largest percentage of donors, the distribution of ABO types reflects that of a donor base in which Caucasian donors comprise the largest group of donors. Additionally, while the percentage of type O products used in the two cohorts was greater than the percentage of type O individuals present in the regional donor population, these differences did not achieve statistical significance (donors 44.1%, ER 37.4%, and nER 44.9%, $P > 0.05$).

4. Discussion

Although the effects of transfusing longer stored RBCs are currently unknown, most authors contend that if clinically significant impacts exist, they are most likely to occur with units stored for greater durations of time and usually greater than 28 days [1–6]. We demonstrate herein that RBC units issued to massively transfused patients within our large tertiary referral center in either an emergent or nonemergent fashion have ages that fall within the same week of storage. Although age differences between the two groups were

statistically significant, an increase in storage duration of less than one storage week is unlikely to be of clinical significance, as even current randomized trials assessing outcomes based on RBC age have chosen to randomize groups separated by at least 8–12 days of storage [12, 16]. Review of the interquartile ranges and greatest length of storage indicates no disproportionate distribution of RBC unit age. Individuals for whom the MTP were activated did not receive older RBC units in any analysis except for the likely insignificant observation that they may receive between 1 and 4 units greater than 28 days. Together, these data suggest that massive transfusion, specifically MTP activation, does not result in the delivery of substantially older RBC units.

An interesting observation from this analysis was that ABO type influences the age of RBCs in patients who underwent massive transfusion. Analysis of type O RBCs revealed minimal differences between ER and nER groups, and since type O units constituted 63.3% of the total units transfused, this likely influenced the cumulative results. In both the ER and nER groups, the ages of non-type O RBCs issued were considerably older than type O units. Thus, in the setting of ER of non-type O units (in a scenario where a massively hemorrhaging patient had an available ABO typing), there was a significant increase in the mean age of RBC units issued, with all non-type O blood groups being over 30 days. Given the relative frequency with which RBCs are transfused in our busy tertiary referral Level I trauma center, it is likely that type O units do not reach older ages prior to their frequent utilization in these populations, whereas the other less frequently transfused non-type O units are more likely to be stored for longer durations prior to issue.

Our analysis of the frequency of donor ABO types from the regional blood donor center suggests that type O RBCs are not disproportionately available to our hospital relative to the use of these type O products in the ER and nER cohorts, further supporting the notion that these units are utilized more rapidly and thus would not be expected to reach ages as old as non-type O RBCs. In confirmation of these observations, when we compared the age of RBCs transfused to non-type O patients before and after the transfusion of type-specific units in the ER group, the median age of issued units increased by more than 2 weeks.

A possible explanation for the significantly younger ages of non-type O RBCs in the nER cohort could be unique RBC special need requirements based on differences in the patient populations between these two groups. As the nER group was composed of patients who were more likely to be on medical services, they would be expected to have a greater likelihood of requiring leukoreduced and/or irradiated RBCs, in addition to antigen-negative RBCs due to previous alloimmunization from transfusion or pregnancy, all of which take more time to acquire or prepare. Almost invariably, all of these special conditions are waived in the setting of ER of ≥10 RBC units, where the need for immediate transfusion in massive quantity exceeds the need for any unique RBC products. While only a hypothesis, it may be that those non-type O units which are leukoreduced, are irradiated, or lack certain antigens are in fact younger than units which are not manipulated, perhaps because these units are utilized more frequently and do not have an opportunity to reach older ages (similar to type O RBCs).

Our study has a number of limitations. The retrospective design does not control for all potential confounding variables. It is also important to note that this was a single-center analysis at a large tertiary academic medical center and the results might not be applicable to other institutions, particularly those that have different policies for issuing RBC units in emergency requests. Due to limitations in the available dataset, we were unable to calculate the difference in the average age of RBCs issued before and after receipt of type-specific blood for individuals with blood type O. However, in this study, as type O units were much younger than non-type O units, it is unlikely that there would have been as significant of an increase in RBC unit age in type O patients compared to the non-type O individuals. Finally, it is important to note that this study was not designed to assess outcome measures associated with RBC storage age. Rather, it was designed to be a descriptive analysis of the age of RBCs utilized during massive transfusion and the effects of ABO type on the age of units distributed. The clinical implications of storage age have yet to be determined in ongoing randomized trials [12, 16].

In summary, the anecdotal belief that massively transfused patients, specifically those for whom the MTP was activated, receive older RBC units is not supported by these data. However, when non-type O RBCs are utilized, the age of transfused units increases markedly and enters the range in which it is hypothesized that there may be a clinically significant effect of the storage lesion [11, 12]. Further research into RBC storage age and outcomes may consider ABO type analysis in their study designs.

Disclosure

Jay S. Raval and Matthew D. Neal are co-senior authors.

Conflict of Interests

The authors declare that there is no conflict of interests regarding the publication of this paper.

References

[1] G. Zallen, P. J. Offner, E. E. Moore et al., "Age of transfused blood is an independent risk factor for postinjury multiple organ failure," *The American Journal of Surgery*, vol. 178, no. 6, pp. 570–572, 1999.

[2] J. A. Weinberg, G. McGwin Jr., R. L. Griffin et al., "Age of transfused blood: an independent predictor of mortality despite universal leukoreduction," *The Journal of Trauma*, vol. 65, no. 2, pp. 279–282, 2008.

[3] P. C. Spinella, C. L. Carroll, I. Staff et al., "Duration of red blood cell storage is associated with increased incidence of deep vein thrombosis and in hospital mortality in patients with traumatic injuries," *Critical Care*, vol. 13, no. 5, p. R151, 2009.

[4] Z. Murrell, J. S. Haukoos, B. Putnam, and S. R. Klein, "The effect of older blood on mortality, need for ICU care, and the length of ICU stay after major trauma," *American Surgeon*, vol. 71, no. 9, pp. 781–785, 2005.

[5] M. E. Keller, R. Jean, W. W. LaMorte, F. Millham, and E. Hirsch, "Effects of age of transfused blood on length of stay in trauma patients: a preliminary report," *Journal of Trauma*, vol. 53, no. 5, pp. 1023–1025, 2002.

[6] P. J. Offner, E. E. Moore, W. L. Biffl, J. L. Johnson, and C. C. Silliman, "Increased rate of infection associated with transfusion of old blood after severe injury," *Archives of Surgery*, vol. 137, no. 6, pp. 711–717, 2002.

[7] S. R. Leal-Noval, M. Muñoz-Gómez, V. Arellano-Orden et al., "Impact of age of transfused blood on cerebral oxygenation in male patients with severe traumatic brain injury," *Critical Care Medicine*, vol. 36, no. 4, pp. 1290–1296, 2008.

[8] E. C. Vamvakas, "Meta-analysis of clinical studies of the purported deleterious effects of "old" (versus "fresh") red blood cells: are we at equipoise?" *Transfusion*, vol. 50, no. 3, pp. 600–610, 2010.

[9] H. A. Phelan, A. L. Eastman, K. Aldy et al., "Prestorage leukoreduction abrogates the detrimental effect of aging on packed red cells transfused after trauma: a prospective cohort study," *The American Journal of Surgery*, vol. 203, no. 2, pp. 198–204, 2012.

[10] R. W. Taylor, J. O'Brien, S. J. Trottier et al., "Red blood cell transfusions and nosocomial infections in critically ill patients," *Critical Care Medicine*, vol. 34, no. 9, pp. 2302–2308, 2006.

[11] D. J. Triulzi and M. H. Yazer, "Clinical studies of the effect of blood storage on patient outcomes," *Transfusion and Apheresis Science*, vol. 43, no. 1, pp. 95–106, 2010.

[12] J. Lacroix, P. Hébert, D. Fergusson et al., "The Age of Blood Evaluation (ABLE) randomized controlled trial: study design," *Transfusion Medicine Reviews*, vol. 25, no. 3, pp. 197–205, 2011.

[13] S. M. Cohn, M. Derosa, A. Kumar et al., "Impact of the age of transfused red blood cells in the trauma population: a feasibility study," *Injury*, vol. 45, no. 3, pp. 605–611, 2014.

[14] L. M. McDaniel, M. D. Neal, J. L. Sperry et al., "Use of a massive transfusion protocol in nontrauma patients: activate away," *Journal of the American College of Surgeons*, vol. 216, no. 6, pp. 1103–1109, 2013.

[15] U.S. Department of Health and Human Services, "The 2011 National Blood Collection and Utilization Survey Report," Department of Health and Human Services, Washington, DC, USA, 2011, http://www.bloodsurvey.org/.

[16] M. E. Steiner, S. F. Assmann, J. H. Levy et al., "Addressing the question of the effect of RBC storage on clinical outcomes: the Red Cell Storage Duration Study (RECESS) (Section 7)," *Transfusion and Apheresis Science*, vol. 43, no. 1, pp. 107–116, 2010.

8

Phenotypic Profile of Rh and Kell Blood Group Systems among Blood Donors in Cote d'Ivoire, West Africa

L. Siransy Bogui,[1,2] **B. Dembele,**[1,3] **Y. Sekongo,**[1,2] **S. Abisse,**[1,2] **S. Konaté,**[1] **and M. Sombo**[2,4]

[1] *National Blood Transfusion Center, 52 boulevard de Marseille, BP 15 Abidjan, Cote d'Ivoire*
[2] *Laboratory of Immunology, UFR of Medical Sciences, BP 34 Abidjan 01, Cote d'Ivoire*
[3] *Laboratory of Immunology, UFR of Pharmaceutical and Biological Sciences, BP 34 Abidjan 01, Cote d'Ivoire*
[4] *Hospital and University Centre of Cocody, BP 1843 Abidjan 08, Cote d'Ivoire*

Correspondence should be addressed to L. Siransy Bogui; lsiransy@gmail.com

Academic Editor: Silvano Wendel

Few countries in sub-Saharan Africa make systematic searches for antigens C, c, E, and e of the Rh and Kell system antigens in the donor and recipient, thereby exposing transfused patients. *Purpose and Objectives.* In this paper, we propose to determine the red cell Rh and Kell blood groups among blood donors from traditional techniques to improve medical care of transfused patients. This study will allow us to assess the frequency of blood group antigens in these systems. *Study Design and Methods.* We carried out a study on the red cell typing in the blood donor population of the National Blood Transfusion Center in Abidjan. This study was performed on 651 blood donors. *Results.* For the Rh system, the antigen frequencies of D, c, e, C, and E are, respectively, 92.93%, 99.85%, 99.85%, 21.97%, and 13.82%. K antigen is found in 0.77% of donors. *Discussion and Conclusion.* Although the frequencies of the most immunogenic antigens are lower than in the white race, lack of preventive measures makes the immunological risk high in Africa. Furthermore, Africa is full of specificities that are important to note for a better care of our patients.

1. Introduction

In Cote d'Ivoire and in other African countries [1, 2], most of transfusions are done only based on ABO and D antigens. Although blood transfusions can save life, they are not without risk. Blood transfusion can carry immediate or delayed immunological risks; the most common and most serious is the hemolytic transfusion reaction by antibody incompatibility. Knowledge about the frequency of red cells antigens phenotypes in Ivorian population is important for the creation of a donor data bank and to minimize risks of alloimmunization. This requires the determination of the immunological characteristics of blood products and blood recipients by performing immunohematology analysis such as phenotyping in Rh and Kell blood group systems. Currently, there are thirty-three major blood group systems [3], but analyses recommended in the usual situation are ABO, Rh, and Kell typing and detecting red cell antibodies.

Unfortunately, in sub-Saharan countries, few practice this systematic search for antigens C, c, e, E, and K in the donor and recipient, thereby exposing the transfused patient to high risk of alloimmunization [4].

Very few studies are available, reporting antigens frequencies of Rh and Kell blood groups in sub-Saharan countries.

This study is the first report on the frequency of blood groups system Rh and Kell in blood donors in Cote d'Ivoire. This work will perform Rh and Kell red cell typing among blood donors by traditional techniques to implement this into the routine for blood donors and recipients. It also allows us to determine the frequency of the major Rh and Kell blood group antigens and phenotypes commonly found among blood donors from Cote d'Ivoire to improve transfusion practices.

2. Materials and Methods

It was a retrospective study conducted at the Laboratory of Immunohaematology of the National Blood Transfusion Center of Abidjan, the capital of Cote d'Ivoire.

2.1. Blood Donors. We analyzed grouping data in Rh and Kell blood group systems from 651 volunteer regular blood donors coming to the national blood on one year. The blood donors have an age range from 18 to 60 years.

Those excluded from donating blood fell within the following categories:

(i) taking drugs for high blood pressure or heart failure;

(ii) having Hb below 11 g/dL (for females) or 12 g/dL (for males);

(iii) testing positive for HBsAg, HCV, and HIV antibodies and syphilis;

(iv) having had jaundice, liver disease, epilepsy, diabetes, duodenal or gastric ulcer, asthma, tuberculosis, or other pathology;

(v) taking self-injected drugs;

(vi) having sickle cell disease;

(vii) being a prostitute and/or homosexual;

(viii) having severe weight loss within the last six months.

2.2. Methods. For optimal results, the determination was performed using a tube freshly drawn into ethylenediaminetetraacetate according to manufacturer's instructions. The techniques are direct agglutination of the antigens with slide technique for Rh system antigens and indirect antiglobulin technique by tube technique for Kell system antigens. Rh phenotyping was done using five monoclonal monospecific antisera: anti-D, anti-E, anti-C, anti-c, and anti-e while Kell phenotyping was performed with anti-K according to manufacturer's instructions. All reagents were supplied by Orgenics PBS, Eurobio.

Positive and negative control red cells and Coombs' control cells were also performed as controls. Data were entered and analyzed with Epi Info version 6.1.

3. Results

We determined blood group antigens in 651 donors with sex ratio 3.6 in favor of men.

605 blood donors representing 92.93% of the blood donors were found to be RhD positive while 46 blood donors representing 7.07 were found to be RhD negative (Figure 1).

The c and e antigens have the highest frequency with 99.83%. C and E antigen were less frequent with 21.97% and 13.82%, respectively (Table 1).

Seven phenotypes were detected among the blood donors (Table 2). The most frequent phenotype among the RhD positive was R_0r 65.12% followed by R_1r 20% and R_2r 12.73%. Among the RhD negative, the most frequent was rr (80.43%).

In the Kell blood group system, 5 blood donors (0.77%) were typed as K antigen positive and 645 (98.08%) as k antigen positive antigens. Accordingly, the K−k+ phenotype was the most common in these donors (98.92%).

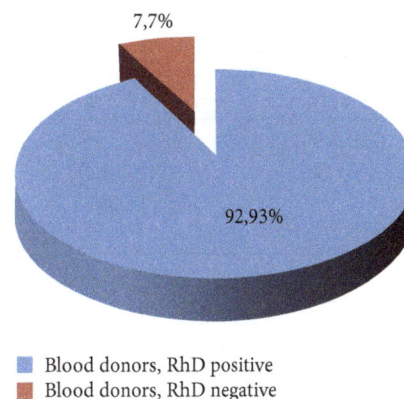

FIGURE 1: Prevalence of RhD antigen in blood donors.

4. Discussion

Our study focused on 651 regular and volunteer blood donors who have made donations at the National Blood Transfusion Center. The techniques used were the traditional techniques of agglutination on slide or in tube (indirect antiglobulin). Although recent years have been marked by the appearance of microtechnology, we wanted to show that, even with traditional techniques, such typing can be performed in a department with limited resources. The findings in our study will introduce plan for better care of the patients.

4.1. The Rh System. After ABO blood group, the Rh system is the most important in transfusion medicine. In Cote d'Ivoire, the blood transfusions are done only regarding ABO and RhD antigens exposing patients to high alloimmunization. Akre [4] found that 62.8% of patients suffering from sickle cell disease and transfused were immunized against Rh and Kell antigens systems. Rh was involved in 44.44% while Kell was involved in 27.78% in sickle cell patients transfused against 38% for both in France [12]. The most frequent alloantibodies were anti-E, anti-C, and anti-KEL1 developed after transfusion of standard red cell units.

In our study, the frequency of D antigen was 92.93%. This is comparable with the findings in the north of Cote d'Ivoire [3] and in the black population [13]. It is higher in other sub-Saharan Africa countries [1, 2, 5] and non-sub-Saharan Africa countries [7–10] (Table 3). Frequencies are lower in the US, France, and Nigeria where the authors found respective prevalence of 85.4%, 85%, and 81.5% [6, 11, 12].

The prevalence of the RhD negative is 7.7%. These results agree with the work of Seka [14] who found 7.28% and the work of Cabannes [15, 16] that quoted values ranging from 1.70 to 9.3% in sub-Saharan Africa.

The frequencies of c and e antigens in our study are high (99, 85%) (Table 1) while the frequencies of C and E antigens are lower, respectively, 21.97% and 13.82%. Among whites, European, and Asian people, e antigen is the most popular, and then comes C antigen [17]. As regards to C and E antigens, frequencies are higher than in our study (C 70% and E 26%) [5, 9, 12, 17]. Among RhD negative donors, E antigen is absent.

TABLE 1: Rh and Kell antigens frequency among 651 Ivorian blood donors.

Antigens	RhD negative donors		RhD positive donors		Total	
	n	%	n	%	n	%
c+	46	100	604	99,83	650	99,85
e+	46	100	604	99,83	650	99,85
C+	9	19,57	134	22,15	143	21,97
E+	0	0	90	14,88	90	13,82
k					650	99,84
K					5	0,77
Kp^a					4	0,61
Kp^b					539	82,80

TABLE 2: Rh and Kell phenotypes frequencies in Cote d'Ivoire blood donors ($n = 651$).

Antigens	Phenotypes	Genotypes		Number	Frequency %
		Wiener	Fischer race		
Rh positive donors				605	
D+C−E−c+e+	R_0r	R^0r R^0R^0	Dce/dce Dce/Dce	394	65,12
D+C+E−c+e+	R_1r	R^1r R^1R^0 R^0r'	DCe/Dce DCe/Dce Dce/dCe	121	20,00
D+C−E+c+e+	R_2r	R_2r R^2R^0	DcE/dce DcE/Dce	77	12,73
D+C+E+c+e+	R_1R_2	R^1R^2 R^1r'' R^2r' R^Zr R^0R^z R^0r^y	DCe/DcE DCe/dcE DcE/dCe DCE/dce Dce/DCE Dce/dCE	12	7,00
D+C+E+c−e−	R_zR_z	R^zR^z R^zr^y	DCE/DCE DCE/dCE	1	0,17
Rh negative donors				46	
D−C−E−c+e+	rr	rr	dce/dce	37	80,43
D−C+E−c+e+	$r'r$	$r'r$	dCe/dce	9	19,57
Kell					
K−k+				645	99.08
K+k+				5	0.77
K−k−(k0)				1	0,15

TABLE 3: Antigens frequencies of Rh blood group compared with published results.

Antigen	Our study (n)	Our study (%)	North Cote d'Ivoire [3]	Mauritania [1]	Guinea [5]	Cameroun [2]	Nigeria [6]	Antananarivo [7]	Morocco [8]	India [9]	Iran [10]	USA [11]
D+	605	92,93	92.5	94,2	95,9	95	81,5	98,9	90,5	94,4	90,2	85.4
D−	46	7,70	7.5	5,77	4,06	6	18,5	1,1	9,5	5,64	9,8	14.6
c+	650	99,85				97,5					73,9	
e+	650	99,85				97,5					97,9	
C+	143	21,97				95					75,9	
E+	90	13,82				92,5					29,5	

In the Rh system, seven phenotypes on eighteen known [13] were identified in our population (Table 2). The phenotype most frequently encountered is the phenotype R_0r (65.12%) regarding RhD positive blood donors and rr 80.43% among RhD negative blood donors. This profile is different from that observed in the whites where the phenotype R_1r or R_1R_1 is the most popular [12, 13]. R_zR_z was found in one donor.

4.2. The Kell System. The importance of this system is due to the K antigen, which has strong immunogenicity. It is among the most immunogenic system after the Rh system.

In the Kell system, k antigen was found in 98.92% of blood donors which is comparable with frequency in whites.

The prevalence of K antigen was found to be 0.92% of donors enrolled in the study, contrary to France where 9% of individuals are K+ [12] and to Germany where 4% express the K antigen [18].

The most common phenotype was K−k+ which is also common in white people. The antigens Kp^a and Kp^b were found, respectively, at frequencies of 0.61% and 82.80% in our sample, against 0.2% and 99.8% in whites [17].

5. Conclusion

Immunohematology data on blood donors are very few in West Africa. The ABO and D antigens are the main examination; other investigations are not performed.

Furthermore, Africa is full of its own specificities that are important to note for better care of patients by improving routine tests like phenotyping red cells, screening, and identifying red cells antibodies.

Research in that field should benefit from common work from West Africa national blood transfusion centers to enhance safety in transfusion medicine.

Conflict of Interests

The authors declare that there is no conflict of interests regarding the publication of this paper.

References

[1] C. T. Hamed, M. A. Bollahi, I. Abdelhamid et al., "Frequencies and ethnic distribution of Rh(D) blood group in Mauritania," *International Journal of Immunogenetics*, vol. 39, pp. 151–154, 2012.

[2] S. H. Mandengue, G. Lehman Leopold, P. Assomo-Ndemba, and M. Mbangue, "Distribution des antigènes des systèmes ABO, rhésus, Kell, MNSs et Duffy chez des drepanocytaires et donneurs de sang bénévoles à Douala (Cameroun): risques de réactions transfusionnelles," *Médecine d'Afrique Noire*, vol. 50, no. 1, pp. 22–24, 2003.

[3] A. Santovito, C. Burgarello, P. Cervella et al., "Erythrocyte polymorphisms in five ethnic groups of Northern Côte d'Ivoire," *International Journal of Immunogenetics*, vol. 36, no. 3, pp. 189–191, 2009.

[4] D. P. Akre, J. Seka-Seka, S. R. Dasse et al., "Alloimmunisation anti érythrocytaire post transfusionnelle chez les drépanocytaires au CHU de Cocody Abidjan," *International Journal of Pharma and Bio Sciences*, vol. 9, no. 2, pp. 64–70, 2008.

[5] A. Loua, M. R. Lamah, N. Y. Haba, and M. Camara, "Frequency of blood groups ABO and rhesus D in the Guinean population," *Transfusion Clinique et Biologique*, vol. 14, no. 5, pp. 435–439, 2007.

[6] A. G. Falusi, O. G. Ademowo, C. A. Latunji et al., "Distribution of ABO and RH genes in Nigeria," *African Journal of Medicine and Medical Sciences*, vol. 29, no. 1, pp. 23–26, 2000.

[7] Z. A. Randriamanantany, D. H. Rajaonatahina, F. E. Razafimanantsoa et al., "Phenotypic and allelic profile of ABO and Rhésus D blood group system among blood donor in Antananarivo," *International Journal of Immunogenetics*, vol. 39, no. 6, pp. 477–479, 2012.

[8] A. Benahadi, R. Alami, and S. Boulahdid, "La distribution des antigènes de groupe sanguins ABO et Rhésus au Maroc," *Transfusion Clinique et Biologiqu*, vol. 20, no. 3, p. 313, 2013.

[9] N. Agarwal, R. M. Thapliyal, and K. Chatterjee, "Blood group phenotype frequencies in blood donors from a tertiary care hospital in north India," *Blood Research*, vol. 48, no. 1, pp. 51–54, 2013.

[10] M. R. Keramati, H. Shakibaei, M. I. Kheiyyami et al., "Blood group antigens frequencies in the northeast of Iran," *Transfusion and Apheresis Science*, vol. 45, no. 2, pp. 133–136, 2011.

[11] G. Garratty, S. A. Glynn, and R. McEntire, "ABO and Rh(D) phenotype frequencies of different racial/ethnic groups in the United States," *Transfusion*, vol. 44, no. 5, pp. 703–706, 2004.

[12] I. Mendel, Bases Immunologiques de la transfusion sanguine, http://efs-alsace.fr/.

[13] G. Daniels, *Human Blood Group*, John Willey & Sons, Hoboken, NJ, USA, 2nd edition, 2002.

[14] S. S. Joseph, *Contribution à l'étude des groupes sanguins érythrocytaires en Côte d'Ivoire. Inventaire et repartition selon les ethnies [Thèse médecine]*, Faculté de Médecine, Abidjan, Côte d'Ivoire, 1985.

[15] R. Cabannes, "Hématologie des ethnies de Côte d'Ivoire. Son apport à la connaissance des populations de ce pays," *Médecine d'Afrique Noire*, vol. 28, pp. 65–72, 1981.

[16] R. Cabannes, A. Senarail, F. Pene, A. Sangare, F. Sombo Mambo, and P. Kple Faget, "Etude hémotypologique des populations de l'afrique de l'Ouest. Référence particulière aux populations ivoiriennes et aux Peulh de l'afrique de l'Ouest," *Annales de l'Université d'Abidjan. Série B, Médecine*, vol. 13, pp. 11–16, 1979.

[17] M. A. Kahar and R. D. Patel, "Phenotype frequencies of blood group systems (Rh, Kell, Kidd, Duffy, MNS, P, Lewis, and Lutheran) in blood donors of south Gujarat, India," *Asian Journal of Transfusion Science*, vol. 8, no. 1, pp. 51–55, 2014.

[18] F. F. Wagner, D. Kasulke, M. Kerowgan, and W. A. Flegel, "Frequencies of the blood groups ABO, Rhesus, D category VI, Kell, and of clinical relevant high-frequency antigens in South-Western Germany," *Infusionstherapie und Transfusionsmedizin*, vol. 22, no. 5, pp. 285–290, 1995.

9

A Comparison Study of the Blood Component Quality of Whole Blood Held Overnight at 4°C or Room Temperature

Shichun Wang, Tiantian Wang, Yahan Fan, Shan Huang, Zhongmei Yi, Ruiqing Li, and Shuming Zhao

Department of Blood Transfusion, Southwest Hospital, The Third Military Medical University, No. 30 Street Gaotanyan, Chongqing 400038, China

Correspondence should be addressed to Shuming Zhao; shumingzhao@yahoo.com

Academic Editor: Erwin Strasser

Background. The use of plasma frozen within 24 hrs is likely to increase. Whole blood (WB) and buffy coats (BCs) can be held for a few hrs or overnight before processing. *Methods.* Twenty-four bags of WB for plasma and 12 bags for platelet (PLT) concentrates were collected. The fresh frozen plasma (FFP) was prepared within 6 hrs. I-FP24 and II-FP24 samples were prepared either from leukodepleted WB that was held overnight or from WB that was held overnight before leukodepletion. The PLT concentrates (PCs) were prepared from BCs within 6 hrs (PC1) and within 18 to 24 hrs (PC2). The typical coagulation factors and some biochemical parameters were determined. *Results.* Compared to the FFP samples, the levels of FVII and FVIII in the I-FP24 and II-FP24 samples decreased significantly. The pH, Na^+, LDH, and FHb levels differed significantly between II-FP24 and FFP. Compared to PC1, PC2 exhibited lower pH, pO_2, and Na^+ levels, a higher PLT count, and increased pCO_2, K^+, Lac, and CD62P expression levels. *Conclusion.* FP24 is best prepared from WB that was stored overnight at 4°C and then leukodepleted and separated within 24 hrs. PCs are best produced from BCs derived from WB that was held overnight at room temperature.

1. Introduction

An important step in safeguarding the quality and safety of the blood supply is recruiting volunteer donors from low-risk populations and producing qualified blood and blood components. Volunteer donor recruitment is a challenging proposition worldwide. In China, it was particularly difficult before 1998. Traditional Chinese culture believes that the loss of even a small amount of blood has a substantial detrimental health effect. Some people also believe that blood donation is a disloyal action against one's ancestors. Old cultural beliefs, combined with inadequate efforts to mobilize volunteer donors, have led to a chronic shortage of blood products in some areas of China [1]. Therefore, many blood centers have tried to prepare more blood components, such as platelet (PLT) concentrates (PCs), from whole blood (WB) to meet the need for blood products.

WB units are generally held at ambient temperatures (20–24°C) when PCs will be prepared within 6 hrs of the blood collection. The United States Food and Drug Administration

(FDA) guidelines during the early 1980s allowed the preparation of components at 20 to 24°C within 8 hrs of collection and a 5-day storage period for PCs. The impetus for extending the time to 8 hrs reflected an increased production demand for PCs and the limitations of the 6 hr period with respect to the collection of a large percentage of WB units at mobile drives, which were sometimes quite distant from the component production laboratories. Currently, because of the overnight holding practice, component manufacturing, including PLT preparation, can be logistically facilitated with related cost savings. Many countries have converted to overnight-hold blood processing because of these advantages [2]. Recently, the Canadian Blood Services has adopted the overnight hold approach to prepare PCs from buffy coats [3].

Currently, the most commonly used plasma product is fresh frozen plasma (FFP), which can be obtained from a plasmapheresis collection or donated WB. FFP must be prepared and frozen within 6 or 8 hrs from the time of collection, according to the usage of different anticoagulants for WB storage. These requirements for FFP preparation

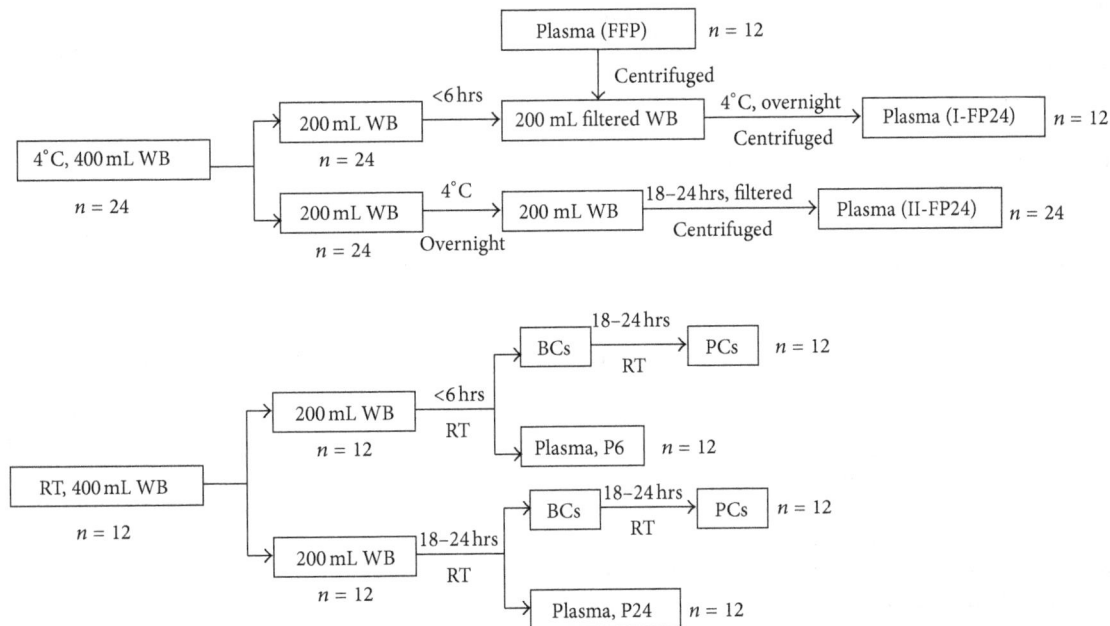

FIGURE 1: Experimental algorithm for the plasma and PCs production validation with WB held overnight ($n = 24/12$ units in each arm). The plasma was frozen as soon as possible after preparation.

could limit the number of WB units that can be processed into FFP because of the blood collections from blood-collecting vehicles. WB stored overnight at 4°C can be used to manufacture plasma and concentrated red blood cells but not for PCs because of the deleterious effect of 4°C storage on PLT quality. PLTs do not tolerate refrigeration and disappear rapidly from circulation if subjected to chilling before transplantation [4–6]. Thus, WB used for PC separation must be stored at room temperature. Currently, PC preparation according to the BC removal method is widely practiced [7–9] and is associated with significantly better PLT recoveries and less PLT activation immediately after preparation [10]. However, it is also inexpedient for PCs that are prepared during the immediate processing of fresh WB. In addition, an overnight hold of BC is good for the PC quantity and quality [11]. There are numerous operational and economic advantages to blood services from ambient WB storage within 24 hrs because of the reduced restrictions on blood processing for PC separation within 8 hrs of collection.

The aim of this study was to compare the quality, as measured by the coagulation factor levels, of plasma prepared from WB that was processed within 8 hrs after collection and storage at 4°C, within 18–24 hrs of storage at 4°C, or within 18–24 hrs of storage at ambient temperature, and the quality of PCs from the BCs processed either from fresh WB or from WB that was held overnight at room temperature.

2. Materials and Methods

2.1. Study Design. The blood component quality of WB that was stored overnight was evaluated; the frame paragraph of these experiments is shown in Figure 1. Briefly, 400 mL WB samples were collected from normal volunteer donors according to standard procedures in the blood donation law of the People's Republic of China (24 bags used for plasma preparation were stored at 4°C, and 12 bags used for PCs preparation were stored at room temperature). The study protocol was approved by the Southwest Hospital Human Research and Ethics Committee. Each WB sample (400 mL ± 10%) was collected into blood collection packs that contained a CPD anticoagulant (Nigale Biomedical Co., Ltd., Sichuan, China), and then equal volumes were divided between 2 units (200 mL/unit). The blood components were processed in a 2-step centrifugation protocol (2,600 rpm or 1,642 ×g for 15 min, followed by 1,000 rpm or 263 ×g for 6 min in a J6-MC centrifuge; Beckman, Miami, FL, USA). The plasma was removed, and the packed RBCs were resuspended in one of the additive solutions SAG-M (100 mL) (Nigale Biomedical Co., Ltd, Sichuan, China). The FFP was prepared within 6 hrs from 1/2 ($n = 12$) of the leukodepleted WB with a WB in-line leukocyte blood filter (Nigale Biomedical Co., Ltd., Sichuan, China). The I-FP24 (I-FP24, 6 hrs/18–24 hrs) were prepared from leukodepleted blood held overnight ($n = 12$) using a WB in-line leukocyte blood filter (Nigale Biomedical Co., Ltd, Sichuan, China) from WB within 6 hrs, or II-FP24 (II-FP24, 18–24 hrs/18–24 hrs) from WB held overnight and then leukodepleted using a WB in-line leukocyte blood filter (Nigale Biomedical Co., Ltd, Sichuan, China) ($n = 24$). One batch of PCs was prepared from BCs (stored overnight) obtained from fresh WB (fresh/stored, $n = 12$, control group, PC1), and the other batch of PCs was prepared from BCs obtained from WB that was stored overnight at room temperature (stored/fresh, $n = 12$, experimental group, PC2). At the same time, plasma from the 2 groups was prepared, including P6 ($n = 12$) from the PC1 group and P24 ($n = 12$) from the PC2 group. All plasma samples were stored in a −30°C freezer before testing, and all PCs were tested after separation. The typical coagulation factors (FV, FVII, FVIII, Fib) and some biochemical indicators (K$^+$, Na$^+$, Cl$^-$, TP, lactic dehydrogenase [LDH], glucose [GLU], FHb, pH) were observed in all plasma samples. The PLT count and the lactate, pCO$_2$, pO$_2$, HSR, pH, GLU, and CD62P expression levels were measured in all PCs.

2.2. In Vitro Assays. In general, the following methods were used.

2.2.1. WB Collection and Processing. WB was collected in disposable plastic blood bag (110414, Nigale Biomedical Co., Ltd, Sichuan, China) and then refrigerated in a blood refrigerator (HXC-158, Haier, Shanghai, China) or held at room temperature. The plasma from WB which was held at 4°C was prepared by a 2-step centrifugation (3500 rpm or 3128 ×g for 10 min, J6-MC, Beckman, Miami, USA), frozen in freezer (MDF-U538, Sanyo, Osaka, Japan), thawed in plasma thawer (KJX III, Szmic, Suzhou, China) at 37°C. PCs were prepared by a 2-step centrifugation (2600 r.p.m. or 1642 ×g for 15 min followed by 1000 r.p.m. or 263 ×g for 6 min, J6-MC, Beckman, Miami, USA).

2.2.2. Coagulation Factors. The clotting factor activity levels were determined with an automatic blood coagulation analyzer (CA1500, Sysmex, Kobe, Japan), and the assay reagents included coagulation factors Fib, FVII, FVIII, APTT, and PT (537991, 500725A, 546529A, 537485A, 545363, Dade Behring Marburg, Marburg, Germany) and coagulation factors FV (503587A, Chengdu Xiehe Biotechnology Co., Ltd., Chengdu, China).

2.2.3. Biochemical Parameters. The glucose and LDH levels were measured using dry chemistry on a chemistry analyzer (AU2700, Olympus, Shimadzu Tokyo, Japan). The FHb level was measured by a 3-wavelength method (380 nm, 415 nm, 450 nm) on a microplate reader (1500-992, Thermo Fisher Scientific, Waltham, MA, USA). The Tris-HCl solution (62.4 mmol/L, pH 8.0) was prepared as the reagent. Briefly, the instrument was zeroed, and the plasma sample was diluted to a 3 mL as Tris-HCl solution : plasma = 9 : 1 (2700 μL : 300 μL) and measured the absorbance against the Tris-HCl solution as blank. The level of FHb is calculated as the formula: FHb (mg/L) = $[1.68 \times A_{415} - 0.84 (A_{380} + A_{450})] \times 1000$ mg/L.

2.2.4. Quantity and Quality of PCs. The PLT counts were obtained using an automated cell analyzer (KX-21N, Sysmex, Kobe, Japan). The pH, pO$_2$, pCO$_2$, glucose, and lactate levels were measured with a blood gas analyzer (ABL715, Radiometer, Copenhagen, Denmark), or pH was measured with a pH meter (PB-21, Sartorius AG, Goettingen, Germany). The glucose and LDH levels were measured using dry chemistry with a chemistry analyzer (AU2700, Olympus, Shimadzu, Tokyo, Japan). The level of HSR and the PAgT were measured with a spectrophotometer (7200, Unic, Bern, Switzerland) and an adhesion meter (HY-I, Beijing Hongrunda instrument

Co., Ltd, Beijing, China). The PLT surface CD62P expression was measured with flow cytometry (FACSCalibur, Beckman Coulter, Miami, FL) and fluorescein isothiocyanate (FITC) or phycoerythrin-labeled monoclonal antibodies (CD41 FITC (Lot: 555469), CD62-P PE (Lot: 348107), and Mouse IgG-1 PE (Lot: 555748), BD, USA).

2.3. Statistical Analysis. All test unit groups were compared with their respective reference groups. The results are expressed as the mean ± standard deviation (SD) and the median (range). Data were analyzed with the SPSS software program (version 13.0, SPSS Inc., Chicago, IL, USA). Comparisons were performed with a two-sample *t*-test with a 95% confidence interval (CI) or a one-way analysis of variance (ANOVA) and Dunnett's test to identify the differences between each storage method. A P value < 0.05 was considered to be significant.

3. Results

3.1. Plasma Appearance Observations. All frozen plasma samples were warmed to 37°C in a water bath on the third day after collection, and no precipitation emerged.

3.2. Effect of Overnight Holding on In Vitro Plasma Quality. The clotting factor analysis of plasma processed under various conditions is shown in Table 1. The plasma was processed approximately 6 hrs after collection or at 18–24 hrs in groups I-FP24 and II-FP24. Compared to FFP, I-FP24 decreased by 22.6%, 29.38%, 32.89%, and 40.71%, including significantly lower FV, FVII, and FVIII levels (P < 0.05); in II-FP24, the decreases were 1.9%, 12.60%, 14.91%, and 32.86%, including significantly lower FVIII levels (P < 0.05). Compared to FFP and I-FP24, II-FP24 had higher levels of K$^+$, LDH, and FHb. The effect of overnight holding of WB at room temperature on the in vitro plasma quality was also analyzed. Compared to P6, P24 had higher levels of Na$^+$, K$^+$, and FHb and lower levels of Cl$^-$, pH, and FVIII. Differences in the pH, Na$^+$, LDH, and FHb levels were observed between the II-FP24 and P24 samples.

3.3. Effect of Overnight Holding of WB at Room Temperature on In Vitro PC Quality. All PCs had PLT counts well above the current acceptance level of 2.0×10^{10}/U. Compared to the control group, PC2 had a higher PLT count ($3.49 \pm 1.19 \times 10^{10}$/U versus $2.78 \pm 1.49 \times 10^{10}$/U), which was 25.54% higher than that of PC1 and 74.50% higher than that of the current acceptance level. The PLT in vitro functional parameters were not significantly different, but differences were observed with respect to CD62P expression (11.93 ± 0.18 versus 10.06 ± 0.28, P < 0.05) and some biochemical indicators (lower pH, pO$_2$ and Na$^+$ levels and higher pCO$_2$, K$^+$, and Lac levels; Table 2).

4. Discussion

Blood collection, processing, and storage conditions significantly influence the quality of blood components, and consequently, these processes are closely regulated to maximize

TABLE 1: Clotting factor levels and some biochemical parameters of plasma prepared from WB stored under different conditions (mean ± SD, median, and range).

WB hold time/components preparation (hrs)	WB stored at 4°C			WB stored at 22°C	
	<6/ <6	< 6/18–24	18~24/18–24	<6	18–24
Plasma	FFP, $n = 12$	I-FP24, $n = 12$	II-FP24, $n = 24$	P6, $n = 12$	P24, $n = 12$
Fib (g/L)	2.08 ± 0.16 2.04 (1.88– 2.26)	1.61 ± 0.43 1.48 (1.18–2.14)	2.04 ± 0.40 2.15 (1.34–2.43)	1.78 ± 0.59 1.97 (1.55–2.24)	1.79 ± 0.59 2.01 (1.52–2.19)
FV (%)	86.57 ± 18.73 92.39 (61.25–107.36)	61.14 ± 13.76* 60.64 (44.98–81.61)	75.66 ± 6.07 78.65 (67.16–81.61)	81.21 ± 6.54 78.65 (73.78–92.39)	87.59 ± 8.84 83.96 (75.78–104.14)
FVII (%)	91.71 ± 25.53 92.58 (60.52–113.00)	61.55 ± 11.45* 61.50 (44.53–75.19)	78.03 ± 19.08 71.96 (49.45–108.49)	80.32 ± 17.37 77.98 (50.92–115.29)	80.84 ± 17.29 81.02 (48.71–108.49)
FVIII (%)	97.65 ± 25.99 107.60 (63.81–128.34)	57.90 ± 7.35* 55.80 (51.26–70.31)	65.56 ± 13.93▲ 61.37 (45.48–92.65)	77.98 ± 11.60 78.59 (48.95–92.65)	66.30 ± 10.16△ 65.06 (43.88–84.37)
TP (g/L)	57.24 ± 0.81 57.40 (56.30– 58.10)	56.80 ± 4.50 57.30 (51.80–61.80)	58.96 ± 3.17 59.00 (53.90–63.90)	58.91 ± 2.94 59.10 (54.80–66.40)	59.78 ± 3.14 59.10 (56.00–66.60)
pH	7.21 ± 0.10 7.17 (7.12–7.38)	7.22 ± 0.09 7.20 (7.11–7.34)	7.24 ± 0.06 7.25 (7.17–7.36)	7.36 ± 0.07 7.35 (7.30–7.53)	7.18 ± 0.04△ 7.18 (7.12–7.24)
Na^+ (mmol/L)	156.78 ± 0.88 157.00 (155.50–157.60)	154.94 ± 3.81 154.00 (151.40–159.00)	156.61 ± 2.01 156.35 (153.80–161.20)	156.05 ± 2.77 156.20 (149.70–160.00)	159.25 ± 3.24△ 159.20 (153.10–163.50)
K (mmol/L)	3.30 ± 0.21 3.35 (3.02–3.53)	3.96 ± 0.22* 4.03 (3.61–4.20)	4.33 ± 0.28▲• 4.39 (3.71–4.69)	3.45 ± 0.21 3.44 (3.19–3.84)	4.25 ± 0.27△ 4.28 (3.67–4.69)
Cl^- (mmol/L)	70.26 ± 2.59 69.90 (67.30–73.20)	70.32 ± 3.72 70.20 (65.80–74.50)	70.92 ± 3.21 71.10 (64.80–75.70)	71.93 ± 1.95 71.95 (68.50–74.80)	69.05 ± 2.23△ 70.20 (65.10–72.20)
LDH (IU/L)	105.75 ± 20.56 91.00 (90.00–134.00)	100 ± 6.78 96.00 (94.00–110.00)	145.70 ± 26.00▲• 151.00 (110.00–175.00)	103.58 ± 22.07 99.50 (67.00–150.00)	120.83 ± 24.39★ 108.00 (81.00–161.00)
GLU (mmol/L)	24.18 ± 1.24 24.58 (22.11–25.39)	22.78 ± 0.61 22.55 (22.12–23.71)	22.72 ± 1.18 22.92 (21.21–24.38)	23.09 ± 1.38 22.78 (21.02–25.48)	21.93 ± 1.48 21.79 (19.89–25.21)
FHb (mg/L)	16.34 ± 7.88 10.02 (1.23–29.91)	43.54 ± 19.76* 44.39 (20.81–73.03)	129.96 ± 34.33▲• 129.94 (71.02–177.17)	22.15 ± 19.51 13.71 (1.67–66.56)	27.46 ± 29.11★ 14.40 (3.89–89.74)

*$P < 0.05$ versus FFP; ▲$P < 0.05$ versus FFP.
△$P < 0.05$ versus P6; ★$P < 0.05$ versus II-FP24.
•$P < 0.05$ versus I-FP24.

safety and efficacy. The current FDA regulations require that WB units held at room temperature must be processed within 8 hrs after collection, or alternatively, the WB units must be refrigerated and processed within 24 hrs [12]. The Council of Europe (COE) guidelines specify that WB units can be held for up to 24 hrs at room temperature provided that the units are rapidly cooled to 20–22°C immediately after collection. The Chinese guidelines require that the WB units are stored at 4°C as soon as possible after collection and are processed within 8 hrs. Overnight room temperature WB holding has both logistical advantages and some disadvantages that

potentially affect the quality of components, particularly red blood cells (RBCs). In recent years, Chinese blood centers have tried to improve the national blood supply and safety. In China, WB units for clinical use are collected at blood centers. More than 400 blood centers are operated at 3 levels: provincial, regional, and county. Local government health offices oversee blood center operations. The WB unit donation models in China have changed from paid donors before 1998 to employer-organized donors after the new blood donation law took effect in 1998, and in most areas of China, donors are now volunteers [1]. The blood donation law bans all paid WB

TABLE 2: In vitro quality variables of PCs collected under various conditions (mean ± SD, median, and range).

	PC1 ($n = 12$)	PC2 ($n = 12$)
PLTs (×10^{10}/U)	2.78 ± 1.49 2.6 (1.11–6.58)	3.49 ± 1.19 3.33 (2.11–5.60)
pH	7.12 ± 0.05 7.13 (7.03–7.17)	6.90 ± 0.04* 6.89 (6.84–6.99)
pCO$_2$(mmHg)	34.61 ± 3.01 35.45 (29.80–39.20)	49.19 ± 5.07* 47.90 (43.80–57.50)
pO$_2$ (mmHg)	117.50 ± 10.46 113.00 (101.00–135.00)	94.81 ± 17.50* 95.40 (60.90–117.00)
K$^+$ (mmol/L)	3.01 ± 0.21 2.95 (2.70–3.30)	3.33 ± 0.24* 3.40 (3.00–3.80)
Na$^+$ (mmol/L)	134.73 ± 1.56 135.00 (131.00–137.00)	131.36 ± 2.11* 132.00 (129.00–135.00)
Cl$^-$ (mmol/L)	73.00 ± 2.05 73.00 (69.00–76.00)	73.00 ± 1.73 72.00 (71.00–76.00)
GLU (mmol/L)	19.17 ± 1.13 19.00 (17.80–21.40)	20.14 ± 1.28 20.20 (18.20–22.60)
Lac (mmol/L)	3.25 ± 0.70 3.10 (2.30–4.70)	4.13 ± 0.41* 4.20 (3.60–4.70)
CD62P expression (%)	10.06 ± 0.28 10.06 (9.86–10.25)	11.93 ± 0.18* 11.93 (11.80–12.06)
Adhesion (%)	43.21 ± 2.27 43.21 (41.61–44.81)	40.37 ± 3.66 40.37 (37.78–42.95)
HSR%	1.01 ± 2.68	
Bacterial culture	Neg	Neg

*$P < 0.05$ versus PC1.

donations for clinical use and encourages all Chinese citizens between the ages of 18 and 55 years who meet the health criteria for blood donation to donate blood voluntarily. According to the law, WB units are mostly collected at blood centers or mobile street stations in strategic locations that are run by blood centers. One or 2 units (200 or 400 mL) of WB can be drawn from 1 volunteer, stored in a refrigerator and transported at 4°C by a blood vehicle, and separated into blood components at 4°C within 8 hrs. Currently, most blood centers report that they have already achieved the goal of meeting all of their region's blood needs with volunteer donations.

In early 1999, O'Neill et al. studied the quality of FP24 by measuring clotting factors in plasma obtained from CPD WB after storage at 22°C and 4°C for as long as 24 hrs before frozen storage at −18°C for 1 month. The authors confirmed that plasma separated from WB that had been stored for up to 24 hrs after collection could be used under all conditions that required FFP for transfusion [13]. In 2005, Cardigan et al. also examined the quality of FFP produced from WB stored at 4°C overnight [14]. The authors suggested that there was good retention of relevant coagulation factor activity in plasma produced from WB that had been stored at 4°C for 18 to 24 hrs and that this would be an acceptable product for most patients who required FFP. Several other studies have assessed the stability of FP24 when thawed and stored at 4°C for up to 5 days [15]. The studies discovered that FFP and FP24 contained adequate coagulation factor activities to

maintain hemostatic activity. In China, the guideline requires that the FVIII level in >75% of FFP must be >0.7 IU/mL. Meanwhile, there is no current quality standard for FP24. In our study, the most variable affective factor during WB storage was FVIII, as might be predicted. Compared to FFP, the FVIII level decreased by 32.86% in II-FP24 and by 40.71% in I-FP24. The activity levels of other coagulation factors in I-FP24 and II-FP24 were not significantly different. These results showed that, with the exception of FVIII, FP24 would be an acceptable product for most patients who required FFP. Kleinman et al. conducted a survey in late 2009 to gather detailed information in which 40% of the respondents chose the highest category, indicating that >75% of their plasma was supplied as FP24 [16]. Interestingly, the FV activity increased substantially during the short period of storage, which was also observed in this study and might reflect activation of the contact system during storage [17]. Alhumaidan et al. also found that plasma manufactured after a 24 hr room temperature hold contains coagulation factors comparable to FFP except for a possible reduction of up to 20% in FVIII. Other clotting factors either were unchanged or showed minimal reduction (<15%). This plasma appears suitable as a transfusable product, and extension of liquid storage to 7 days merits consideration [18]. FFP had the best results for the metabolism variables K$^+$, LDH, and FHb. Compared to the other 2 groups, II-FP24 had higher K$^+$, LDH, and FHb levels. This result might be explained by the RBC metabolism in WB stored overnight at 4°C and the increased osmotic fragility that resulted in RBC lysis increasing some parameters in the plasma processed from WB. The differences in several biochemical parameters between the II-FP24 and P24 groups might be caused by the holding of WB at different temperatures, which induced different levels of RBC membrane fragility and deformation properties. Comprehensively, the quality of plasma from the WB that was held overnight at 4°C and then leukodepleted is much better than that of the plasma from leukodepleted WB that was then held overnight. Thus, once filtrated, plasma should be separated as soon as possible.

Although PCs must be prepared within 6 hrs through fresh WB processing, this process is inexpedient because of blood collection from mobile vehicles or from a wide geographic area. Thus, it is important to extend the allowable processing time for PCs. The BC removal method, which is considered as a good PC preparation method, is used in many countries. Some scientists think that overnight BCs holding benefits the quantity and quality of PCs [10]. In this study, the quantity and quality of PCs from BCs and WB that were held overnight were compared. All PCs had PLT counts well above the current acceptance level of 2.0×10^{10}/U. In particular, the PLT counts were much higher in PC2 (25.54% higher than those in PC1 and 74.50% higher than the current acceptance level). Other studies have shown levels that were 18.60%–33.00% higher in the overnight-held PCs [19, 20]. We studied the effect of BCs holding time before the PLT preparation on the quality of PCs and found lower PLT counts with a 0 hr holding time than with 4 or 16 hr holding times. Thus, we concluded that PLT recovery was comparatively affected by immediate BCs processing. This result could be explained by the relatively short rest period of BCs (i.e., the PLTs were still forming aggregates that were easily removed during centrifugation prior to disaggregation). Some biochemical indicators were different between the PC1 and PC2 groups, which could be explained by RBC metabolism in WB during overnight storage and by the lower amount of PLT in the storage bag, thus resulting in a lower total metabolism level in the bag. Although the CD62P expression was significantly different, the levels were still lower [21]. The PLT quantity is actually improved by overnight room temperature hold, and the quality is not affected.

Recently, in a special supplement report to the journal of Transfusion, scientists in 9 major blood product developmental laboratories evaluated the quality of components from WB that was held overnight at room temperature, including RBCs, plasma, and PCs. The scientists concluded that overnight holding of WB before processing had no lasting deleterious effects on the in vitro qualities of the subsequently prepared components and that using different RBC additive solutions did not appear to offer significant advantages in terms of final RBC quality, regardless of the processing method [21, 22]. Furthermore, Dijkstra-Tiekstra and colleagues analyzed the differences between PCs from fresh and overnight-stored blood. Their data showed that PCs are best prepared after a 20 to 24 hr WB hold [23]. Some scientists confirmed that storing WB for 22 ± 2 hrs at 22°C before preparing the PCs could increase the yield of PLTs in a concentrate by 43% while concurrently improving all measures of 7-day poststorage PLT viability [24, 25]. Furthermore, Cardigan and his colleague, who have extensively studied plasma, tested the coagulation factor content of plasma from WB that was stored for 24 hrs at an ambient temperature and indicated that WB storage at ambient temperature for 24 hrs had minimal effects on the plasma coagulation activity and, thus, was an acceptable alternative to producing plasma on the day of blood collection [26]. There are numerous operational and economic advantages of the blood services of ambient WB storage for 24 hrs because of the removal of the requirement to process blood for PLTs or plasma within 6 hrs of collection. Even the partial loss of FVIII in the plasma can be replaced with a biological FVIII product for clinical use when necessary.

5. Conclusion

In this study in which 400 mL WB samples were divided equally, the group data revealed real differences. Overnight WB holding might be a suitable method for blood component processing. FP24 is best prepared from WB that was stored overnight at 4°C, followed by leukodepletion and separation within 24 hrs. PCs are best prepared within 6 hrs from BC that was derived from WB that was held overnight at room temperature.

Abbreviations

FFP: Fresh frozen plasma
FP24:   Plasma frozen within 24 hrs of phlebotomy
BC(s): Buffy coat(s)
HSR: Hypotonic shock response
PC(s): Platelet concentrate(s)
PLT: Platelet
WB: Whole blood
LDH: Lactate dehydrogenase
FHb: Free hemoglobin
hrs: Hours
TP: Total protein
APTT: Activated partial thromboplastin time
PT: Prothrombin time
GLU: Glucose
Lac: Lactic acid.

Conflict of Interests

The authors declare that they have no conflict of interests.

Acknowledgments

The authors thank Zerong Wang, Ronghua Diao, and Fang Lin for their help with sample collection and Hui Guo for laboratory measures and analysis. This project was in part supported by the National Natural Science Foundation of China (NSFC 81270649). Shichun Wang and Tiantian Wang are co-first authors.

References

[1] H. Shan, J. Wang, F. Ren et al., "Blood banking in China," The Lancet, vol. 60, no. 9347, pp. 1770–1775, 2002.

[2] G. Moroff, J. P. AuBuchon, C. Pickard, P. H. Whitley, W. A. Heaton, and S. Holme, "Evaluation of the properties of components prepared and stored after holding of whole blood units for 8 and 24 hours at ambient temperature," Transfusion, vol. 51, supplement S1, pp. 7S–14S, 2011.

[3] K. Serrano, K. Scammell, S. Weiss et al., "Plasma and cryoprecipitate manufactured from whole blood held overnight at room temperature meet quality standards," Transfusion, vol. 50, no. 2, pp. 344–353, 2010.

[4] S. Murphy and F. H. Gardner, "Effect of storage temperature on maintenance of platelet viability—deleterious effect of refrigerated storage," The New England Journal of Medicine, vol. 280, no. 20, pp. 1094–1098, 1969.

[5] K. M. Hoffmeister, T. W. Felbinger, H. Falet et al., "The clearance mechanism of chilled blood platelets," Cell, vol. 112, no. 1, pp. 87–97, 2003.

[6] V. Rumjantseva, P. K. Grewal, H. H. Wandall et al., "Dual roles for hepatic lectin receptors in the clearance of chilled platelets," Nature Medicine, vol. 15, no. 11, pp. 1273–1280, 2009.

[7] R. R. Vassallo and S. Murphy, "A critical comparison of platelet preparation methods," Current Opinion in Hematology, vol. 13, no. 5, pp. 323–330, 2006.

[8] E. Levin, B. Culibrk, M. I. C. Gyöngyössy-Issa et al., "Implementation of buffy coat platelet component production: comparison to platelet-rich plasma platelet production," Transfusion, vol. 48, no. 11, pp. 2331–2337, 2008.

[9] W. P. Sheffield, V. Bhakta, C. Jenkins, and D. V. Devine, "Conversion to the buffy coat method and quality of frozen plasma derived from whole blood donations in Canada," Transfusion, vol. 50, no. 5, pp. 1043–1049, 2010.

[10] W. A. L. Heaton, P. Rebulla, M. Pappelettera, and W. H. Dzik, "Comparative analysis of different methods for routine blood component preparation," *Transfusion Medicine Reviews*, vol. 11, no. 2, pp. 116–129, 1997.

[11] S. Pérez-Pujol, M. Lozano, D. Perea, R. Mazzara, A. Ordinas, and G. Escolar, "Effect of holding buffy coats 4 or 18 hours before preparing pooled filtered PLT concentrates in plasma," *Transfusion*, vol. 44, no. 2, pp. 202–209, 2004.

[12] J. D. Roback, M. R. Combs, B. J. Grossman, and C. D. Hillyer, Eds., *American Association of Blood Banks Technical Manual*, AABB, Bethesda, Md, USA, 16th edition, 2008.

[13] E. M. O'Neill, J. Rowley, M. Hansson-Wicher, S. McCarter, G. Ragno, and C. R. Valeri, "Effect of 24-hour whole-blood storage on plasma clotting factors," *Transfusion*, vol. 39, no. 5, pp. 488–491, 1999.

[14] R. Cardigan, A. S. Lawrie, I. J. Mackie, and L. M. Williamson, "The quality of fresh-frozen plasma produced from whole blood stored at 4°C overnight," *Transfusion*, vol. 45, no. 8, pp. 1342–1348, 2005.

[15] M. H. Yazer, A. Cortese-Hassett, and D. J. Triulzi, "Coagulation factor levels in plasma frozen within 24 hours of phlebotomy over 5 days of storage at 1 to 6°C," *Transfusion*, vol. 48, no. 12, pp. 2525–2530, 2008.

[16] S. Kleinman, B. Grossman, and P. Kopko, "A national survey of transfusion-related acute lung injury risk reduction policies for platelets and plasma in the United States," *Transfusion*, vol. 50, no. 6, pp. 1312–1321, 2010.

[17] E. A. Vogler and C. A. Siedlecki, "Contact activation of blood-plasma coagulation," *Biomaterials*, vol. 30, no. 10, pp. 1857–1869, 2009.

[18] H. Alhumaidan, T. Cheves, S. Holme, and J. Sweeney, "Stability of coagulation factors in plasma prepared after a 24-hour room temperature hold," *Transfusion*, vol. 50, no. 9, pp. 1934–1942, 2010.

[19] P. F. van der Meer, J. A. Cancelas, R. R. Vassallo, N. Rugg, M. Einarson, and J. R. Hess, "Evaluation of the overnight hold of whole blood at room temperature, before component processing: platelets (PLTs) from PLT-rich plasma," *Transfusion*, vol. 51, supplement 1, pp. 45S–49S, 2011.

[20] F. Q. Lu, W. Kang, Y. Peng, and W. M. Wang, "Characterization of blood components separated from donated whole blood after an overnight holding at room temperature with the buffy coat method," *Transfusion*, vol. 51, no. 10, pp. 2199–2207, 2011.

[21] P. F. van der Meer, J. A. Cancelas, R. Cardigan et al., "Evaluation of overnight hold of whole blood at room temperature before component processing: effect of red blood cell (RBC) additive solutions on in vitro RBC measures," *Transfusion*, vol. 51, supplement 1, pp. 15S–24S, 2011.

[22] M. F. Veale, G. Healey, and R. L. Sparrow, "Effect of additive solutions on red blood cell (RBC) membrane properties of stored RBCs prepared from whole blood held for 24 hours at room temperature," *Transfusion*, vol. 51, supplement 1, pp. 25S–33S, 2011.

[23] M. J. Dijkstra-Tiekstra, P. F. van der Meer, R. Cardigan et al., "Platelet concentrates from fresh or overnight-stored blood, an international study," *Transfusion*, vol. 51, supplement 1, pp. 15S–24S, 2011.

[24] S. J. Slichter, J. Corson, M. K. Jones, T. Christoffel, E. Pellham, and D. Bolgiano, "Platelet concentrates prepared after a 20- to 24-hour hold of the whole blood at 22°C," *Transfusion*, vol. 52, no. 9, pp. 2043–2048, 2012.

[25] L. McMillian, V. Hornsey, A. Morrison, O. Drummond, and C. Prowse, "Storage of whole blood for up to 24H and its effect on platelet concentrates," *Transfusion Medicine*, vol. 19, supplement 1, article 20S, 2009.

[26] R. Cardigan, P. F. van der Meer, C. Pergande et al., "Coagulation factor content of plasma produced from whole blood stored for 24 hours at ambient temperature: results from an international multicenter BEST Collaborative study," *Transfusion*, vol. 51, supplement 1, pp. 50S–57S, 2011.

10

High Rates of Hepatitis B and C and HIV Infections among Blood Donors in Cameroon: A Proposed Blood Screening Algorithm for Blood Donors in Resource-Limited Settings

Florent Fouelifack Ymele,[1,2] **Basile Keugoung,**[2,3] **Jeanne Hortense Fouedjio,**[1,4]
Nadege Kouam,[5] **Sandrine Mendibi,**[4] **and Jacqueline Dongtsa Mabou**[6]

[1] *Yaoundé Central Hospital, P.O. Box 31186, Yaoundé, Cameroon*
[2] *Research, Education and Health Development Associates Group (REHDAG), Dschang, Cameroon*
[3] *Ministry of Public Health, Yaoundé, Cameroon*
[4] *Faculty of Medicine and Biomedical Sciences, University of Yaoundé I, P.O. Box 1364, Yaoundé, Cameroon*
[5] *Institute for Training and Demographic Research, P.O. Box 5644, Yaoundé, Cameroon*
[6] *Yaoundé Central Hospital, Blood Bank Unit, P.O. Box 31186, Yaoundé, Cameroon*

Correspondence should be addressed to Florent Fouelifack Ymele, yfouelifack@gmail.com

Academic Editor: Maria Rios

Background. Infections with human immunodeficiency virus (HIV), hepatitis B (HBV), and hepatitis C virus (HCV) are currently major public health problems. *Methods.* A retrospective study was conducted from January to June 2008 at the Blood Bank of the Central Hospital, Yaoundé (Cameroon). The objective was to study the prevalence of HIV, HBV, and HCV and their coinfections among blood donors. *Results.* A total of 4650 donors were identified, and the sex ratio (male/female) was 14/1. The median age of donors was 28 years (range: 16 to 69 years). Among blood donors, HBV, HIV, and HCV infection prevalences were 12.14% ($n = 565$), 4.44% ($n = 206$), and 1.44% ($n = 67$), respectively. Coinfection with HIV and HBV was observed among 0.77% donors, followed by hepatitis B and C co-infection (0.21%) and HIV and HCV coinfection (0.06%). Co-infection with HIV-HBV-HCV was encountered in 2 donors. The HIV, HBV, and HCV infections lead to a destruction of one out of six sets of blood collected. *Conclusion.* There is a need to review policies for blood collection from donors, by modifying the algorithm of blood donors testing. Pretesting potential donors using rapid tests could help to avoid collection and destruction of (infected) blood.

1. Introduction

Infections due to the human immunodeficiency virus (HIV), hepatitis B virus (HBV), and hepatitis C virus (HCV) are major public health problems worldwide [1]. In sub-Saharan Africa, these infections are frequent among the general population and blood donors [2, 3]. In 2010, 68% of the 34 million of people infected with HIV were living in sub-Saharan Africa [4]. Between 1983 and 2001, the Central African region had the highest HCV prevalence worldwide with a prevalence of 6% and this prevalence was 13.8% in Cameroon [5]. The seroprevalence of hepatitis B S antigen among blood donors in Cameroon was 10.7% in 2003 [2].

The HIV, HBV, and HCV coinfections are severe and frequent in sub-Saharan Africa. In a systematic review, the mean prevalence rates of HBV and HCV among HIV-positive people were 15% and 7%, respectively [6]. Indeed, these viruses have the same mode of transmission through sexual intercourse, mother-to-child, and blood transfusion. Furthermore, their coinfection has more negative effects. The influence of HIV on HBV is characterized by a more frequent evolution towards chronicity, an increased viral replication rate, a viral reactivation leading to fibrosing cholestatic hepatitis, and an increased progression towards fibrosis and liver cirrhosis [7–9]. On the other hand, the HBV infection aggravates the progression towards AIDS and an increased in vitro replication of HIV [10]. Unfortunately, access to treatment against these viruses is not always accessible for most people in developing countries. Even though significant improvement has been achieved, in 2010, only 41% of HIV positive eligible people had access to antiretroviral therapy in sub-Saharan Africa [4]. Therefore, screening for these three viruses is imperative before any blood transfusion.

Studies have shown that in sub-Saharan Africa, international models and standards for organizing blood banks and blood donation were not affordable and might even be unsustainable. Consequently, these models and standards should be adapted to resource poor environments [11]. Even though improvement has been achieved, many challenges remain unsolved to ensure blood safety especially in rural areas [12]. Tagny and colleagues [13] revealed that in sub-Saharan Africa, there were several problems undermining the blood safety including the low implementation of national policies for transfusion, organizational dysfunctions, inadequate financing, and the lack of adequate blood screening equipment. Despite these shortcomings, measures are urgently needed to ensure blood safety and to avoid the spread of infectious agents and the deterioration of blood donors and of blood recipients' health. Therefore, the safety of not only blood recipients but also of blood donors should guide the blood safety procedures.

Few studies have been carried out in recent years on the coinfections with HIV, HBV, and HCV among blood donors in Cameroon, but none has analyzed the procedures used for ensuring blood safety. Knowing the prevalence of these viruses among blood donors will underpin the extent to which these infections are present in Cameroon. Additionally, identifying safety issues in blood donation procedures will guide health actors to urgently develop and implement efficient strategies for ensuring blood safety.

Therefore, the objectives of this study are to determine the prevalence of HIV, HBV, and HCV and their coinfections among blood donors at the Yaounde Central Hospital and to propose an efficient screening algorithm of blood donors for resources limited settings.

2. Material and Methods

We carried out a retrospective study from January to June 2008 at the Yaounde Central Hospital. Data was collected from the registers of the blood bank and was filled in a data collecting form. Observation was used to describe the blood donation procedures at the blood bank. All blood donors registered at the blood bank during the study period were included in the study.

Data retrieved included the demographic characteristics of donors: age, sex, residence, and the results of HIV, HBV, and HCV serologies.

Data on blood donors and the results of all performed tests on their blood were entered on Microsoft Excel 2007 spreadsheets by one investigator then controlled by a second investigator. Data was analyzed using the SPSS 19 software. Bivariate analysis was used to find correlation between characteristics of donors and studied infections. The following indicators were assessed: (i) the distribution of

blood donors per age and sex; (ii) the number and ratio of persons infected by HIV, HBV, and HCV viruses and of persons coinfected by two or three viruses; lastly (iii) the ratio of blood donors infected by HIV, HBV, and HCV by age group. Tables and figures were constructed.

Medians, means, and ratios were calculated. The chi-square test was used to compare means. The difference was considered statistically significant for P value < 0.05. All data was aggregated to ensure confidentiality. We did not meet or interact with donors or patients.

3. Results

Of the 4650 donors recruited for the study, the sex of 4645 (99.9%) donors was available. The age of 4630 (99.6%) donors was available while HIV, HBV, HCV, and syphilis tests were conducted in 4641 (99.8%) donors.

3.1. Procedures for Blood Donation and Safety Procedures. The Yaounde Central Hospital Blood Bank is the largest and the most used in Cameroon. Current procedures of screening blood donors consist of two types of blood donations—voluntary or benevolent donation and family donation. Benevolent donations represent less than 25% of all blood donations in Cameroon in general [4]. In this case, blood is collected during public sensitization campaigns from voluntary donors.

Regarding family blood donation, a family that has a patient in need of blood transfusion brings its blood donors found within the family or not. Two donors are required by the hospital for each set of no infected blood that will be provided to the patient. Counselling is not done to the donor and in general, donors do not return to the blood bank to have information about the results of the tests performed on their collected blood.

In both cases, data on the blood donor are registered and include name, age, sex, profession, and telephone number. Blood is collected from donors and tests are carried out later on to check if the blood is safe and to categorize the blood group. These tests consist of blood group and Rhesus, the haemoglobin electrophoresis, and the screening of infections using HIV serology, HBV antigen S test, HCV serology, and syphilis serology (TPHA and VDRL). If one or more of these infection tests is positive, the collected blood set is destroyed.

3.2. Demographic Characteristics. Out of the 4645 blood donors, 4337 (93.37%) donors were males while 308 (6.67%) donors were females giving a male-to-female sex ratio of 14 : 1. The age of blood donors varied from 16 to 69 years with a median age of 28 years. The majority of donors (55%) had between 20 and 29 years of age (see Figure 1).

3.3. Seroprevalence of HIV, HBV, and HCV and their Coinfections in Blood Donors. The results of the laboratory tests were available for 4644 (99.98%) blood donors, of which 564 (12.14%) were infected with the HBV, 206 (4.44%) with the HIV, and 67 (1.46%) with the HCV (see Table 1). HBV infection was most frequent in men ($P = 0.02$). A total of

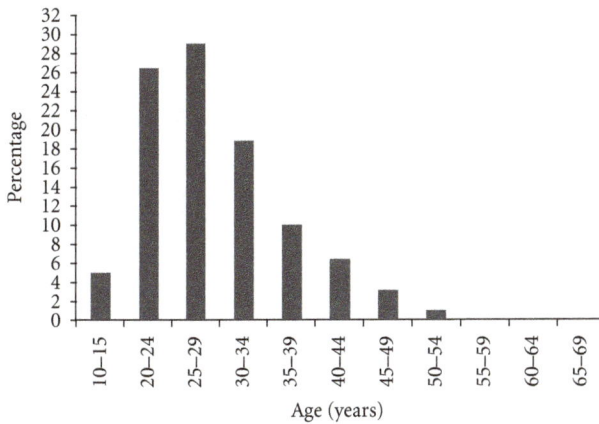

FIGURE 1: Distribution of blood donors by age group. Each row represents the proportion of the number of donors in the age group among the 4645 blood donors.

837 (18%) sets of blood were destroyed due to infection by at least one of the three viruses.

Coinfections were not very common in blood donors. A total of 36 (0.78%) cases of HIV and HBV coinfections were recorded, followed by HBV-HCV coinfection with a prevalence of 0.22% and a prevalence of 0.06% for HIV and HCV coinfection. The coinfection with the three viruses was 0.04% among blood donors (see Table 2).

3.4. Cross-Distributions between Ages and Infections. HIV, HBV, and HCV infections were found in all age groups (see Figure 2). The prevalence of HIV and HCV increased with the age of the donors. On the contrary, HBV infection prevalence decreased with the age of the donors.

4. Discussion

The seroprevalence of HIV infection in blood donors (4.43%) was lower than the HIV seroprevalence of 5.5% found in the adult population between 15 and 49 years in 2004 during the National Demographic Survey [14]. This could be explained by the fact that families search for "physically healthy" blood donors.

Regarding HBV infection, the prevalence seems to be increasing with time. In 1993, Ndumbe and Skalsky [15] found a HBV prevalence of 6.7% while Mbanya et al. [2] recorded a prevalence of 10.7% in Cameroon in 2001, compared to 12.14% in our study. They conducted their study among blood donors in a hospital at Yaoundé but they had a sample size (252 blood donors) 18 times much lower than in our study. In 2006, hepatitis B vaccination was introduced in the Expanded Program of Immunization of Cameroon but only for children below one year of age. Other studies have shown the high endemicity of HBV in other sub-Saharan African countries but with various prevalences [16–21]. Blood transfusion is the major route of transmission of HCV. In a study carried out in Nigeria on blood donors and sickle cell patients, the prevalence of HCV was recorded at 14% by Mutimer et al. [22]. In developed countries, the risk of HCV infection through transfusion is low and was

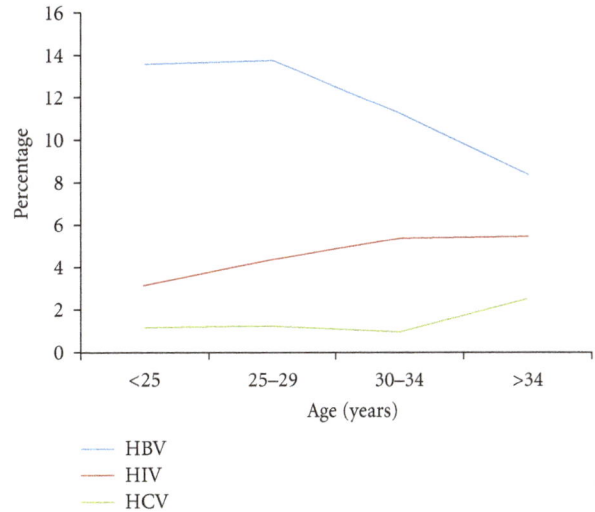

FIGURE 2: Prevalence of HIV, HBV, and HCV infections in blood donors according to age. The proportion of blood donors with a positive test was calculated over the total number of blood donors in the age group.

estimated at 1 on 3000 transfusions due to its low prevalence among the general population and the adequate checkup [23].

Regarding coinfections, the prevalences of HIV-HBV and HIV-HCV were much lower than results obtained by Laurent et al. [24] and Mbanya et al. [2] in 2001 at Yaounde. Indeed, Laurent et al. found among HIV-positive patients, 8.3% and 12.4% coinfections with HBV and HCV, respectively. But these results were obtained from 169 HIV-positive people eligible for antiretroviral therapy, thus at a more advanced stage of the HIV infection.

The presence of HIV, HBV, and HCV coinfections increases the risk of disease in blood donors. Moreover, collection of blood from an infected donor could increase the progression to a symptomatic or disease stage. In fact, the loss of 500 mL of blood reduces the haemoglobin level by about 1 g as well as leucocytes and antibodies of the donor. De Cock and colleagues argued that some approaches to fight against HIV/AIDS and other infectious diseases were often poorly adapted to adequately address the disease [25].

The HIV/AIDS National Control Programme is in charge of HIV/AIDS and other sexually transmitted diseases in Cameroon. However, it mainly focuses on HIV/AIDS. This could be explained by the HIV/AIDS "exceptionalism" but neglecting other sexually transmitted infections such as HBV and HVC could lead to the spread of both these diseases and even HIV. Secondly, processing infection screening tests in parallel and on sets of blood already collected leads to wastage of screening tests and to a loss of blood collected from infected donors.

Consequently, we proposed new strategies for improving efficiency and management of blood donors in resource-limited settings and ensuring blood safety (Figure 3). Firstly, the screening tests should be performed in series. The next test will only be carried out if the previous one is negative. The order in which the tests should be processed will be based on the prevalence of the infections found in the

TABLE 1: Prevalence of HIV, HBV, and HCV among blood donors.

Sex	HIV test			HBV test			HCV test			Total positive
	Positive (%)	Negative (%)	Total (%)	Positive (%)	Negative (%)	Total (%)	Positive (%)	Negative (%)	Total (%)	
Male	192 (4.43)	4144 (85.57)	4336 (100)	544 (12.55)	3792 (87.45)	4336 (100)	65 (1.49)	4271 (98.50)	4336 (100)	800 (18.5)
Female	14 (4.55)	294 (95.45)	308 (100)	20 (6.49)	288 (93.51)	308 (100)	2 (0.65)	306 (99.35)	308 (100)	37 (12)
Total	**206 (4.44)**	4438 (95.56)	4644 (100)	**564 (12.14)**	4080 (87.86)	4644 (100)	**67 (1.46)**	4577 (98.56)	4644 (100)	837 (18)
P value	0.923			0.02			0.227			

In Table 1, the results of HIV, HBV, and HCV tests are presented by blood donor sex. The proportion of blood donors with a positive test was compared by sex group using the chi-square test.

TABLE 2: Seroprevalence of HIV, HBV, and HCV coinfections according to sex among blood donors.

Sex	Co-infection VIH-VHB			Co-infection VIH-VHC			Co-infection VHB-VHC			Co-infection VIH-VHB-VHC		
	Positive (%)	Negative (%)	Total (%)	Positive (%)	Negative (%)	Total (%)	Positive(%)	Negative (%)	Total (%)	Positive (%)	Negative (%)	Total (%)
Male	32 (0.74)	4303 (99.26)	4335 (100)	3 (0.07)	4333 (99.93)	4336 (100)	9 (0.21)	4326 (99.79)	4336 (100)	2 (0.05)	4333 (99.95)	4335 (100)
Female	4 (1.30)	304 (98.70)	308 (100)	0 (0.00)	308 (100.00)	308 (100)	1 (0.32)	307 (99.68)	308 (100)	0 (0.00)	308 (100.00)	308 (100)
Total	36 (0.78)	4607 (99.22)	4643 (100)	3 (0.06)	4644 (99.94)	4644 (100)	10 (0.22)	4633 (99.78)	4644 (100)	2 (0.04)	4641 (99.96)	4643 (100)
P value	0.279			0.644			0.668			0.706		

In Table 2, the results of coinfections with HIV, HBV, and HCV among blood donors are presented by blood donor sex. The proportion of blood donors with a positive coinfection was compared by sex group using the chi-square test.

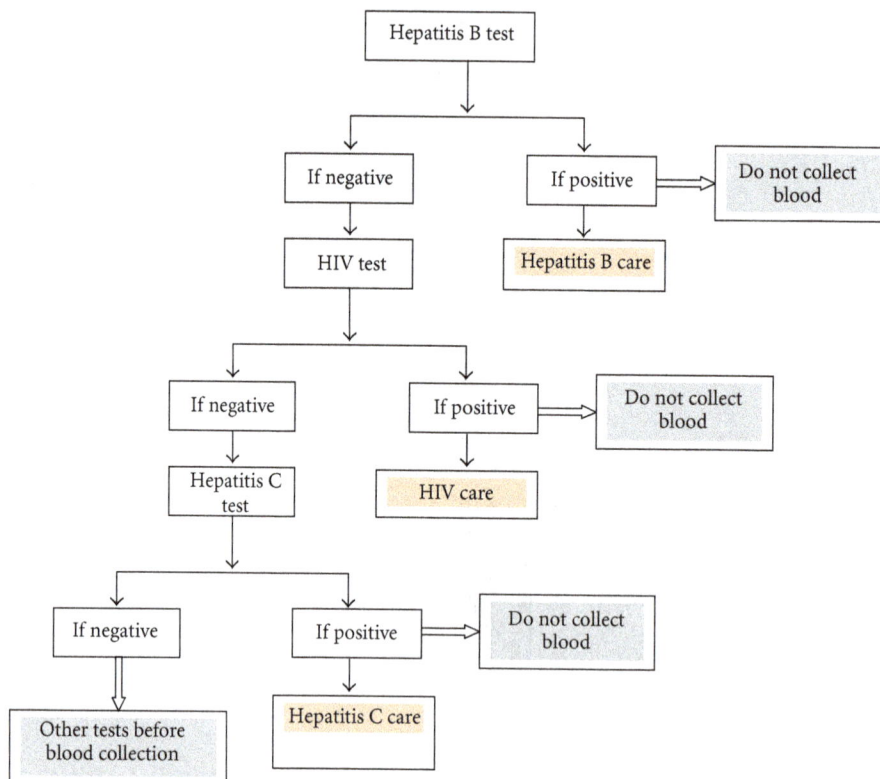

FIGURE 3: New algorithm for blood donors infections screening.

country starting from the most prevalent infection and finishing with the least frequent one. With regard to the Cameroon context, the HBV test will be performed first, followed by the HIV test, and finally the HCV test. Other tests such as syphilis test can be performed depending on the local epidemiology. This strategy is more efficient in the sense that it avoids the wastage of materials, reagents, and time and is done on a small sample of blood.

Secondly, blood will be collected only if all the tests are negative, avoiding blood collection from infected donors. This has the advantages of saving time and reducing workload for processing all the tests. The time saved should be used to improve counselling of infected donors, and prepare them for future clinical followup and care.

The implementation of this algorithm requires a new approach towards blood donation. This approach includes counselling of blood donors, carrying out rapid tests and communicating the results to donors, and putting in place strategies for the care of infected blood donors. This strategy even goes beyond efficiency and encompasses moral and ethical considerations to offer quality health care to people willing to save other lives through blood donation while being themselves in urgent need of care.

5. Conclusion

HIV, HBV, and HCV infections are frequent among blood donors in Cameroon. Collecting sets of blood and carrying out screening tests later are not efficient. Serial tests should be processed on blood samples using rapid tests, and sets of blood should be collected only from donors with negative tests. Lastly, strategies should be put in place to take care of infected blood donors.

Conflict of Interests

The authors declare no conflict of interests.

References

[1] UNAIDS, *2009 Aids Epidemic Update*, WHO, Geneva, Switzerland, 2004.

[2] D. N. Mbanya, D. Takam, and P. M. Ndumbet, "Serological findings amongst first-time blood donors in Yaoundé, Cameroon: is safe donation a reality or a myth?" *Transfusion Medicine*, vol. 13, no. 5, pp. 267–273, 2003.

[3] H. Jager, K. Nseka, B. Goussard et al., "Voluntary blood donor recruitment: a strategy to reduce transmission of HIV-1, hepatitis-B and syphilis in Kinshasa, Zaire," *Infusionstherapie*, vol. 17, no. 4, pp. 224–226, 1990.

[4] WHO, *Global HIV/AIDS Response: Epidemic Update and Health Sector Progress Towards Universal Access, Progrss Report 2011*, WHO, Geneva, Switzerland, 2011.

[5] V. Madhava, C. Burgess, and E. Drucker, "Epidemiology of chronic hepatitis C virus infection in sub-Saharan Africa," *The Lancet*, vol. 2, no. 5, pp. 293–302, 2002.

[6] R. E. Barth, Q. Huijgen, J. Taljaard, and A. I. M. Hoepelman, "Hepatitis B/C and HIV in sub-Saharan Africa: an association between highly prevalent infectious diseases. A systematic review and meta-analysis," *International Journal of Infectious Diseases*, vol. 14, no. 12, pp. e1024–e1031, 2010.

[7] S. J. Rossi, D. Pharm, A. Paul, M. D. Volberding, L. Teresa, and M. D. Wright, "Does hepatitis C virus infection increase the risk of HIV disease progression?" *Journal of the American Medical Association*, vol. 288, no. 2, pp. 241–243, 2002.

[8] M. S. Sulkowski, R. D. Moore, S. H. Mehta, R. E. Chaisson, and D. L. Thomas, "Hepatitis C and progression of HIV disease," *Journal of the American Medical Association*, vol. 288, no. 2, pp. 199–206, 2002.

[9] C. L. Cooper, E. Mills, B. O. Wabwire, N. Ford, and P. Olupot-Olupot, "Chronic viral hepatitis may diminish the gains of HIV antiretroviral therapy in sub-Saharan Africa," *International Journal of Infectious Diseases*, vol. 13, no. 3, pp. 302–306, 2009.

[10] R. J. Burnett, G. Francois, M. C. Kew et al., "Hepatitis B virus and human immunodeficiency virus co-infection in sub-Saharan Africa: a call for further investigation," *Liver International*, vol. 25, no. 2, pp. 201–213, 2005.

[11] J. P. Allain, S. Owusu-Ofori, and I. Bates, "Blood transfusion in sub-Saharan Africa," *Transfusion Alternatives in Transfusion Medicine*, vol. 6, no. 1, pp. 16–23, 2004.

[12] A. F. Fleming, "HIV and blood transfusion in Sub-Saharan Africa," *Transfusion and Apheresis Science*, vol. 18, no. 2, pp. 167–179, 1997.

[13] C. T. Tagny, D. Mbanya, J. B. Tapko, and J. J. Lefrère, "Blood safety in Sub-Saharan Africa: a multi-factorial problem," *Transfusion*, vol. 48, no. 6, pp. 1256–1261, 2008.

[14] INS & ORC Macro, "Cameroon demographic and health survey," Maryland 2004, http://www.measuredhs.com/pubs/pdf/SR107/SR107.pdf.

[15] P. M. Ndumbe and J. Skalsky, "Hepatitis C virus infection in different populations in Cameroon," *Scandinavian Journal of Infectious Diseases*, vol. 25, no. 6, pp. 689–692, 1993.

[16] B. F. Igbida, M. M. Abidemi, and J. Z. Awortu, "Sero-epidemiology of transfusion-transmissible infectious diseases among blood donors in Osogbo, south-west Nigeria," *Blood Transfusion*, vol. 7, no. 4, pp. 293–299, 2009.

[17] H. I. Awadalla, M. H. Ragab, M. A. Osman, and N. A. Nassar, "Risk factors of viral hepatitis B among Egyptian blood donors," *British Journal of Medicine and Medical Research*, vol. 1, no. 1, pp. 7–13, 2011.

[18] D. N. Noah, R. Njouom, A. Bonny, P. Pirsou, J. Meli, and M. B. Sida, "HBs antigene prevalence in blood donors and the risk of transfusion of hepatitis B at the central hospital of Yaounde, Cameroon," *Open Journal of Gastroenterology*, vol. 1, pp. 23–27, 2011.

[19] F. B. Sinoussi, J. C. Chermann, and F. Rey, "Isolation of a T-lymphotropic retrovirus from a patient at risk for acquired immune deficiency syndrome (AIDS)," *Science*, vol. 220, no. 4599, pp. 868–871, 1983.

[20] A. Ado, S. Alhassan, U. G. Chonoko, and A. U. Samaila, "Seroprevalence of hepatitis B surface antigen (Hbsag) among blood donors attending Ahmadu Bello University Teaching Hospital (Abuth), Zaria, Nigeria," *Bayero Journal of Pure and Applied Sciences*, vol. 3, no. 1, pp. 20–22, 2010.

[21] Y. Foupouapouognigni, S. A. Sadeuh Mba, E. B. à Betsem et al., "Hepatitis B and C virus infections in the three Pygmy groups in Cameroon," *Journal of Clinical Microbiology*, vol. 49, no. 2, pp. 737–740, 2011.

[22] D. J. Mutimer, A. Olomu, S. Skidmore et al., "Viral hepatitis in Nigeria—sickle-cell disease and commercial blood donors," *Quarterly Journal of Medicine*, vol. 87, no. 7, pp. 407–411, 1994.

[23] D. Moradpour, A. Cerny, M. H. Heim, and H. E. Blum, "Hepatitis C: an update," *Swiss Medical Weekly*, vol. 131, no. 21-22, pp. 291–298, 2001.

[24] C. Laurent, A. Bourgeois, E. Mpoudi-Ngolé et al., "High rates of active hepatitis B and C co-infections in HIV-1 infected Cameroonian adults initiating antiretroviral therapy," *HIV Medicine*, vol. 11, no. 1, pp. 85–89, 2010.

[25] K. M. De Cock, D. Mbori-Ngacha, and E. Marum, "Shadow on the continent: public health and HIV/AIDS in Africa in the 21st century," *The Lancet*, vol. 360, no. 9326, pp. 67–72, 2002.

11

Assessment of Intraoperative Blood Loss during Oral and Maxillofacial Surgical Procedures in a Nigerian Tertiary Health Care Center

Babatunde O. Akinbami[1] and Bisola Onajin-Obembe[2]

[1] Department of Oral and Maxillofacial Surgery, University of Port Harcourt Teaching Hospital, Choba,
 PMB 6173 Port Harcourt, 500004 Rivers State, Nigeria
[2] Department of Anaesthesia, University of Port Harcourt Teaching Hospital, PMB 6173 Port Harcourt, 500004 Rivers State, Nigeria

Correspondence should be addressed to Babatunde O. Akinbami; akinbamzy3@yahoo.com

Academic Editor: Silvano Wendel

Background. Reports on estimated amount of blood loss in maxillofacial surgical procedures will guide clinicians through units of blood required for each procedure. The aim of the study was to assess the amount of blood loss and duration of surgery. *Methods.* All cases of maxillofacial surgical procedures done under GA in the MFU theatre, from January 2007 to December 2013, were included in the study. Pre- and postoperative haematocrit values, number of units of whole blood requested and used, amount of blood loss, and duration of surgery were recorded. *Results.* 139 patients were analyzed, of which 75 (54.0%) were males and 64 (46.0%) were females. Fifty-six (40.3%) cases involved soft tissues. Eighty-three cases involved hard tissues. Age range was 2 months to 78 years; mean ± (SD) was 21.3 ± (18.5) years. Isolated unilateral cleft lip had the lowest mean value of estimated blood loss of 10.4 ± 10.8 mLs and also the lowest duration of surgery of 58 (76) minutes. There was no significant relationship between both parameters for cleft lip. Fractures of the mandible had mean blood loss of 352 mLs and duration was 175 min. *Conclusion.* In this study, there was significant relationship between estimated blood loss and duration of surgery for mandibular and zygomatic complex fractures.

1. Introduction

Intraoperative blood loss is one of the causes of death during surgical procedures [1]. Acute anaemia can also result from excessive blood loss and this can affect healing of tissues after surgery [1]. Maxillofacial surgical procedures can be classified as minor, intermediate, major, or supramajor cases based on the type and duration of the procedures [2–9]. These procedures may be associated with excessive blood loss from the facial microvasculature and major blood vessels within the operation field of the surgeon [3, 10–14]. Quite often, the lesions have also invaded the walls of the vessels [3] or lie close to these vessels, thereby making them vulnerable to injury during surgery with consequent loss of blood. Furthermore, a significant amount of bleeding can occur during dissection of the capillary-rich skin, subcutaneous tissue, and muscles in the maxillofacial region. Various strategies for preventing

excessive blood loss have been applied to maintain haemostasis and these also include the use of hypotensive anaesthesia and tranexamic acid [4].

Patients may be required to donate varying number of units of blood prior to surgery which may or may not be used. The potential blood loss and estimated number of blood products required should therefore be predetermined using many factors [7]. These include haemoglobin or hematocrit levels, body weight of the patient especially for paediatric cases, extent of the lesion, age, and gender as well as the type and extent of procedure. The experience of the surgeon and possibly the duration of surgery must also be considered. Madsen et al. [15] evaluated intraoperative blood loss by thromboelastography (TEG) and they stated that it was an objective method of assessing and predicting intraoperative blood loss.

Much attention has been given to blood loss following general and orthognathic surgeries in the literature, but little work has been done on other maxillofacial procedures [5–9, 15–20]. The aim of the study was therefore to assess the amount of blood loss and the number of units of whole blood required for oral and maxillofacial procedures and also to evaluate any relationship between the amount of blood loss and duration of surgery.

2. Methods and Patients

Ethical approval to carry out the study (UPTH/ADM/90/S.II/VOL.X/371) was provided by the University of Port Harcourt Hospital's Ethics and Research Committee (Chairperson Professor Anthony Okpani) on January 27, 2014. All cases of maxillofacial surgical procedures done under GA in the MFU theatre, from January 2007 to December 2013, were included in the study. Patients' demographics and haematological profile retrieved from the case files and theatre records by the house officer and cross-checked by one of the consultants (B. O. A) were documented in a retrospective review chart. Data included the extent, diagnosis of lesion, and medical comorbidities. Pre- and postoperative haematocrit values, number of units of whole blood requested, cross-matched, and used, procedure, amount of blood loss, and duration of surgery were recorded. All cases done under local anaesthesia in the clinic were excluded from the study. The cases were divided into two groups which were diseases or procedures on soft and hard tissues. The total blood loss estimation was done by calculating the amount of blood in the suction bottle and adding this to the estimated value from all the blood soaked gauze.

Data obtained was analyzed with SPSS (SPSS Inc., Chicago, IL) version 16. Means and standard deviation of haematocrit values, estimated blood loss, and duration of surgery for each category of disease were determined and the means within groups and between the two groups were compared with paired sample t-test. Linear regression analysis was used to analyze the association between blood loss and duration of surgery. R coefficients and significance values were determined. P values equal to or less than 0.05 were considered significant.

3. Result

A total of 139 patients were analyzed, out of which 75 (54.0%) were males and 64 (46.0%) were females; age range was 2 months to 78 years; mean ± (SD) was 21.3 ± (18.5) years. Fifty-six (40.3%) cases involved soft tissues. Isolated cleft palate 19 (13.7%) and cleft lip 18 (12.9) constituted the highest number of cases seen. Range and mean haematocrit values of soft tissue lesions are reflected in Table 1. Cases of malignant soft tissue tumours presented with the lowest preoperative haematocrit and cases of soft tissue tumours had the highest mean value. Up to 3 units of blood were requested for malignant tumours, but we mostly used 2 units for the less extensive resections. Lowest preoperative haematocrit level taken for elective surgery was 21% and this was in cleft lip.

Eighty-three cases involved hard tissues. Range and mean haematocrit values of bony lesions are reflected in Table 2. Cases with multiple fractures presented with the lowest preoperative haematocrit and cases of cysts/fibroosseous lesions had the highest mean value. Up to 3 units of blood were requested for resection and reconstruction in mandibular tumours, but we mostly used 2 units.

Isolated unilateral cleft lip had the lowest mean value of estimated blood loss of 10.4 ± (10.8) mLs and also the lowest duration of surgery of 58 (76) mins. There was no significant relationship between both parameters for cleft lip (Table 3). Comparison of mean values of blood loss and duration between isolated cleft lip and isolated palates gave $P > 0.05$. Complete cleft of primary and secondary palate recorded blood loss of 400 mLs with a mean duration of 4 hrs 23 mins, but the correlation coefficient, 0.327, was not significant, with a $P > 0.05$.

The association between blood loss in benign soft tissue tumours, 360 mls, and duration of surgery, 2 hrs 10 mins, was the least significant, $P > 0.05$. For fractures of the mandible blood loss was 352 mls and duration was 175 min, significance: $P < 0.05$ (Table 4). Zygomatic complex fractures recorded blood loss of 248 mLs and duration of 185 mins, significance: $P < 0.05$.

In mandibular tumours, blood loss was 1214 mls and duration was 5 hrs 30 min. There was no relationship between both parameters. In maxillary tumours treated by hemimaxillectomy, mean blood loss was 627 mLs and duration was approximately 2 hrs; the relationship was not significant with P value as reflected in Table 4. Comparison of mean values of blood loss and duration between mandibular and maxillary tumours gave $P > 0.05$.

When the mean blood loss in the two groups was compared, there was significant difference, R coefficient of 0.935, $P < 0.05$. By comparison of means of duration of surgery, R coefficient was 0.817 and $P < 0.05$ also showed significant differences between the two groups.

4. Discussion

Intraoperative blood loss can be predicted by preoperative thromboelastography which measures the interaction between coagulation factors, platelets, and fibrinolytic agents. Parameters measured included the clot formation time, maximal clot firmness, fibrinolytic resistance of clot, and α angle. Madsen et al. [15] separated their patients into 2 groups based on intraoperative bleeding volume (≤400 mLs and >400 mL); they found no significant associations between routine anticoagulant tests and intraoperative blood loss. When the TEG results for the two groups were compared, there was significant association between clot formation time, maximum clot firmness, and alpha angle, but the fibrinolytic resistance of blood clot was not related to intraoperative blood loss and they concluded that alpha angle greater than 67 degrees was suggestive of blood loss of 400 mls or less with 95% certainty, but such predictions may not reflect actual values.

Eipe and Ponniah [18] opined that differences in pre- and postoperative haematocrit values and deductions of

TABLE 1: Age, gender, hematocrit values, and blood requirements of fifty-six (56) patients with 56 procedures on soft tissues.

Diagnosis	Number of procedures	Age range	Male (%)	Female (%)	Range, mean (SD) pre-PCV	Number of units requested	Number of units used	Range, mean (SD) post-PCV
Cleft lip	18	2 months–35 years	9 (6.6)	9 (6.6)	21–35, 31.4 (4.1)	1	0	27–29, 28 (1.4)
Cleft palate	19	10 months–28 years	4 (2.9)	15 (11.0)	28–38, 33.9 (3.6)	1	0	27–30, 28.3 (1.5)
Cleft lip and palate	4	5 months–20 years	2 (1.5)	2 (1.5)	25–35, 30.3 (5.0)	1	0	24–32, 28.7 (4.2)
Soft tissue tumors	9	4 months–33 years	6 (4.4)	3 (2.2)	33–46, 39.5 (9.2)	2	1	23–44, 33.5 (14.8)
Malignant soft tissue tumors	3	26–32 years	2 (1.5)	1 (0.7)	25–32, 28.5 (4.9)	3	3	34–40, 37.0 (4.2)
Palatal salivary gland tumors	3	26–41 years	3 (2.2)	0 (0)	30–35, 32.5 (3.5)	1	0	—
Total	56	—	26 (18.7)	30 (21.6)	—	—	—	—

TABLE 2: Age, gender, hematocrit values, and blood requirements of eighty-three (83) patients with 83 procedures on bony tissues.

Diagnosis	Number of procedures	Age range (years)	Male (%)	Female (%)	Range, mean (SD) pre-PCV	Number of pints requested	Number of pints used	Range Mean (SD) post-PCV
Fractures of the mandible	17	2–65	14 (10.1)	3 (2.2)	31–38, 33.3 (3.3)	1	1	38–44, 41.0 (4.2)
Zygomatic fractures	6	8–38	4 (2.9)	2 (1.5)	21–44, 29.5 (6.0)	1	0	29–32, 30.5 (2.1)
NOE and Le Fort fractures	6	4–27	3 (2.2)	3 (2.2)	28–35, 31.5 (4.9)	0	0	—
Multiple fractures	3	24–35	2 (1.5)	1 (0.8)	20–31, 25.5 (7.8)	2	2	—
Mandible tumors	24	10–78	11 (8.1)	13 (9.6)	25–44 35.5 (5.2)	3	2	25–42, 34.0 (6.2)
Maxillary tumors	16	6–60	9 (6.5)	7 (5.0)	25–36, 34.3 (2.1)	2	1	32–38, 35 (4.2)
Cysts and fibroosseous	6	11–27	3 (2.2)	3 (2.2)	35–38, 36 (1.7)	2	1	28–42, 35 (9.9)
TMJ ankylosis and dislocation	5	11–64	3 (2.2)	2 (1.5)	25–42, 33.5 (12.0)	1	1	30–35, 33 (2.6)
Total	83		49 (36.0)	34 (25)	—	—	—	—

TABLE 3: Estimated blood loss, duration of surgery, and *P* values of fifty-six (56) patients with 56 procedures on soft tissues.

Diagnosis	Treatment	Estimated blood loss Mean (SD) (mLs)	Duration of surgery Mean (SD) (mins)	R coefficient	Significance level P value 0.05
Unilateral cleft lip	Millard's repair	10.4 (10.8)	58 (76)	0.191	0.464
Cleft palate	Palatoplasty	142 (139)	127 (48)	0.081	0.749
Complete cleft lip and palate	Millard's repair/palatoplasty	400 (265)	263 (58)	0.327	0.788
Benign soft tissue tumors	Excision	360 (164)	130 (82)	0.130	0.835
Malignant soft tissue tumors	Excision	1950 (778)	360 (81)	1.000	0.009
Palatal salivary gland tumors	Excision	367 (293)	83 (40)	0.985	0.109

P level < 0.05.

TABLE 4: Estimated blood loss and duration of surgery and *P* values of eighty-three (83) patients with procedures on bony tissues.

Diagnosis	Treatment	Estimated blood loss Mean (SD) (mLs)	Duration Mean (SD) (mins)	R coefficient	Significance level
Fractures of the mandible	ORIF and IMF	352 (351)	175 (75)	0.585	0.014
Zygomatic complex fractures	Zygomatic bone elevation, antral support, and ORIF	248 (185)	185 (112)	0.966	0.034
NOE and Le Fort fractures	Nasal bone reduction, ORIF, canthopexy, and internal suspension	370 (421)	287 (53)	0.873	0.325
Multiple fractures	Zygomatic bone elevation, internal suspension, and IMF	350 (50)	293 (11)	1.000	0.009
Mandible tumors	Resection and reconstruction	1214 (661)	328 (95)	−0.061	0.843
Maxillary tumors	Resection/hemimaxillectomy	627 (471)	127 (61)	0.550	0.125
Cysts and fibroosseous lesions	Enucleation/excision	530 (327)	103 (28)	0.804	0.103
TMJ ankylosis/dislocation	Interposition arthroplasty	550 (303)	210 (82)	0.715	0.285

P level < 0.05.

blood loss by the Gross formula are invaluable; the formula stated that actual blood loss equals blood volume multiplied by the difference in pre- (initial) and postoperative (final) hematocrit values and divided by mean of both hematocrit values; blood volume was calculated by multiplying body weight in kilograms by 70 mL/kg; however, the values are usually difficult to correlate with exact intraoperative loss due to intraoperative blood transfusion and crystalloid infusions as well as postoperative blood losses/fluid dilutions [18]. Hence clinical estimates of intraoperative blood loss are quite useful and this is done before irrigating wounds with any fluid.

In the operating room, considering the controversy surrounding the use of a discrete concentration of haemoglobin as a transfusion trigger for managing acute blood loss, the anaesthetists mainly depend on the clinical estimation of blood loss which includes checking for pallor and the trends of the patient's oxygen saturation, capillary perfusion, blood pressure, and heart rate patterns. Therefore, each patient was assessed individually and blood transfusion was patient-specific.

In this study, the higher blood loss as well as the longer duration of surgery recorded during operations on hard tissues when compared with soft tissues was likely due to the significant amount of blood loss while dissecting the soft tissue overlying bone before resecting the affected bone itself.

Although our result showed that operations for the excision of malignant soft tissue tumours recorded the highest amount of blood loss and the longest duration of surgery on the whole, this was mainly due to the large dimensions and extent of the tumours involved. Revascularization of abnormally proliferating cells and local spread of the lesion also contributed to increasing bleeding episode seen in our patients.

It is not surprising that, in the hard tissue category, the amount of blood loss and duration of surgery were particularly highest for mandibular tumours undergoing resection and reconstruction of the jaw. The association between these primary and secondary outcome variables was quite significant for mandibular and zygomatic complex fractures but not for tumours of the jaws. Treatment of these fractures involves the dissection and detachment of soft tissues and reflection of the mucoperiosteum overlying the bones and these result in appreciable bleeding. Open reduction and internal fixation of these bone segments are actually major surgeries especially when multiple sites are involved and the number of fracture sites will determine the duration of surgery and amount of blood loss. Our findings will serve as baseline studies for comparison with future studies on intraoperative blood loss from surgical management of facial fractures.

Bell et al. [2] in their study on reconstruction of severely atrophic mandible documented a median blood loss of 300 mLs with an interquartile range of 150–1100 mLs whereas we had an average of 1214 mLs with a range of 300–2800 mls. While the study carried out by Pogrel et al. [4] documented a longer duration of operation for vascularized bone grafts (VBG), they however documented equal blood loss (1,100 mLs) during reconstruction of mandible with vascularized and nonvascularized bone grafts. The main reason why our patients bled more may be accounted for by the extent of the benign and locally aggressive nature of ameloblastomas of the mandible seen in our environment. Also contributing to the bleeding were the bone grafts harvested from both anterior and posterior iliac crests. These were used for covering large continuity defects. On the contrary, the relatively less bleeding seen in operations involving maxillary tumours may be due to the fact that most of the tumors were removed by intraoral approach. For maxillary tumours, resections were performed, after which the defect was covered with Sofra-Tulle-wrapped gauze while rehabilitation was accomplished with obturators. However, the amount of blood loss during maxillary tumour resection will also depend on the size and extent of the lesions.

We always use infiltration of adrenaline 1 : 200,000 for up to 15 min prior to the wound incision in addition to hypotensive anaesthesia for major surgeries and these contribute to reduction in blood loss. The meta-analysis of Hardwicked et al. has proven that adrenaline infiltration can reduce bleeding during reduction mammoplasties [21] and the outcome, safety, and efficacy do not depend on the extent/size of the lesions or the tissues involved [22]. Experience has shown that a wider nasal floor mucosa repair in the palate causes more bleeding which is further exacerbated by the diffuse and multiple blood supply of the palate when compared to the skin of the lip.

The American College of Physicians [23] recommended that RBC transfusions should be done unit by unit and reassessment should be done between each transfusion. According to Tartter and Barron [24] excessive intraoperative blood transfusion during surgeries for colorectal malignancies, without reevaluating the haemoglobin concentration in between transfusions, resulted in 90% of the unnecessary transfusions. In our center, the anaesthetists habitually request for a few more units of blood than required which may not be used. This is due to the correct assumption that most maxillofacial procedures are associated with excessive blood loss. On the contrary, our evaluation showed that the highest number of units needed during surgeries for extensive malignant lesions was 3 units while reconstructive surgery for benign tumours of the mandible required 2 units of whole blood. Essentially, blood transfusion may be indicated in cases where the preoperative

haemoglobin value used as the transfusion trigger was less than 8 mg/dL.

The lowest preoperative packed cell volume taken for elective surgery in our study was 21%. The benefits of performing operations on patients with low PCV or haematocrit values should be weighed against the risks while blood must be made available in case intraoperative transfusion is required. Notwithstanding, the decision to operate despite a low preoperative haematocrit value as in this case was guided by the favourable anticipated amount of blood loss and duration of surgery.

Apart from maintaining haemostasis, care must be taken to prevent excessive blood losses by avoiding major blood vessels. The approach of lesions via avascular planes, as well as subperiosteal dissections for noninvasive lesions, and safety margin sacrifice of tissues in infiltrative lesions are excellent techniques for preventing intraoperative bleeding. Considering that blood transfusion has potential complications [25–29] and that blood is also a limited resource, inappropriate use of blood must be discouraged. Blood wastage can be avoided by paying more attention to the expected blood loss and using preset criteria for homologous blood administration [23, 30, 31].

In maxillofacial patients, allogenic transfusion can be minimized by intraoperative isovolaemic haemodilution [32]. Unfortunately, autologous blood transfusion and intraoperative blood salvage, commonly used for intracavity operations such as abdominal and thoracic operations, may not be technically amenable to maxillofacial surgeries in our centre. The initiatives taken by the National Blood Transfusion Committees and the use of patient blood management guidelines [33], according to Goodnough and Shander [34], have shown that patient's outcome can be improved by evidence-based transfusion practices, minimization of blood loss, and optimization of patient red blood cell mass.

To provide flexibility, as well as avoid the complications and cost of transfusion, the authors prefer the group and save policy rather than the type and cross-match protocol for lesions with expected blood loss of 500 mls or less. This blood can then be made available and cross-matched for use in case of unexpected high loss [16, 17, 23].

In conclusion, in this study, there was significant relationship between estimated blood loss and duration of surgery for mandibular and zygomatic complex fractures. The number of units of whole blood requested for was a little higher than the blood loss estimates except for malignant soft tissue tumours, multiple fractures, mandible fractures, and TMJ disorders. The decision was based on precaution, considering the fact that blood may not be available if needed. Multiple factors may be responsible for blood loss during maxillofacial operations, but much still has to do with the physiological status and normal clotting mechanisms of the patients, nature of the lesions, and the use of anaesthetic and surgical control measures.

Conflict of Interests

The authors declare that there is no conflict of interests regarding the publication of this paper.

Authors' Contribution

Babatunde O. Akinbami and Bisola Onajin-Obembe contributed equally to this work.

Acknowledgment

The authors hereby acknowledge Dr. Rahul Mongia, House Officer in the Department of Oral and Maxillofacial Surgery, for his effort in the collation of the required data.

References

[1] ASA Task Force, "Practice guidelines for blood component therapy," *Anaesthesiology*, vol. 84, article 32, 1996.

[2] R. B. Bell, G. H. Blakey, R. P. White, D. G. Hillebrand, and A. Molina, "Staged reconstruction of the severely atrophic mandible with autogenous bone graft and endosteal implants," *Journal of Oral and Maxillofacial Surgery*, vol. 60, no. 10, pp. 1135–1141, 2002.

[3] K. F. W. Messmer, "Acceptable haematocrit levels in surgicalpatients," *World Journal of Surgery*, vol. 11, pp. 41–46, 1987.

[4] M. A. Pogrel, S. Podlesh, J. P. Anthony, and J. Alexander, "A comparison of vascularized and nonvascularized bone grafts for reconstruction of mandibular continuity defects," *Journal of Oral and Maxillofacial Surgery*, vol. 55, no. 11, pp. 1200–1206, 1997.

[5] B.-K. Choi, E.-J. Yang, K. S. Oh, and L.-J. Lo, "Assessment of blood loss and need for transfusion during bimaxillary surgery with or without maxillary setback," *Journal of Oral and Maxillofacial Surgery*, vol. 71, no. 2, pp. 358–365, 2013.

[6] A. Piñeiro-Aguilar, M. Somoza-Martín, J. M. Gandara-Rey, and A. García-García, "Blood loss in orthognathic surgery: a systematic review," *Journal of Oral and Maxillofacial Surgery*, vol. 69, pp. 885–892, 2011.

[7] D. Rummasak, B. Apipan, and P. Kaewpradup, "Factors that determine intraoperative blood loss in bimaxillary osteotomies and the need for preoperative blood preparation," *Journal of Oral and Maxillofacial Surgery*, vol. 69, no. 11, pp. e456–e460, 2011.

[8] W. B. Kretschmer, G. Baciut, M. Bacuit, W. Zoder, and K. Wangerin, "Intraoperative blood loss in bimaxillary orthognathic surgery with multisegmental Le Fort I osteotomies and additional procedures," *British Journal of Oral and Maxillofacial Surgery*, vol. 48, no. 4, pp. 276–280, 2010.

[9] K. Ueki, K. Marukawa, M. Shimada, K. Nakagawa, and E. Yamamoto, "The assessment of blood loss in orthognathic surgery for prognathia," *Journal of Oral and Maxillofacial Surgery*, vol. 63, no. 3, pp. 350–354, 2005.

[10] Expert Working Group, "Guidelines for red blood cell and plasma transfusion for adults and children," *Canadian Medical Association Journal*, vol. 56, pp. 1–24, 1997.

[11] G. A. Nuttall, B. C. Brost, R. T. Connis et al., "Practice guidelines for perioperative blood transfusion and adjuvant therapies: an updated report by the American society of anesthesiologists task force on perioperative blood transfusion and adjuvant therapies," *Anesthesiology*, vol. 105, no. 1, pp. 198–208, 2006.

[12] M. F. Murphy, T. B. Wallington, P. Kelsey et al., "Guidelines for the clinical use of red cell transfusions," *British Journal of Haematology*, vol. 113, no. 1, pp. 24–31, 2001.

[13] J. C. Marshall, "Transfusion trigger: when to transfuse?" *Critical Care*, vol. 8, no. 2, pp. S31–S33, 2004.

[14] J. L. Carson, P. A. Carless, and P. C. Hébert, "Outcomes using lower vs higher hemoglobin thresholds for red blood cell transfusion," *Journal of the American Medical Association*, vol. 309, no. 1, pp. 83–84, 2013.

[15] D. E. Madsen, J. Ingerslev, J. J. Sidelmann, J. J. Thorn, and J. Gram, "Intraoperative blood loss during orthognathic surgery is predicted by thromboelastography," *Journal of Oral and Maxillofacial Surgery*, vol. 70, no. 10, pp. e547–e552, 2012.

[16] M. Fenner, P. Kessler, S. Holst, E. Nkenke, F. W. Neukam, and A. I. Holst, "Blood transfusion in bimaxillary orthognathic operations: need for testing of type and screen," *British Journal of Oral and Maxillofacial Surgery*, vol. 47, no. 8, pp. 612–615, 2009.

[17] H. Malik, H. Bishop, and J. Winstanley, "Audit of blood transfusion in elective breast cancer surgery—do we need to group and save pre-operatively?" *Annals of the Royal College of Surgeons of England*, vol. 90, no. 6, pp. 472–473, 2008.

[18] N. Eipe and M. Ponniah, "Perioperative blood loss assessment-how accurate?" *Indian Journal of Anaesthesia*, vol. 50, pp. 35–38, 2006.

[19] M. T. Hallissey, M. C. Crowson, R. S. Kiff, J. W. L. Fielding, and R. D. Kingston, "Blood transfusion: an overused resource in colorectal cancer surgery," *Annals of the Royal College of Surgeons of England*, vol. 74, no. 1, pp. 59–62, 1992.

[20] R. Cartotto, M. A. Musgrave, M. Beveridge, J. Fish, and M. Gomez, "Minimizing blood loss in burn surgery," *Journal of Trauma—Injury, Infection and Critical Care*, vol. 49, no. 6, pp. 1034–1039, 2000.

[21] J. T. Hardwicke, R. W. Jordan, and J. M. Skillman, "Infiltration of epinephrine in reduction mammaplasty: a systematic review of the literature," *Plastic and Reconstructive Surgery*, vol. 130, no. 4, pp. 773–778, 2012.

[22] A. O. Ogbemudia, A. Bafor, and L. West-Osemwengie, "Reactionary haemorrhage reduction with adrenaline infiltration in proximal tibial osteotomy: a randomized clinical study of safety and efficacy," *Archives of Orthopaedic and Trauma Surgery*, vol. 132, no. 1, pp. 21–24, 2012.

[23] "Practice strategies forelective red blood cell transfusion," *Annals of Internal Medicine*, vol. 116, no. 5, pp. 403–406, 1992.

[24] P. I. Tartter and D. M. Barron, "Unnecessary blood transfusions in elective colorectal cancer surgery," *Transfusion*, vol. 25, no. 2, pp. 113–115, 1985.

[25] D. R. Spahn and M. Casutt, "Eliminating blood transfusions: new aspects and perspectives," *Anesthesiology*, vol. 93, no. 1, pp. 242–255, 2000.

[26] H. J. Nielsen, "Detrimental effects of perioperative blood transfusion," *British Journal of Surgery*, vol. 82, no. 5, pp. 582–587, 1995.

[27] M. A. Popovsky, H. C. Chaplin Jr., and S. B. Moore, "Transfusion-related acute lung injury: a neglected, serious complication of hemotherapy," *Transfusion*, vol. 32, no. 6, pp. 589–592, 1992.

[28] D. Stainsby, H. Jones, D. Asher et al., "Serious hazards of transfusion: a decade of hemovigilance in the UK," *Transfusion Medicine Reviews*, vol. 20, no. 4, pp. 273–282, 2006.

[29] L. B. Seeff, F. B. Hollinger, H. J. Alter et al., "Long-term mortality and morbidity of transfusion-associated non-A, non-B, and type C hepatitis: a National Heart, Lung, and Blood Institute Collaborative Study," *Hepatology*, vol. 33, no. 2, pp. 455–463, 2001.

[30] A. Shander, A. Hofmann, S. Ozawa, O. M. Theusinger, H. Gombotz, and D. R. Spahn, "Activity-based costs of blood transfusions in surgical patients at four hospitals," *Transfusion*, vol. 50, no. 4, pp. 753–765, 2010.

[31] B. Mozes, M. Epstein, I. Ben-Bassat, B. Modan, and H. Halkin, "Evaluation of the appropriateness of blood and blood product transfusion using preset criteria," *Transfusion*, vol. 29, no. 6, pp. 473–476, 1989.

[32] E. C. Vamvakas and M. A. Blajchman, "Transfusion-related mortality: the ongoing risks of allogeneic blood transfusion and the available strategies for their prevention," *Blood*, vol. 113, no. 15, pp. 3406–3417, 2009.

[33] National Blood Authority Australia, "Patient blood management guidelines," http://www.nba.gov.au/guidelines/review.html.

[34] L. T. Goodnough and A. Shander, "Patient blood management," *Anesthesiology*, vol. 116, no. 6, pp. 1367–1376, 2012.

12

Motivational Differences between Whole Blood and Apheresis Donors in Quebec, Canada: A Questionnaire-Based Survey in a Voluntary Nonremunerated Context

Johanne Charbonneau, Marie-Soleil Cloutier, and Élianne Carrier

Research Chair of Social Aspect of Blood Donation, INRS-Centre Urbanisation Culture Société, 385 Sherbrooke Street East, Montreal, QC, Canada H2X 1E3

Correspondence should be addressed to Marie-Soleil Cloutier; marie-soleil.cloutier@ucs.inrs.ca

Academic Editor: Erwin Strasser

Background. Finding ways to recruit apheresis donors is crucial. The aim of this study was to provide a quantitative analysis of the motivations of regular plasma/platelets donors (PPDs) in comparison with those of regular whole blood donors (WBDs), in a voluntary and nonremunerated context. *Study Design and Methods.* Motives to donate blood and demographic characteristics were collected through questionnaires completed by 795 WBDs and 473 PPDs. Chi-square tests were completed to determine which motivations stand out across the two blood donor groups. *Results.* The motivator selected by the highest percentage was "my blood can save lives." Comparison of WBDs and PPDs showed that 12 out of 23 items were statistically significantly different from one group to another. *Conclusion.* The belief that helping others is in their nature is more prevalent among PPDs. In this sense, their profile is unique. Four other motivators distinguish this group from the WBDs: "I think there is a strong need for blood products," "it gives me a sense of pride," "I like to have goals," and "I receive telephone reminders." These motivators point to the role the ongoing support provided by blood collection agencies (BCAs) plays with PPDs.

1. Introduction

Finding effective ways to recruit blood donors is crucial for blood collection agencies (BCAs) given the rising demand for blood due to an aging population, strict donor deferral criteria, new therapeutic treatments, and the limited shelf life of blood products [1–3]. In addition, the demand for plasma-derived therapeutic products—particularly polyvalent intravenous immune globulin (IVIg)—is projected to increase in the future [4, 5]. However, apheresis components (plasma and platelets) are still procured from compensated donors in many high-income countries, such as Germany and the United States. This later country alone provides 55% of the world's supply of plasma derivatives [6]. As is the case in many countries, in the province of Quebec (Canada), the organization responsible for blood product supply, Héma-Québec, is attempting to increase its degree

of self-sufficiency by appealing to nonremunerated volunteer donors [7]. Demand for IVIg in Quebec has increased by 8.3% annually since 2003 [8]. In 2013-2014, the rate of IVIg self-sufficiency was 14.5%. There are currently only five fixed collection sites equipped for apheresis donation in the province, two of which opened recently (in 2013). According to the most recent annual report, Héma-Québec will open new permanent blood centers devoted to the collection of plasma for fractionation in the next few years [8]. There are also plans for a fractionation plant to open in 2019 [9].

In such a context, recruitment to the plasmapheresis panel becomes a crucial issue. Apheresis donation differs in many ways from whole blood donation. Whereas a whole blood donor may donate once every 56 days, a plasma donor may donate every 6 days and a platelet donor every 14 days. In addition, plasma and platelet donation processes last longer due to the return of saline and red blood cells (RBC) to the donor: a minimum of 45 minutes for plasmapheresis and up to three hours for plateletpheresis as compared to up to 15 minutes for whole blood donation.

Despite the obvious need to recruit more apheresis donors, there is very little literature on their motivations. The meta-analysis review produced by Bednall and Bove in 2011 [10] on self-reported motivators for donating blood showed that only seven samples out of 92 included plasma or platelet donors. With only a single exception, all of the studies reported in their analysis were conducted in countries where remuneration for plasmapheresis or plateletpheresis is available.

Analyses of apheresis donors have focused primarily on their socioeconomic profile [11, 12], the conversion process from whole blood donation to apheresis donation [13–17], barriers (deterrents) or reasons given for discontinuing the practice [18–21], and, of course, the motivations of such donors, which have sometimes been compared to those of whole blood donors [11–13, 22–29].

Of the original eleven studies on donor motivators we identified, five had been conducted in the United States and the others in Australia or Europe (Germany, Austria, Belgium, France, or The Netherlands). In the three studies in which donors were remunerated [11, 26, 28], payment was the chief motivator for donation. Of the eight remaining studies, only three compared the motivations of apheresis donors with those of whole blood donors [12, 22, 27]. Retained samples for the eight studies ranged in size from 9 [23] to 2028 participants [22]. Three of the studies focused on platelet donors and the others on plasma donors. As might be expected, in smaller surveys, researchers chose to study motivations via semistructured interviews. In other studies, focus groups or mixed methods approaches with open- and closed-ended questions were used. Some researchers focused on the reasons behind the first apheresis donation, while others also explored general motivations (or the benefits donors perceived [13]). The number of answer choices given to participants in the four questionnaire surveys [22, 26–28] was quite limited (4, 6, 9, and 12). Finally, the analyses often focused on the primary motivator. However, qualitative studies on smaller sample using open-ended questions have shown the practice of blood donation to be associated with numerous motivators [23, 25], including personality traits, social influences, ongoing support by blood center staff, and the sort of practical accommodations agencies are able to provide donors with [30]. Moreover, the relative importance of different motivators changes over a donor's career [31]. Aside from the transition from extrinsic to intrinsic motivations [32, 33], the motivational dynamic is also linked to different events over the course of the donor's life [30]. For example, practicalities become a priority when donors must balance their donation practice with more demanding family and professional commitments.

In the studies selected by Bednall and Bove [10] as well as in those we found, the motivators most frequently cited by plasma and platelet donors were prosocial, even though such motivators would appear to reflect concerns that are more collectivistic (duty, obligation, and solidarity) than individualistic (altruism) in nature. Some studies highlighted the importance of the interpersonal relationships developed with collection staff and other donors [12, 13, 23, 25]. Other motivators associated with the specific conditions of apheresis donation were noted: the ease of developing a routine (due to the possibility of making an appointment) and the ability to increase one's number of donations or develop a sense of belonging to a special group, a blood donation "elite," more rapidly. However, of the four studies that explored the range of apheresis donors' motivations in greater depth [13, 23–25], two made no comparisons with whole blood donors' motivations.

In short, studies discussed so far have numerous limitations. As noted by Bednall and Bove [10], few researchers have attempted to study apheresis donation in the context of volunteer nonremunerated donation. Samples have often been small, and few studies have compared the motivations of apheresis donors with those of regular whole blood donors. Analysis of motivations has itself often been limited in scope, due either to the restricted number of answer choices provided or to the researcher's decision to focus on the primary motivator. Bednall and Bove [10] also pointed out that most studies have focused on prosocial motivations and personal norms and shown little interest in social influences.

In response to these gaps in the literature, this study seeks to provide a thorough quantitative analysis of the motivations of apheresis donors (plasma/platelets) in comparison with regular whole blood donors, in the context of a voluntary and nonremunerated system.

2. Materials and Methods

2.1. Sample Selection. Sampling was done by accessing and extracting information from Héma-Québec's donor information system (Progesa, Mak System, Paris, France). Since 1987, this computerized database includes personal information on date of birth, sex, address of residence, dates of all previous donations, types of donations, previous and current deferrals, and screening test results for all donors. Two (a third group of lapsed donors were also recruited for this survey but were not used in the present analysis.) groups of donors were defined on the basis of their donation history: current whole blood donors (WBD) were those who had given two allogenic donations during their previous history and one donation during the 6 months preceding the survey, and plasma and platelets donors (PPDs) were those who had given three plasma or platelets donations during their previous history and one during the six months preceding the survey. Two other criteria were taken into account to extract a random sample of donors to whom the survey was sent: age (to be between 18 and 55 years at the time of the sample extraction) and sex (women were oversampled for PPD, since they are less often donors).

The initial targeted number of respondents was 750 subjects (50% men and 50% women): 500 regular WBDs and 250 regular PPDs. To achieve this target, 2000 WBDs were randomly selected from the database but the potential group of PPDs was smaller: the Progesa database contained 1968 donors who met our criteria (453 women and 1515 men). From this pool, all the women were selected and 547 men were randomly selected to achieve our target of 1000 mailed questionnaires. Participants' residential postal codes were used as geographical markers to ensure the sample's geographical representativeness. Sampling was conducted on March 25, 2014.

2.2. Questionnaire Development. Data were collected with a self-administered mailed questionnaire (see appendix). The survey was developed specifically for the study, which had a twofold topic: (1) motivators for blood donation and (2) the practical aspects of the blood donation experience. (When, where, and how long donors give blood; what forms of transportation they use; what activities precede or follow their visits to blood drives; what was the overall trajectory of their last visit; has their practice changed over the past few years and why; and diverse time pressure considerations.)

The first question concerned motivators for blood donation. Several sources were used in selecting and formulating the proposed answer choices (see Table 1). To begin with, our research team had completed four qualitative surveys of blood donors between 2009 and 2012 [30] (the methods used in the four surveys are presented in further detail in Charbonneau et al. [30]), conducting 136 interviews with WBDs and/or PPDs. We were inspired by the interdisciplinary perspective chosen by Piliavin and Callero [31] to study the career of blood donors. Our approach, incorporating sociological and psychological theories [34], sought to identify individual and social factors associated with the experience of giving blood. Although they had different objectives, all four surveys allowed for exploration of the reasons that had led donors to start their practice and to continue it, or not, over time. Respondents who remembered their first blood donation initially mentioned contextual elements that had contributed to it; those with long donor careers spoke of the circumstances that had enabled them to continue their practice. However, 85% of donors cited general motivations for their actions and always mentioned more than one. Although a respondent might say that a specific motivator was "the most important" (to meet the need for blood products, e.g.), later in the interview the same respondent would mention another "primary" motivator (e.g., the collection centre was close-by), when it came to mind in the course of the discussion. This multiplicity of motivators has been observed in other surveys [23, 25]; as suggested by Caillé [35], it lends itself to a combination of selfish reasons (egotism), selfless reasons (altruism and goodwill), and social obligations (social pressure), while always incorporating a number of institutional aspects (direct solicitation or ease of access to collection centers). Thus, in the present survey, respondents were given the opportunity to choose five answers out of 22 when asked about motives for donating blood. Furthermore, they were permitted to add their own reasons (the analysis of open-ended responses will be published later). They were not, however, asked to indicate a chief motive or to rate their answers.

In order to select answer choices for the present survey, we also reviewed the survey tools used by other researchers to study blood donation motivators, as well as of the results presented in 24 separate studies (see Table 1). Some statements— "someone close to me has received one or more blood transfusions in the past," "it is my civic duty/a way to help out the community," "I think there is a strong need for blood products"—have figured in a large number of studies. Others have been used less frequently—"I like to have goals (20, 50, 100, 200 donations, etc.)," "it is an activity that encourages you to monitor and take care of your health"—but were added because they tend to be cited more frequently in surveys with apheresis donors; this was also the case for "I join people that I know (donors, staff) at the blood drive."

The second part of the questionnaire was also written based on the results of our previous qualitative studies. We also consulted other studies on the same topics before making the final decision as to the choice of questions. Questions on demographic characteristics (age, sex, education level, employment status, marital status, number of children, country of origin, postal code, and blood type) were also included, but they will be the subject of further analysis and are therefore only briefly exposed here.

The first version of the questionnaires was submitted to a pretest, involving 16 donors in four focus groups. Each focus group was designed to target a specific population (2 WBD groups, 1 PPD group, and 1 lapsed blood donors' group) and conducted in a different setting (Downtown Montreal (2), Southern Montreal Suburb, and Quebec City).

Groups ranged in size from 3 to 6 participants (27 to 53 years old; 7 women, 9 men). During each focus group, participants were first asked to complete the questionnaire. Each participant's responses were then shared with the group and discussed at length, one question at a time. The average focus group took approximately 1.5 hours. Each participant was given 20 CAN$ at the end of the focus group as a token of appreciation.

After the last focus group, the research team revised the questionnaire based on the participants' criticisms, comments, and suggestions. For the question on motivations, out of the original 24 statements, 11 remained the same, seven were reformulated, two were partially truncated, four were grouped together into two, and one was eliminated, while two new answer choices were added.

The final version of the questionnaire consisted of 25 questions and took approximately 20 minutes to complete. Two separate questionnaires were produced: one for the WBDs and one for the PPDs, where subjects were asked if they would like to participate in a qualitative follow-up survey (data to be analysed later). The questionnaires were first developed in French and then translated in English.

2.3. Survey Procedures. An introductory letter signed by an executive officer at Héma-Québec was included in the mailing package, along with a letter explaining the study signed by the head researcher, the questionnaire, the consent form, and a prestamped return envelope. Questionnaires were anonymous (no individual identifiers retained) but return envelopes were supplied with a code, permitting the questionnaire to be tracked back to the original database.

TABLE 1: Question on motivators for donating blood.

Time use and blood donation questionnaire	References	Motivator categories (Bednall and Bove [10])
Question 1 "which of the following elements motivate you to donate blood?" (check off up to five answers)		
A blood drive is being held near where I live or near my workplace/place of study	[18, 40]	Convenience of collection site
		Prosocial motivation
My blood can save lives	[18, 41, 42]	Altruism
It is a positive thing to do and requires little effort	[12, 18, 25, 40, 43]	
It is my civic duty/a way to help out the community	[18, 24, 25, 31, 40, 42, 44, 45]	Collectivism (community)
I give thinking that a member of my family or a close friend could need blood someday	[18, 23, 27, 40, 46]	Collectivism (family and friends)
		Personal values
Helping other people is in my nature*	[18, 25, 44, 47]	Personal moral norms
My religious practice or convictions have encouraged me to donate	[18, 25]	Religiosity
I think there is a strong need for blood products	[12, 13, 18, 25, 40, 42, 45]	Perceived need for donation
		Indirect reciprocity
Someone close to me has received one or more blood transfusions in the past	[13, 18, 24, 25, 27, 40, 45]	Upstream
It gives me confidence that others will give if I need it later	[18, 23, 24, 40, 46]	Downstream
I like to have goals (20, 50, 100, 200 donations, etc.)**	[24]	Intrinsic motivation
It gives me a sense of pride	[18, 25, 27]	Self-esteem
		Marketing communication
I receive telephone reminders from Héma-Québec	[18, 25, 27]	Direct marketing
When I see posters and advertising	[18]	Advertising
I join people that I know (donors, staff) at the blood drive	[13, 19, 20, 23, 25]	Blood drives
		Incentives
It is an activity that encourages you to monitor and take care of your health	[13]	Perceived health benefits
It gives me energy in the following days	[12, 18, 42]	
I have a rare and sought-after blood type	[40, 44, 48]	Learn blood type
I feel recognition from people around me ***	[13, 18, 25]	Recognition
		Social norms
Blood donation is a tradition in my family	[13, 18, 23, 25, 46]	Descriptive norm
My coworkers also give blood	[46]	
I like to be accompanied	[23]	Subjective norm
Another reason (specify):		

* Also: intrinsic motivation (indirect reciprocity).
** Also: recognition (incentives).
*** Also: subjective norm (social norm).

The research ethics committees of the local university and Héma-Québec approved the study. Questionnaires were mailed based on language preference information in the donor information system (French = 6562 and English = 436). The initial questionnaire mail-out began on April 25, 2014. There were two successive waves in total (1000 PPD questionnaires mailed in May; 2000 WBD questionnaires mailed in July-August). We received the last completed questionnaire on January 28, 2015.

To avoid the possibility of analysis results being skewed due to the 22 answer choices to the motivation question being consistently presented in the same order, three versions of the questionnaire with different answer choice orders were produced and mailed out, with each version going to one-third of the two groups (WBD and PPD).

Of the 3000 questionnaires dispatched, 1361 were returned fully or partially completed. Forty-three (43) questionnaires were also returned owing to incorrect addresses, or because recipients had moved or were deceased. Ninety-three (93) questionnaires were eliminated from our analysis because they were returned without the consent form or had too much missing data. The response rate was 40% for the WBD group and 48% for the PPD group. As has been found elsewhere [36, 37], response rates were higher among women, especially for WBDs (46% versus 34% for men). Older donors (50–56 years old) had the highest response rates (11% for WBDs and 15% for PPDs) while the 30- to 39-year-old group had the lowest response rates both for WBDs (8%) and PPDs (9%), although differences with other age groups were small. Analyses of motivations were performed using 1268 admissible questionnaires (795 WBDs and 473 PPDs).

2.4. Statements' Classification and Statistical Analysis. For the purpose of this analysis, we classified the motivations' statements in the categories identified by Bednall and Bove in their meta-analysis [10] (see Table 1). These authors developed a taxonomy based on established terminology from both psychology [38] and marketing [39] literature. Sixteen out of 22 items from our questionnaire were easily classified in this taxonomy because our statement was referring to the same definition or example shown in Bednall and Bove's list. Three items fell under more than one category. For example, "helping other people is in my nature" could be classified as both a prosocial (altruistic) motivator and an intrinsic motivator. Likewise, "I like to have goals"—an item that, although not specifically mentioned in the list of Bednall and Bove [10], is more frequently cited by apheresis donors—may be interpreted as an intrinsic motivator that may be highly influenced by the recognition mechanisms established by BCAs. "I feel recognition from people around me" may belong as much in the social norms category, if friends and family members, as in the incentives category, express such recognition if it comes from BCAs instead. Three other answer choices were difficult to classify under the categories proposed by Bednall and Bove [10]. Saying that donating blood "is an activity that encourages monitoring and taking care of your health" does not entirely coincide with the notion of perceived health benefits. Also, while giving blood "is

a positive thing to do and requires little effort" may be considered an altruistic motivator, the idea of a low cost charitable act also reveals a slightly egotistical nature. In the first version of the questionnaire, two separate statements were proposed, but the focus groups' participants suggested grouping them together. Finally, giving blood because the donor knows that "I have a rare and sought-after blood type" also lends itself to multiple interpretations (pride, a sense of obligation, and a need for recognition). This particular answer choice was not included in the Bednall and Bove [10] list, which instead contained "to learn my blood type," a reflection of the fact that their meta-analysis also included studies on motivators for first donations. For the purpose of this analysis, each item was classified into only one category (which is shown in Table 1).

Data entry on ACCESS began in July 2014, alternating with mail-out of the final wave of questionnaires. Descriptive statistics were carried out for each question and demographic variable. Next, Chi-Two tests were completed to determine which motivations stood out across the three groups. Analyses were performed with SAS version 9.4.

3. Results

The final sample had more women in the WBD (58% women) but proportions of women and men were equivalent in the PPD group, as we had oversampled women (Table 2). Age groups were similar for WBDs and PPDs, with 25% of respondents belonging to the 18- to 29-year-old category, respectively, 22% and 19% of WBD and PPD respondents belonging to the 30- to 39-year-old category, almost a quarter of respondents to the 40- to 49-year-old (23% for WBDs and 25% for PPDs) a third to the 50- to 56-year-old age groups (30% for WBDs and 32% for PPDs). In terms of education and marital status, both groups were well educated (between 36% and 40% of respondents had university degrees) and the majority of respondents were married (63% and 64%). WBD respondents came mostly from Montreal (39% against 22% for PPDs) and elsewhere in Quebec (43% against 19% for PPDs). In part due to the small number of collection sites in the province, most PPDs came from the Quebec City region (59%). Only the gender and the region of origin variables were statistically different between the two groups.

Table 3 presents the proportion of respondents in the whole sample and the two subsamples (WBDs and PPDs) that selected each of the motivators. The motivator indicated by the highest percentage was "my blood can save lives," with 81% of all respondents having included this motivation in their list and more WBDs (83%) than PPDs (77%). Comparison of WBDs and PPDs according to their reported motivators shows that results for 12 motivators were statistically significantly different from one group to another.

A greater proportion of WBDs selected "it is a positive thing to do and requires little effort" (62%), "I give thinking that a member of my family or a close friend could need blood someday" (47%), and "a blood drive is being held near where I live or near my workplace/place of study" (34%) as significant motivators. Three other motivators were more often cited by

TABLE 2: Proportions of WBD and PPD respondents for each sociodemographic variable.

	Total n = 1268	%	WBDs n = 795	%	PPDs n = 473	%	Sign. (p)
Women	696	55	458	58	238	50	p < 0,05
Men	572	45	337	42	235	50	
18–29 years	317	25	200	25	117	25	
30–39 years	265	21	176	22	89	19	n.s.
40–49 years	300	24	182	23	118	25	
50–56 years	386	30	237	30	149	31	
Elementary/High School	295	23	199	25	96	20	
CÉGEP	498	39	311	39	187	40	n.s.
University	473	37	283	36	190	40	
Single	363	29	218	28	145	31	
Married, common law	804	64	506	65	298	63	n.s.
Divorced, separated, widowed	81	7	51	7	30	6	
Respondent from the Quebec City region	419	33	141	18	278	59	
Respondent from the Montreal region	416	33	311	39	105	22	p < 0,0001
Respondent from another region	433	34	343	43	90	19	

TABLE 3: Proportions of WBD and PPD respondents for each selected motivators.

Motivators	All donors (n = 1268)	WBDs (n = 795)	PPDs (n = 473)	P
My blood can save lives	81%	83%	77%	<0,05
It's a positive thing to do and requires little effort	58%	62%	52%	<0,001
Helping other people is in my nature	53%	49%	61%	<0,0001
I give thinking that a member of my family or a close friend could need blood someday	44%	47%	40%	<0,05
I think there is a strong need for blood products	41%	38%	47%	<0,01
It gives me a sense of pride	38%	33%	45%	<0,0001
It's my civic duty/a way to help out the community	31%	32%	28%	NS
A blood drive is being held near where I live or near my workplace/place of study	24%	34%	8%	<0,0001
I receive telephone reminders from Héma-Québec	22%	18%	28%	<0,0001
I like to have goals (20, 50, 100, 200 donations, etc.)	17%	13%	23%	<0,0001
I have a rare and sought-after blood type	16%	17%	14%	NS
Someone close to me has received one or more blood transfusions in the past	16%	16%	16%	NS
It gives me confidence that others will give if I need it later	11%	12%	11%	NS
It's an activity that encourages you to monitor and take care of your health	8%	8%	9%	NS
Other reason	7%	6%	8%	NS
I feel recognition from people around me	6%	6%	7%	NS
Blood donation is a tradition in my family	6%	6%	6%	NS
It gives me energy in the following days	4%	5%	3%	<0,05
When I see posters and advertising	4%	5%	1%	<0,0001
My coworkers also give blood	2%	2%	1%	<0,05
I join people that I know (donors, staff) at the blood drive	2%	1%	2%	NS
My religious practice or convictions have encouraged me to donate	1%	1%	1%	NS
I like to be accompanied	0%	1%	0%	NS

TABLE 4: Proportions of WBD and PPD respondents for each of Bednall and Bove's motivator categories [10].

Motivator categories*	All donors (n = 1268)	WBDs (n = 795)	PPDs (n = 473)	p from Chi-Two
Convenience of collection sites	24%	34%	8%	<0,0001
Prosocial motivation	97%	97%	97%	NS
Personal values	54%	50%	61%	<0,0001
Perceived need for donation	41%	38%	47%	<0,01
Indirect reciprocity	60%	56%	67%	<0,0001
Marketing communication	25%	22%	30%	<0,01
Incentives	31%	31%	29%	NS
Social norms	15%	15%	14%	NS

*See Table 1 for the list of motivators in each category.

WBDs compared to PPDs, despite a lower proportion overall: "it gives me energy the following days" (5%), "when I see posters and advertising" (5%), and "my coworkers also give blood" (2%).

PPDs reported several motivators in greater proportions to WBDs. The highest proportion of PPD respondents was for the "Helping other people is in my nature" (61%) motivator. Almost half of them stated that "I think there is a strong need for blood products" (47%) and "it gives me a sense of pride" (45%) were important motivators. Finally, PPDs choose "I receive telephone reminders from Héma-Québec" (28%) and "I like to have goals" (23%) in greater proportions than WBDs.

Table 4 presents the proportion of respondents for each of Bednall and Bove [10] motivator categories. These categories combine all the motivators shown in Table 2. The category with the highest percentage is the "prosocial motivation" with 97% of both WBD and PPD respondents having selected at least one motivation in this category. The comparison of WBDs and PPDs according to their reported proportions of motivators in each category shows that results were statistically significantly different for five categories, four of them having higher proportions for PPDs. The only category where WBDs rated motivators in greater proportions is the "convenience of collection site" (34% against only 8% for PPDs). Approximately two-thirds of PPD respondents chose motivators in the "personal values" (61%) and "indirect reciprocity" (67%) categories, the highest proportions for both categories as compared to the WBDs (resp., 50% and 56%). Two other categories were higher for PPDs: the "perceived need for donation" (47%) and the "marketing communication" motivators (30%).

4. Discussion

Despite the growing demand for plasma-derived therapeutic products and several countries' desire to reduce their dependency on imported products, little research has been conducted to date on the behaviour of apheresis donors. This study sought to provide an analysis of the motivations of apheresis donors (plasma/platelets) in comparison with regular whole blood donors, in the context of a voluntary and nonremunerated system.

The results confirm those of other researchers who have highlighted the importance of prosocial motivations for blood donors. The greatest number of respondents, regardless of donor type, chose the altruistic motivation of "my blood can save lives." Previous studies [22–25, 41, 42] have mentioned the importance of this motivation in blood donors. Although this formulation is not the one most commonly used in questionnaires for measuring prosocial altruistic motivation, it tends to be employed spontaneously by donors when answering open questions and in interview surveys [22, 23, 25, 30]. It also highlights the role of BCAs, which have long used it as a catchy promotional slogan. Whether given simply by reflex or because it is considered a socially desirable answer [10, 31], this response, which is strongly inspired and encouraged by the BCAs themselves, clearly promotes the utilitarian aspect of blood which does in fact save lives, in a very concrete fashion [30, 49].

If one applies the categories proposed by Bednall and Bove [10], one notes that almost all respondents (97%) mentioned one "prosocial motivation" or another. Motivations associated with "indirect reciprocity" were selected by the second highest percentage of respondents (60%). Donors were motivated to choose this category primarily due to someone close to them having received a transfusion. "Personal values" ("helping others is in my nature") was the last category selected by more than 50% of respondents.

4.1. Different Motivations by Donor Type. The five answers selected by the highest percentages of respondents show that WBDs and PPDs are associated with different motivator groupings. Using the categories proposed by Bednall and Bove [10], we observe that for the two donor types the reasons for donating blood combine prosocial motivations, personal values, and the perception of need. But PPDs exhibit a greater range of motivators, encompassing indirect reciprocity in their grouping. Differences between the two profiles are also readily apparent when we analyze several of the possible motivators.

The second most popular motivator among WBDs is the belief that giving blood "is a positive thing to do and requires little effort." Considering blood donation to be a positive gesture is also a prosocial altruistic motivation. However, the second part of the sentence lends itself to multiple interpretations. Given the fact that a very small proportion of the population gives blood, stating that donating blood is an act that requires very little effort may be a way of contradicting all those who cite numerous reasons for never giving blood. Further, from the perspective of an interpretation inspired by the sociology of gift-giving [50, 51], denying the effort demanded by this gesture is an expected reflex in the giving cycle, as it neutralizes the donor's sense of superiority towards the donation's recipient. However, emphasizing how little effort is required may also be interpreted as a reference to other types of charitable activities that call for a much more intensive form of commitment. From this perspective, blood donation suddenly seems to be a means of giving oneself a clear conscience "at little cost" to oneself [30]. Giving blood—which could take no more than fifteen minutes—once a year because a drive is held at one's workplace or place of study may be considered a fairly simple form of community service. However, our analysis reveals that a large proportion of apheresis donors also chose this statement, even though their practice is far more demanding in terms of frequency, distance traveled, and length of procedure [13].

Among PPDs, the second most popular motivator is the belief that "helping others is in my nature." In their comparison of WBDs and plasma donors, Veldhuizen and van Dongen [27] suggested that "different donor profiles for whole blood and plasma donors already exist before the very first donation experience" (p. 1684). They observed that cognitive attitude was a better predictor of intention in future plasma donors than in WBDs and that "even before the first donation experience, future plasma donors were more motivated, felt more able to donate, and also expressed more positive attitudes toward donating blood" (p. 1683). In short, our results are in line with previous observations that suggest that PPDs are more "driven by self" [13, 24].

Four other motivators distinguish PPDs from WBDs: "I think there is a strong need for blood products," "It gives me a sense of pride," "I like to have goals," and "I receive telephone reminders from Héma-Québec." These motivators point to the role BCAs' ongoing support plays with PPDs. Staff members are the ones who let donors know that there is a strong need for plasma, that the act of donating plasma or platelets is rare, and also that these donors may feel being part of an elite [13, 25]. Blood collections have all, in their own way, developed recognition programs for major donors, which permit PPDs to enjoy high visibility, especially when they reach specific donation targets (100, 200, 500, etc.) Special gifts may mark the most memorable moments [52]. BCAs have also developed services that phone donors to remind them when the prescribed period between two donations is almost up, and to appeal directly to certain donors for targeted types of donations; many PPDs count on these reminders. These motivators call to mind Healy's assertion that "blood can be seen not as something that individuals donate but as something that organizations collect" [53, p.71]. These observations would tend to encourage the adoption of a sociological institutionalist approach [54–57], with its proposal that the institutional context gives rise to the conditions surrounding the practice of blood donation, as well

as the rhetoric of altruistic donation, and that organizations contribute to defining a set of available and widely accepted reasons for donation, among which donors are able to pick and choose.

However, one could make the equally strong argument that BCAs' strategies are effective with a specific population that is particularly receptive to their messages, as is reflected in the previously cited results of Veldhuizen and van Dongen [27]. The results of their study suggest that plasma donors appear to be more conscientious than WBDs, having a personality-type generally characterized by the aim for achievement. The particular importance of indirect reciprocity for PPDs ("it gives me a sense of pride," "I like to have goals") also underscores the unique nature of a blood donation practice that is far more demanding than whole blood donation. When the personal cost is high, beliefs in personal benefits are more important for promoting actions [15, 44]. In short, donors who engage in this type of donation practice seem driven more by benevolence than by altruism [58].

What may be most surprising about our results is the low score the statement "I join people that I know (donors, staff) at the blood drive" obtained with the PPD group, as previous studies have emphasized the fact that such donors especially appreciate the possibility of developing personal bonds with collection staff and other donors who are present at the same time as them [13, 23, 25]. The low score may be due to the formulation of the statement chosen to express this phenomenon.

4.2. Recommendations. Some suggestions for recruiting and retaining plasma/platelet donors may be developed from these results. As we have observed, BCAs play a key role in supporting PPDs practices. In recent decades, there have been numerous studies in the field of behavioural psychology to determine the psychosocial factors that prompt individuals to develop a blood donation practice and maintain it over the long term [34]. Much less attention has been given to the influence of broader factors influencing blood donation, including the BCAs role [54]. First of all, collection staff is certainly in the best position to identify WBDs who display those characteristics most likely to promote conversion to apheresis donation, especially those individuals who seem interested in rapidly increasing their number of blood donations and who show considerable pride in reaching specific targets. Except for Schneider et al.'s [24], no study has so far pointed out the importance of achieving goals for PPDs.

Collection staff should also be strongly encouraged to spread information on apheresis donation, for example, by reminding people of the fact that the need is likely to grow while the country is far from self-sufficient as it is. As Kalargirou et al. [49] pointed out, this is not usually the strategy chosen by BCAs, which prefer focusing on altruism. Reminding PPDs that the organization is proud of them and that there are fewer apheresis donors than WBDs, making them truly special people, should also encourage donors. It is thus very important that recognition programs be maintained for this type of donor.

For its part, whole blood donation certainly benefits from the fact that it can be offered at mobile drives located as near as possible to donors' daily activities, which makes it a positive gesture that requires little effort. With attention given to the planning and development of new fixed centers for plasma, BCAs may be tempted to reduce the number of mobile drive locations. Some donors could then discontinue their practice if they are no longer able to find a place where they can give blood in their immediate environment.

4.3. Limitations. Our data have some limitations that must be discussed. First, our study was conducted on a sample of blood donors in Quebec, Canada, who may differ from blood donors in other countries. Moreover, we chose to restrict our study to donors between the ages of 18 and 55 years. The survey also tries to better understand the integration of blood donation into daily life and especially any barriers to the practice and reasons for its discontinuation among women in their thirties and forties: this is why our sample is age-specific. In addition, a complementary study using semistructured interviews was conducted to better understand the motivations and blood donation practice of PPDs; this second study involved an older population (up to 70 years of age) and results are to be published later. One should keep this possible bias in mind when discussing our data.

We should also point out the fact that we decided to place plasma and platelet donors together in the same group. While the growing need for blood products primarily concerns plasma derivatives, we believe that plasma and platelet donation practices and motivations are sufficiently similar for these two types of donors to be grouped together. Indeed, we know that donors increasingly make both plasma and platelet donations. It should also be noted that this grouping helped increase the number of potential respondents in our survey.

Our results were also constrained by the fact that motivations were self-reported, which may have biased results in favour of socially desirable answers [10, 13, 31]. Another of our study's limitation is that we did not specifically explore the motivations for first donations as other studies have done. This was because our previous studies [30] had demonstrated the difficulty of collecting reliable information on this topic when the first donation was several years prior, but it may account for why motivations associated with donors' social context—in particular, the influence of family—are less prominent in our results. We should also mention the nonstandard formulation of the statements chosen to represent the different motivators, which makes comparison of our results with those of other studies in the same domain somewhat difficult. Finally, we must remind the difficulty we had to classify some statements in the taxonomy of Bednall and Bove. Our results are directly influenced by the choices of classification we made.

5. Conclusion

At a time when numerous countries are seeking to develop increased self-sufficiency in plasma-derived products, it is extremely important to acquire a better understanding of the motivations of apheresis blood donors, especially in a context of voluntary nonremunerated context. Previous studies presented a detailed analysis of motivations for a small number of donors, or an analysis of motivations for a large number of donors, but only offering a very limited answer choice list. Our analysis is the first to combine a wide selection of blood donation motivators with a quantitative approach, therefore enabling the comparison of a large number of WBDs (795) and PPDs (473). Moreover, our survey permitted us to produce one of the very rare comparisons of WBDs, and PPDs in the domain. The decision not to have donors prioritize a single motivation permitted us to obtain a better understanding of the blend of motivators [30] that cause individual donors to give blood. These results offer points for BCAs to ponder in developing new blood donor recruiting and retention strategies.

Conflict of Interests

The authors declare that they have no conflict of interests relevant to the publication of this paper.

References

[1] S. A. Ali, *Beliefs about the effect of using blood donation payments: survey results from Norway [M.S. thesis]*, Department of Health Economics and Health Management, The Faculty of Medicine, Universitetet I Oslo, Oslo, Norway, 2013.

[2] M. C. Carter, J. Wilson, G. S. Redpath, P. Hayes, and C. Mitchell, "Donor recruitment in the 21st century: challenges and lessons learned in the first decade," *Transfusion and Apheresis Science*, vol. 45, no. 1, pp. 31–43, 2011.

[3] A. Drackley, K. B. Newbold, A. Paez, and N. Heddle, "Forecasting Ontario's blood supply and demand," *Transfusion*, vol. 52, no. 2, pp. 366–374, 2012.

[4] B. O. Mahony and A. Turner, "The Dublin Consensus Statement on vital issues relating to the collection of blood and plasma and the manufacture of plasma products," *Vox Sanguinis*, vol. 98, no. 3, part 2, pp. 447–450, 2010.

[5] P. Robert, "Global plasma demand in 2015," *Pharmaceuticals, Policy and Law*, vol. 11, no. 4, pp. 359–367, 2015.

[6] A. Farrugia, J. Penrod, and J. M. Bult, "Payment, compensation and replacement—the ethics and motivation of blood and plasma donation," *Vox Sanguinis*, vol. 99, no. 3, pp. 202–211, 2010.

[7] WHO Expert Group, "Expert consensus statement on achieving self-sufficiency in safe blood and blood products, based on voluntary non-remunerated blood donation (VNRBD)," *Vox Sanguinis*, vol. 103, no. 4, pp. 337–342, 2012.

[8] Héma-Québec, *Rapport annuel 2013-2014*, 2014.

[9] A. Dubuc, *Green Cross construira une usine de 200 millions au Québec*, La Presse, Montréal, Canada, 2014.

[10] T. C. Bednall and L. L. Bove, "Donating blood: a meta-analytic review of self-reported motivators and deterrents," *Transfusion Medicine Reviews*, vol. 25, no. 4, pp. 317–334, 2011.

[11] L. Anderson, K. Newell, and J. Kilcoyne, "'Selling blood': characteristics and motivations of student plasma donors," *Sociological Spectrum*, vol. 19, no. 2, pp. 137–162, 1999.

[12] C. J. Julius and S. R. Sytsma, "Comparison of demographics and motivations of highly committed whole blood and platelet donors," *Journal of Clinical Apheresis*, vol. 8, no. 2, pp. 82–88, 1993.

[13] L. L. Bove, T. Bednall, B. Masser, and M. Buzza, "Understanding the plasmapheresis donor in a voluntary, nonremunerated environment," *Transfusion*, vol. 51, no. 11, pp. 2411–2424, 2011.

[14] G. Godin and M. Germain, "Predicting first lifetime plasma donation among whole blood donors," *Transfusion*, vol. 53, supplement 5, pp. 157S–161S, 2013.

[15] G. Godin and M. Germain, "How to motivate whole blood donors to become plasma donors," *Journal of Blood Transfusion*, vol. 2014, Article ID 752182, 6 pages, 2014.

[16] M. Kuriyan and S. Wells, "Matching blood donations to type-specific product needs: a recruitment technique," *Journal of Clinical Apheresis*, vol. 10, no. 1, pp. 23–26, 1995.

[17] K. L. Bagot, B. M. Masser, K. M. White, and L. C. Starfelt, "Recruiting and retaining plasmapheresis donors: a critical belief analysis," *Transfusion and Apheresis Science*, vol. 52, no. 3, pp. 350–357, 2015.

[18] K. L. Bagot, L. L. Bove, B. M. Masser, T. C. Bednall, and M. Buzza, "Perceived deterrents to being a plasmapheresis donor in a voluntary, nonremunerated environment," *Transfusion*, vol. 53, no. 5, pp. 1108–1119, 2013.

[19] A. Pagliariccio, G. Guermandi, M. Marinozzi, and M. Piani, "Can better information increase hemapheresis?" *Transfusion and Apheresis Science*, vol. 28, no. 2, pp. 149–153, 2003.

[20] J. Ringwald, N. Lange, C. Rabe et al., "Why do some apheresis donors donate blood just once?" *Vox Sanguinis*, vol. 93, no. 4, pp. 354–362, 2007.

[21] S. Yuan, A. Ziman, B. Smeltzer, Q. Lu, and D. Goldfinger, "Moderate and severe adverse events associated with apheresis donations: incidences and risk factors," *Transfusion*, vol. 50, no. 2, pp. 478–486, 2010.

[22] S. A. Glynn, J. W. Smith, G. B. Schreiber et al., "Repeat whole-blood and plateletpheresis donors: unreported deferrable risks, reactive screening tests, and response to incentive programs," *Transfusion*, vol. 41, no. 6, pp. 736–743, 2001.

[23] A. Henrion, *L'Énigme du Don de Sang. Approche Ethnographique d'un Don entre Inconnus*, Faculté de Philosophie et Lettres, Université de Liège, Liège, Belgium, 2003.

[24] T. Schneider, O. Fontaine, and J. J. Huart, "Ethiques, motivations des donneurs d'aphérèse plasmatique," *Transfusion Clinique et Biologique*, vol. 11, no. 3, pp. 146–152, 2004.

[25] L. S. Szymanski, B. Cushna, B. C. H. Jackson, and I. O. Szymanski, "Motivation of plateletpheresis donors," *Transfusion*, vol. 18, no. 1, pp. 64–68, 1978.

[26] M. Trimmel, H. Lattacher, and M. Janda, "Voluntary whole-blood donors, and compensated platelet donors and plasma donors: motivation to donate, altruism and aggression," *Transfusion and Apheresis Science*, vol. 33, no. 2, pp. 147–155, 2005.

[27] I. Veldhuizen and A. van Dongen, "Motivational differences between whole blood and plasma donors already exist before their first donation experience," *Transfusion*, vol. 53, no. 8, pp. 1678–1686, 2013.

[28] C. Weidmann and H. Kluter, "Blood collection and donor motivation in Germany," *ISBT Science Series*, vol. 8, no. 1, pp. 238–241, 2013.

[29] J. F. Cataldo, E. Cohen, and J. B. Morganti, "Motivation of voluntary plasmapheresis donors," *Transfusion*, vol. 16, no. 4, pp. 375–379, 1976.

[30] J. Charbonneau, M. Cloutier, A. Quéniart, and N. Tran, *Le don de sang: un geste social et culturel*, P.U.L. Santé et Société, 2015.

[31] J. A. Piliavin and P. L. Callero, *Giving Blood: The Development of an Altruistic Identity*, Johns Hopkins University Press, Baltimore, Md, USA, 1991.

[32] E. L. Deci and R. M. Ryan, *Intrinsic Motivation and Self-Determination in Human Behavior*, Plenum, New York, NY, USA, 1985.

[33] L. Goette, A. Stutzer, and B. M. Frey, "Prosocial motivation and blood donations: a survey of the empirical literature," *Transfusion Medicine and Hemotherapy*, vol. 37, no. 3, pp. 149–154, 2010.

[34] J. Charbonneau, *Approches psychologiques et sociologiques du don de sang*, Institut National de la Recherche Scientifique, Montreal, Canada, 2014.

[35] A. Caillé, *Anthropologie du Don. Le Tiers Paradigme*, Desclée de Brouwer, Paris, France, 2000.

[36] D. L. Moore and J. Tarnai, "Evaluating nonresponse error in mail surveys," in *Survey Nonresponse*, R. M. Groves, D. A. Dillman, J. L. Eltinge, and R. J. A. Little, Eds., pp. 197–211, John Wiley & Sons, New York, NY, USA, 2002.

[37] R. Curtin, S. Presser, and E. Singer, "The effects of response rate changes on the index of consumer sentiment," *Public Opinion Quarterly*, vol. 64, no. 4, pp. 413–428, 2000.

[38] L. G. Tuleya, *Thesaurus of Psychological Index Terms*, American Psychological Association, Washington, DC, USA, 2007.

[39] P. Kotler, L. Brown, S. Adam, and G. Armstrong, *Marketing*, Pearson Education, Frenchs Forest, Australia, 2004.

[40] J. Kuruvatti, V. Prasad, R. Williams, M. A. Harrison, and R. P. O. Jones, "Motivations for donating blood and reasons why people lapse or never donate in Leeds, England: a 2001 questionnaire-based survey," *Vox Sanguinis*, vol. 101, no. 4, pp. 333–338, 2011.

[41] A. Fernández-Montoya, "Altruism and payment in blood donation," *Transfusion Science*, vol. 18, no. 3, pp. 379–386, 1997.

[42] B. H. Shaz and C. D. Hillyer, "Minority donation in the United States: challenges and needs," *Current Opinion in Hematology*, vol. 17, no. 6, pp. 544–549, 2010.

[43] A. H. Misje, V. Bosnes, O. Gåsdal, and H. E. Heier, "Motivation, recruitment and retention of voluntary non-remunerated blood donors: a survey-based questionnaire study," *Vox Sanguinis*, vol. 89, no. 4, pp. 236–244, 2005.

[44] M. E. Hupfer, "Helping me, helping you: self-referencing and gender roles in donor advertising," *Transfusion*, vol. 46, no. 6, pp. 996–1005, 2006.

[45] S. Yuan, M. Hoffman, Q. Lu, D. Goldfinger, and A. Ziman, "Motivating factors and deterrents for blood donation among donors at a university campus-based collection center," *Transfusion*, vol. 51, no. 11, pp. 2438–2444, 2011.

[46] N. Zaller, *To Donate or Not to Donate: An Analysis of Blood Donors and Blood Donation Knowledge, Attitudes and Practices in Northwestern China*, Johns Hopkins University, Baltimore, Md, USA, 2004.

[47] B. M. Masser, K. M. White, M. K. Hyde, and D. J. Terry, "The psychology of blood donation: current research and future directions," *Transfusion Medicine Reviews*, vol. 22, no. 3, pp. 215–233, 2008.

[48] M. Harrington, M. R. Sweeney, K. Bailie et al., "What would encourage blood donation in Ireland?" *Vox Sanguinis*, vol. 92, no. 4, pp. 361–367, 2007.

[49] A. A. Kalargirou, A. I. Beloukas, A. G. Kosma, C. I. Nanou, M. I. Saridi, and A. G. Kriebardis, "Attitudes and behaviours of

Greeks concerning blood donation: recruitment and retention campaigns should be focused on need rather than altruism," *Blood Transfusion*, vol. 12, no. 3, pp. 320–329, 2014.

[50] J. Godbout and A. Caillé, *L'Esprit du Don*, La Découverte, Paris, France, 1992.

[51] M. Mauss, *Essai sur le don: forme et raison de l'échange dans les sociétés archaïques 1923-1924*, Les Presses Universitaires de France, Paris, France, 2004.

[52] J. Charbonneau and A. Quéniart, "The influence of blood collection organizations on blood donation motivations and practices," in *Giving Blood: The Institutional Making of Altruism*, J. Charbonneau and A. Smith, Eds., Routledge, London, UK, 2016.

[53] K. Healy, "Embedded altruism: blood collection regimes and the European union's donor population," *American Journal of Sociology*, vol. 105, no. 6, pp. 1633–1657, 2000.

[54] J. Charbonneau and A. Smith, Eds., *Giving Blood: The Institutional Making of Altruism*, Routledge, London, UK, 2016.

[55] P. J. DiMaggio and W. W. Powell, "The iron cage revisited: institutional isomorphism and collective rationality in organizational fields," *American Sociological Review*, vol. 48, no. 2, pp. 147–160, 1983.

[56] J. W. Meyer and B. Rowan, "Institutionalized organizations: formal structure as myth and ceremony," *The American Journal of Sociology*, vol. 83, no. 2, pp. 340–363, 1977.

[57] W. R. Scott and J. Meyer, "The organization of societal sectors," in *Organizational Environments: Ritual and Rationality*, J. Meyer and W. R. Scott, Eds., Sage Publications, Beverly Hills, Calif, USA, 1983.

[58] E. Ferguson, K. Farrell, and C. Lawrence, "Blood donation is an act of benevolence rather than altruism," *Health Psychology*, vol. 27, no. 3, pp. 327–336, 2008.

13

Estimating the Risk of ABO Hemolytic Disease of the Newborn in Lagos

Alani Sulaimon Akanmu, Olufemi Abiola Oyedeji,
Titilope Adenike Adeyemo, and Ann Abiola Ogbenna

Department of Hematology & Blood Transfusion, Faculty of Clinical Sciences, College of Medicine, University of Lagos,
PMB 12003, Lagos, Nigeria

Correspondence should be addressed to Olufemi Abiola Oyedeji; drfemoyedeji@yahoo.com

Academic Editor: Silvano Wendel

Background. ABO hemolytic disease of the newborn is the most common hemolytic consequence of maternofetal blood group incompatibility restricted mostly to non-group-O babies of group O mothers with immune anti-A or anti-B antibodies. *Aim.* We estimated the risk of ABO HDN with view to determining need for routine screening for ABO incompatibility between mother and fetus. *Materials and Methods.* Prevalence of ABO blood group phenotypes in blood donors at the donor clinic of the Lagos University Teaching Hospital and arithmetic methods were used to determine population prevalence of ABO genes. We then estimated proportion of pregnancies of group O mothers carrying a non-group-O baby and the risk that maternofetal ABO incompatibility will cause clinical ABO HDN. *Results.* Blood from 9138 donors was ABO typed. 54.3%, 23%, 19.4%, and 3.3% were blood groups O, A, B, and AB, respectively. Calculated gene frequencies were 0.1416, 0.1209, and 0.7375 for A, B, and O genes, respectively. It was estimated that 14.3% of deliveries will result in a blood group O woman giving birth to a child who is non-group-O. Approximately 4.3% of deliveries are likely to suffer ABO HDN with 2.7% prone to suffer from moderately severe to severe hemolysis.

1. Introduction

ABO hemolytic disease of the newborn (ABO HDN) is the most common maternofetal blood group incompatibility. Unlike the rhesus disease, it is usually a problem of the neonate rather than the fetus. ABO HDN is restricted almost entirely to group A or B babies born to group O mothers with immune anti-A or anti-B antibodies.

ABO HDN is caused by IgG (immune) maternal antibodies which have the ability to cross the placental barrier. A high titre of these immune antibodies may not present with adverse effects in utero as A and B antigens are present on cells of all other tissues and body fluid and not only on red cells. The presence of these antigens helps to protect the incompatible fetal red cells by neutralizing the transferred maternal antibody with small amounts of antibody reacting directly with the fetal red cells [1]. The red cells which are sensitized by the antibodies are destroyed by macrophages in the fetal spleen with consequent hyperbilirubinaemia [2].

ABO-HDN in literature is described as a condition having a very low incidence in the population and characterized by a benign evolution because of a mild degree of hemolysis [3, 4]. Anaemia is rare with the main clinical problem being jaundice. Severe hemolysis and anaemia requiring exchange blood transfusion have however been reported [5]. Early detection and treatment of neonatal hyperbilirubinaemia is important in prevention of bilirubin-induced encephalopathy in the affected children [6].

The above statements, however, are not valid for all populations. Studies have revealed that statistically, mother and infant are ABO-incompatible in one of every five pregnancies among Caucasians [7, 8]. The incidence of ABO HDN in the United Kingdom is about 2% of all births, but severe hemolytic disease occurs in only 0.03% of births [9]. The incidence of ABO HDN in Blacks [10] is said to be higher than in Caucasians [11–13]. This is due to the higher prevalence and titres of immune anti-A and anti-B antibodies in the Black population [14–18].

TABLE 1: ABO typing of blood donors at the Lagos University Teaching Hospital University Teaching Hospital.

Blood group	O POS.	O Neg.	A POS.	A Neg.	B POS.	B Neg.	AB POS.	AB Neg.	Total
Number of donors	4679	283	2001	97	1677	94	281	26	**9138**
%	51.2	3.1	21.9	1.1	18.4	1.0	3.0	0.3	**100**

POS.: positive.
Neg.: negative.

Routine antenatal antibody screening tests (indirect Coombs test) do not routinely include screening for ABO HDN. Diagnosis is usually made by investigation of a newborn baby who has developed jaundice during the first day of life. Routine screening for ABO incompatibility between mother and fetus is not performed and according to Han et al. it is not cost effective to routinely screen for ABO incompatibility in the Asian population [19].

The prevalence of immune anti-A and anti-B antibodies and the population and gene frequencies of the various ABO blood groups are useful in predicting an estimate of children born by blood group O women married to non-group-O husbands who are at risk of developing ABO HDN.

This study aims at estimating the risk of ABO HDN in our population with a view to determining whether there is the need for routine screening since the incidence of ABO HDN is expected to be higher in Blacks.

2. Subjects and Methods

We determined the prevalence of ABO blood types among 9138 blood donors at Lagos University Teaching Hospital by collating the data of all donors over a one-year period. Arithmetical methods based on Hardy Weinberg equilibrium were then used to determine population prevalence of different ABO genes using the phenotype data obtained from ABO typing of blood donors (Appendix A).

The population prevalence of hemolysins in Lagos [20] in combination with the obtained ABO gene frequencies was used to calculate the likelihood of scenario where a non-blood-group-O baby will be born to a blood group O mother with immune ABO antibodies (Appendix B). These were then used to arrive at an estimate of the incidence of ABO HDN within the population.

3. Results

A total of 9138 blood donors were ABO blood group typed. 4962 (54.3%) were blood group O. Blood group A was slightly more prevalent (23.0%) than blood group B (19.4%). AB blood group constituted only 3.3% (Table 1).

The calculated population prevalence of the A, B, and O genes in Lagos is 0.1416, 0.1209, and 0.7375, respectively (details of calculations are presented in Appendix A).

The calculated probability of a blood group O woman giving birth to a child who is non-group-O phenotype is 14.3% of deliveries in Lagos (details of calculations are presented in Appendix B).

With a prevalence of anti-A and anti-B hemolysins in blood group O individuals of 30.3% and with 18.6% of blood group O donors having significant visual titres, approximately 4.3% of deliveries (30.3% of 14.3% deliveries) are likely to suffer ABO HDN with 2.7% of deliveries (18.6% of 14.3% deliveries) prone to suffer from moderately severe to severe hemolysis.

4. Discussion

The incidence of severe neonatal jaundice within the first few hours of life (bilirubin above 10 mg/100 mL) is fairly common with a significant number requiring exchange transfusions. However, the number of cases that are due to hemolysis from ABO incompatibility between mother and fetus have not yet been established. A 1 in 5 chance of ABO incompatibility between fetal red cells and maternal serum exists but the incidence of ABO HDN elsewhere is said to be uncommon occurring in 2% of all births [5, 9]. Race has however been shown to have an effect on the incidence and severity of ABO HDN with a higher incidence and severity being observed among Blacks [10] and Latin Americans [7]. Thus we can expect the incidence and severity of ABO HDN to be higher in Nigeria.

Blood group O individuals were 54.3% of the donor population which is consistent with those found in an earlier population study by Ahmed et al. in Lagos State [21]. As it can be assumed that sex factor has no influence on ABO gene inheritance and blood group distribution, then 54.3% of females in Lagos can be assumed to be blood group O.

From results obtained in this study using the gene frequencies of the ABO blood group antigens and then calculating the probabilities of a blood group O woman marrying a non-group-O man and having a non-group-O child, the incidence of ABO incompatible pregnancies in the population with the mother being blood group O is 14.3%. This is similar to results obtained by Cariani et al. [7] in Venezuela and what has been reported for anglosaxon countries [22]. This is due to the similar frequency of blood group O in the studied populations.

Anti-A and anti-B hemolysins prevalence in the study population is 30.3% with 18.6% having significant visual titres of 8 and above [20]. From calculations, 4.3% of deliveries in Lagos (30.3% of 14.3% deliveries) are likely to suffer ABO HDN. This is consistent with reports which have found that the incidence of ABO HDN is higher in Blacks than in Caucasians [11–13] and is double that of the figures obtained for the United Kingdom [9]. This higher finding can be explained by the higher prevalence of hemolysins in Black population. Visual titres of hemolysins of 8 and above have been associated with significant in vivo hemolysis [17, 23]. Assuming those with significant visual titre as being capable of leading to severe ABO HDN, potentially 2.7% of deliveries (18.6% of 14.3% deliveries) will have moderately severe to severe ABO HDN. This finding is considerably higher than in the United Kingdom where severe hemolytic disease occurs in only 0.03% of births [9].

Routine screening for ABO incompatibility is presently not performed in Lagos University Teaching Hospital with most babies discharged as soon as possible after delivery. Also, there is no test that is of high predictive value for severe HDN. It can however be suggested that hemolysis from ABO HDN can be more severe amongst Nigerian neonates whose mothers tend to have higher prevalence and titres of immune anti-A and anti-B antibodies from several studies [14–18]. Thus, there may be a case for routine screening for immune antibodies in pregnant blood group O women to monitor fetuses that may be at risk.

As routine testing for hemolysins is not performed in this environment, blood group O women with suspected high immune antibody titre or with a history of ABO incompatibility in a previous pregnancy may also require monitoring of their neonates.

5. Conclusion

The estimated risk of ABO HDN among non-group-O offspring of blood group O women is 4.3% of all deliveries in Lagos University Teaching Hospital. 2.7% of babies ABO incompatible with their mothers are at risk of moderately severe to severe HDN. With this finding, it may not be cost effective to routinely screen for ABO HDN. However, best practices for detecting neonatal jaundice need to be put in place and, if severe neonatal jaundice occurs in a setting of ABO incompatibility, intravenous immunoglobulin which usually avoids the invasive procedure of an exchange transfusion should be considered.

Appendices

A. Arithmetical Calculation of Population Prevalence of ABO Genes from Phenotype Data

From Figure 1, the gene, genotype, and phenotype frequencies of the ABO blood groups can be deduced.

According to Mourant et al. [24], square e-f-g-h in Figure 1 has a breadth and length of unity such that the area of the square is also unity. If along the length and breadth we have genes O, A, and B representing the ABO genes of both parents of a child, the possible genotypes of the offspring are represented in the smaller boxes within the bigger square and these possible genotypes can easily be derived from expansion of binomial $(A + B + O)^2$ to give $(A^2 + B^2 + O^2 + 2AB + 2AO + 2BO)$.

From this expansion, we can estimate the population prevalence of different ABO genotypes in a given population if the prevalence of some of the genotypes is known particularly the genotype that can easily be derived from knowing the prevalence of the phenotype:

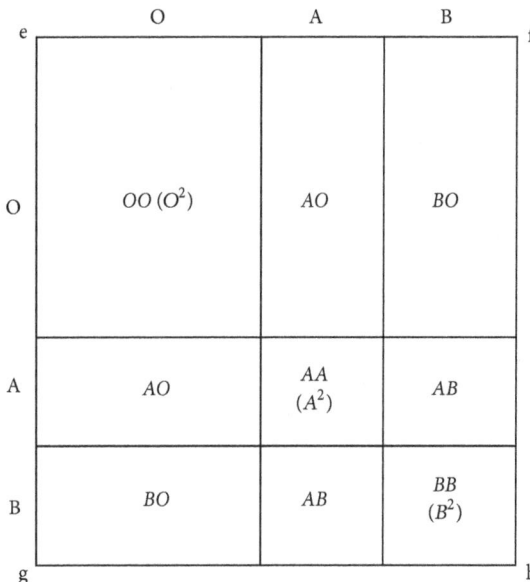

FIGURE 1: Deducing the gene, genotype, and phenotype frequencies of the ABO blood in a population.

Phenotype O has genotype OO (O = OO).

Phenotype A has genotype $AA + AO$ (A = $AA + AO$).

Phenotype B has genotype $BB + BO$ (B = $BB + BO$).

Phenotype AB has genotype AB (AB = AB).

It is conventional to represent genes A, B, and O with letters p, q, and r, respectively.

Thus, genotype AA prevalence is a square of the prevalence of gene A in a given population; that is,

$$AA = A^2 = p^2. \tag{A.1}$$

Similarly,

$$BB = B^2 = q^2, \tag{A.2}$$

$$OO = O^2 = r^2. \tag{A.3}$$

From Figure 1 or the expansion of the binomial $(A + B + O)^2$ to give $(A^2 + B^2 + O^2 + 2AB + 2AO + 2BO)$ prevalence of genotype AO will be given by

$$AO = 2AO = 2pr. \tag{A.4}$$

Similarly,

$$BO = 2BO = 2qr,$$
$$AB = 2AB = 2pq. \tag{A.5}$$

Equations (A.1) to (A.5) shall now be used to calculate the prevalence of the ABO genes in a given population.

A gene occurs in genotypes AA and AO. Thus prevalence of A gene is given by

$$A = (AA + AO) = \left(p^2 + 2pr\right). \tag{A.6}$$

Similarly,

$$B = (BB + BO) = \left(q^2 + 2qr\right). \qquad (A.7)$$

Adding (A.6) and (A.3), we have,

$$(A + O) = p^2 + 2pr$$
$$+ r^2 \; (\text{Hardy Weinberg Equation}). \qquad (A.8)$$

Extracting square root of (A.8),

$$\sqrt{A + O} = (p + r). \qquad (A.9)$$

Since $p + q + r = 1$ (i.e., sum of prevalence of A, B, and O genes in a given population),

$$q = 1 - (p + r) = 1 - \sqrt{A + O}. \qquad (A.10)$$

Similarly,

$$p = 1 - (q + r) = 1 - \sqrt{B + O}. \qquad (A.11)$$

From (A.3), we can derive that prevalence of gene O that is, r, is

$$r = \sqrt{O^2}. \qquad (A.12)$$

Applying the above equations to the prevalence of ABO blood group phenotypes from the record of 9138 blood donors at the Lagos University Teaching Hospital donor clinic we estimate the following.

4962 of 9138 (54.3%) donors were blood group O, 23.0% (2098) were blood group A, 19.4% (1771) were blood group B, and 3.3% (307) were blood group AB.

From (A.11) $p = 1 - \sqrt{B + O}$ and using the values above,

$$p = 1 - \sqrt{0.194 + 0.543} = 1 - \sqrt{0.737} = 1 - 0.8585$$
$$= 0.1415. \qquad (A.13)$$

Therefore population frequency for A gene $= p = 0.1415$.
From (A.10), also using the above values,

$$q = 1 - \sqrt{0.23 + 0.543} = 1 - \sqrt{0.773} = 1 - 0.8792$$
$$= 0.1208. \qquad (A.14)$$

Therefore population frequency for B gene $= q = 0.1208$.
From (A.3), we can say that

$$O^2 = r^2 = 0.543. \qquad (A.15)$$

Therefore population frequency for O gene $= \sqrt{O^2} = \sqrt{0.543} = 0.7369$.
Thus $r = 0.7369$.

A.1. Corrected ABO Gene Frequencies. According to Bernstein [25] the sum total of p, q, and r does not usually sum up to 1. The p, q, and r estimates need to be corrected using a quantity D which is defined as

$$D = 1 - (p + q + r). \qquad (A.16)$$

From addition above, $(p + q + r) = 0.1415 + 0.1208 + 0.7369 = 0.9992$. Consider

$$D = 1 - 0.9992 = 0.0008. \qquad (A.17)$$

The corrected frequencies for $p(p_c)$, $q(q_c)$, and $r(r_c)$, according to Bernstein, are

$$p_c = \frac{p}{1 - D} = \frac{0.1415}{1 - 0.0008} = \frac{0.1415}{0.9992} = 0.1416,$$

$$q_c = \frac{q}{1 - D} = \frac{0.1208}{1 - 0.0008} = \frac{0.1208}{0.9992} = 0.1209, \qquad (A.18)$$

$$r_c = \frac{r}{1 - D} = \frac{0.7369}{1 - 0.0008} = \frac{0.7369}{0.9992} = 0.7375.$$

Thus the calculated gene frequencies were 0.1416, 0.1209, and 0.7375 for the A, B, and O genes, respectively.

B. Calculating Likelihood of Scenario Where a Non-Blood-Group-O Child Is Born to a Blood Group O Mother

For ABO hemolytic disease of the newborn to occur, a blood group O woman must be married to a non-group-O man and have an offspring who is non-blood-group-O.

The probability will be the summation of probability of occurrence of blood group genotypes AA, BB, AO, BO, and AB husband being married to group OO genotype wife resulting in an offspring with non-group-O gene.

Using the gene frequencies calculated above, one has the following.

The probability that an OO genotype woman will be married to AA genotype is the product of frequency of OO genotype and frequency of AA genotype:

$$AA = r^2 \times p^2. \qquad (B.1)$$

Therefore,

$$AA = 0.7375^2 \times 0.1416^2 = 0.010906. \qquad (B.2)$$

Similarly,

$$BB = 0.7375^2 \times 0.1209^2 = 0.007950. \qquad (B.3)$$

The probability that an OO genotype woman will be married to AO genotype man will be given by

$$AO = r^2 \times 2pr. \qquad (B.4)$$

The probability that the child will inherit the A gene from the father is half. Therefore the probability that an AO man and an OO woman will have an AO child will be given by

$$AO = \frac{\left(r^2 \times 2pr\right)}{2} = r^2 \times pr,$$
$$AO = 0.7375^2 \times 0.1416 \times 0.7375 = 0.056800. \qquad (B.5)$$

Similarly,

$$BO = 0.7375^2 \times 0.1209 \times 0.7375 = 0.048497. \qquad \text{(B.6)}$$

The probability that OO genotype woman will be married to AB genotype man and the child will have either A or B gene is given by

$$AB = r^2 \times 2pq,$$
$$AB = 0.7375^2 \times 2 \times 0.1416 \times 0.1209 = 0.018623. \qquad \text{(B.7)}$$

The sum of all the probabilities = 0.142776.

Therefore, 14.3% of deliveries in Lagos University Teaching Hospital University Teaching Hospital will result in a woman whose blood group is O giving birth to a child who has a non-group-O phenotype.

Conflict of Interests

The authors declare that there is no conflict of interests regarding the publication of this paper.

References

[1] R. Ottenberg, "Studies in isoagglutination: I. Transfusion and the question of intravascular agglutination," *The Journal of Experimental Medicine*, vol. 13, no. 4, pp. 425–438, 1911.

[2] A. G. Hadley, "Laboratory assays for predicting the severity of haemolytic disease of the fetus and newborn," *Transplant Immunology*, vol. 10, no. 2-3, pp. 191–198, 2002.

[3] I. Halbrecht, "Icterus precox. Further studies on its frequency, etiology, prognosis and the blood chemistry of the cord blood," *The Journal of Pediatrics*, vol. 39, no. 2, pp. 185–190, 1951.

[4] D. Voak and C. C. Bowley, "A detailed serological study on the prediction and diagnosis of ABO haemolytic disease of the newborn (ABO-HD)," *Vox Sanguinis*, vol. 17, no. 5, pp. 321–348, 1969.

[5] B. K. Gilja and V. P. Shah, "Hydrops fetalis due to ABO incompatibility," *Clinical Pediatrics*, vol. 27, no. 4, pp. 210–212, 1988.

[6] A. Petrova, R. Mehta, G. Birchwood, B. Ostfeld, and T. Hegyi, "Management of neonatal hyperbilirubinemia: pediatricians' practices and educational needs," *BMC Pediatrics*, vol. 6, article 6, 2006.

[7] L. Cariani, E. L. Romano, N. Martinez et al., "ABO-haemolytic disease of the newborn (ABO-HDN): factors influencing its severity and incidence in Venezuela," *Journal of Tropical Pediatrics*, vol. 41, no. 1, pp. 14–21, 1995.

[8] M. S. Kennedy and A. Waheed, "Hemolytic disease of the newborn and fetus," in *Modern Blood Banking and Transfusion Practices*, D. Harmening, Ed., pp. 431–432, F.A. Davis Company, Philadelphia, Pa, USA, 4th edition, 1999.

[9] M. McDonnell, S. Hannam, and S. P. Devane, "Hydrops fetalis due to ABO incompatibility," *Archives of Disease in Childhood: Fetal and Neonatal Edition*, vol. 78, no. 3, pp. F220–F221, 1998.

[10] G. H. Vos, M. Adhikari, and H. M. Coovadia, "A study of ABO incompatibility and neonatal jaundice in black South African newborn infants," *Transfusion*, vol. 21, no. 6, pp. 744–749, 1981.

[11] K. J. Peevy and H. J. Wiseman, "ABO hemolytic disease of the newborn: evaluation of management and identification of racial and antigenic factors," *Pediatrics*, vol. 61, no. 3, pp. 475–478, 1978.

[12] H. N. Kirkman Jr., "Further evidence for a racial difference in frequency of ABO hemolytic disease," *The Journal of Pediatrics*, vol. 90, no. 5, pp. 717–721, 1977.

[13] K. A. Bucher, A. M. Patterson Jr., R. C. Elston, C. A. Jones, and H. N. Kirkman Jr., "Racial difference in incidence of ABO hemolytic disease," *American Journal of Public Health*, vol. 66, no. 9, pp. 854–858, 1976.

[14] A. G. Kulkarni, R. Ibazebe, and A. F. Fleming, "High frequency of anti-A and anti-B haemolysins in certain ethnic groups of Nigeria," *Vox Sanguinis*, vol. 48, no. 1, pp. 39–41, 1985.

[15] K. E. Onwukeme and O. U. Nanna, "Frequency of anti-A and anti-B hemolysins in Nigerians living in Jos," *Nigerian Medical Practitioner*, vol. 20, article 29, 1990.

[16] S. Worlledge, S. E. Ogiemudia, C. O. Thomas, B. N. Ikoku, and L. Luzzatto, "Blood group antigens and antibodies in Nigeria," *Annals of Tropical Medicine and Parasitology*, vol. 68, no. 3, pp. 249–264, 1974.

[17] A. S. David-West, "Blood transfusion and blood bank management in a tropical country," *Clinics in Haematology*, vol. 10, no. 3, pp. 1013–1028, 1981.

[18] H. O. Olawumi and P. O. Olatunji, "Prevalence and titre of alpha and beta haemolysins in blood group 'O' donors in Ilorin," *African Journal of Medicine and Medical Sciences*, vol. 30, no. 4, pp. 319–321, 2001.

[19] P. Han, R. Kiruba, R. Ong, R. Joseph, K. L. Tan, and H. B. Wong, "Haematolytic disease due to ABO incompatibility: incidence and value of screening in an Asian population," *Australian Paediatric Journal*, vol. 24, no. 1, pp. 35–38, 1988.

[20] O. Oyedeji, T. Adeyemo, A. Ogbenna, and A. Akanmu, "Prevalence of anti-A and anti-B hemolysis among blood group O donors in Lagos," *Nigerian Journal of Clinical Practice*, vol. 18, no. 3, pp. 328–332, 2015.

[21] O. A. Ahmed, P. U. Agomo, D. K. Olukoya, and G. J. F. Esan, "The prevalence of ABO blood group antigens and antibodies in Lagos State, Nigeria," *African Journal of Medicine and Medical Sciences*, vol. 22, no. 3, pp. 49–53, 1993.

[22] P. L. Mollison, C. P. Engelfriet, and M. Contreras, *Blood Transfusion in Clinical Medicine*, Blackwell Scientific Publications, Oxford, UK, 8th edition, 1987.

[23] D. G. Saphire, N. S. Rudolph, S. M. Hackleman, and W. H. Stone, "The effect of age on the level of human ABO blood group antibodies," *Aging*, vol. 5, no. 3, pp. 177–184, 1993.

[24] A. E. Mourant, A. C. Kopec, and K. Domaniewska-Sobczak, "Gene frequency calculation," in *The Distribution of Human Blood Groups and Other Polymorphisms*, pp. 47–61, Oxford University Press, London, UK, 2nd edition, 1976.

[25] F. Bernstein, "Forgesetzte Untersuchungen aus der Theorie der Blutgruppen," *Zeitschrift für Induktive Abstammungs- und Vererbungslehre*, vol. 56, pp. 233–272, 1930.

14

Frequencies and Specificities of "Enzyme-Only" Detected Erythrocyte Alloantibodies in Patients Hospitalized in Austria: Is an Enzyme Test Required for Routine Red Blood Cell Antibody Screening?

Dietmar Enko,[1] **Claudia Habres,**[2] **Franz Wallner,**[1]
Barbara Mayr,[2] **and Gabriele Halwachs-Baumann**[1]

[1] *Department of Laboratory Medicine, Central Hospital Steyr, Sierningerstraße 170, 4400 Steyr, Austria*
[2] *University of Applied Sciences for Health Professions Upper Austria, Bachelor Program Biomedical Science,*
 Central Hospital Steyr, Sierningerstraße 170, 4400 Steyr, Austria

Correspondence should be addressed to Dietmar Enko; dietmar.enko@gespag.at

Academic Editor: Arturo Pereira

The aim of this study was to determine the frequencies and specificities of "enzyme-only" detected red blood cell (RBC) alloantibodies in the routine antibody screening and antibody identification in patients hospitalized in Austria. Routine blood samples of 2420 patients were investigated. The antibody screening was performed with a 3-cell panel in the low-ionic strength saline- (LISS-) indirect antiglobulin test (IAT) and with an enzyme-pretreated (papain) 3-cell panel fully automated on the ORTHO AutoVue Innova System. The antibody identification was carried out manually with an 11-cell panel in the LISS-IAT and with an enzyme-pretreated (papain) 11-cell panel. In total 4.05% ($n = 98$) of all patients ($n = 2420$) had a positive RBC antibody screening result. Of them 25.51% (25/98) showed "enzyme-only" detected specific or nonspecific RBC alloantibodies. Rhesus and Lewis system antibodies were found the only specificities of "enzyme-only" RBC alloantibodies: all in all 4.8% (4/98) were detected with anti-E, 3.06% (3/98) with anti-Le^a, 3.06% (3/98) with anti-D after anti-D prophylaxis and 1.02% (1/98) with anti-e. In total, 14.29% (14/98) showed a nonspecific RBC alloantibody result with the enzyme test. The results of the present study demonstrate that a high number of unwanted positive reactions with the enzyme technique overshadows the detection of "enzyme-only" RBC alloantibodies. (Trial Registration: K-37-13).

1. Introduction

Pretransfusion blood grouping, red blood cell (RBC) antibody screening, and compatibility testing are essential to prevent incompatible blood transfusion and alloimmunization. The Nobelist Karl Landsteiner, discoverer of the first human marker locus, published the results of a complete cross testing of the RBCs and sera of six people (including himself) in his 1901 paper [1–3]. Since then numerous other human blood group antigens have been described and categorized. Alloimmunization can cause a hemolytic transfusion reaction in individuals lacking the corresponding blood group antigen on their erythrocytes [4, 5]. RBC alloimmunization correlates with the number of transfusions [6–8], and the immunogenicity of the blood group antigens is crucial [5, 9]. About 25–28 antigens are known to cause hemolytic transfusion reactions and should be detected with the pretransfusion RBC antibody screening test [10]. The Rhesus (Rh), Kell (K), Duffy (Fy), and Kidd (Jk) antigens are some of these clinically significant blood group antigens [11].

Pretransfusion compatibility testing involves ABO grouping, Rh typing, RBC antibody screening, RBC antibody identification, and also cross matching the RBC unit designed to be transfused [12]. Hemagglutination is still the classical method for antigen testing and antibody screening [13]. The indirect antiglobulin test (IAT) is considered to be a reliable and effective method to detect clinically relevant

RBC alloantibodies [14]. In the last few years, pretransfusion testing practices have shifted from tube to gel technology. The gel test is more sensitive than the conventional tube method [15, 16]. It has been well known for a long time that the enzyme treatment of RBCs modifies the erythrocyte surface [17–19] and that some Rh antibodies occur only in the enzyme (papain) technique [20, 21]. The main argument for the use of the enzyme technique in the routine testing would be to detect clinically significant RBC alloantibodies, but published works on this topic are rare [22]. In Austria, hospital blood banks without donation, production and screening facilities, and the so-called "blood-depositories" are mainly managed by specialists for anesthesiology, laboratory medicine, transfusion medicine, and internal medicine [23]. Among the blood-depositories, differences of opinion exist regarding the use of enzyme-pretreated RBCs.

The aim of this study was to determine the frequencies and specificities of "enzyme-only" detected erythrocyte alloantibodies in the routine RBC antibody screening and identification in patients hospitalized in Austria.

2. Materials and Methods

The ethical approval for this study was provided by the Ethical Committee of Upper Austria, Linz, Austria (Trial Registration no.: K-37-13). The study period was from January 17, 2013 to May 17, 2013.

2.1. Patient Material. Blood samples of 2420 hospitalized patients, who underwent routine blood grouping and RBC antibody screening at the Department of Laboratory Medicine in the Central Hospital Steyr (Austria), were investigated. The patients were mainly adults and in very few instances children. Ethylendiamintetraacetic acid (EDTA) plasma was used for the analysis. All the patients were tested for the ABO blood group, the Rh antigen D, and RBC alloantibodies.

2.2. Blood Group Determination. The fully automated ABO/ Rh typing was performed using the gel technique on the ORTHO AutoVue Innova System (Ortho Clinical Diagnostics, Raritan, New Jersey). According to the Austrian Guidelines for Blood Group Serology and Transfusion Medicine (latest version July 2000), the RBC antigens A, B, and Rh D, as well as the presence of isoagglutinins, were tested. All patients with a positive result in the RBC antibody screening were tested for the Rh antigens C, c, E, and e.

2.3. RBC Antibody Screening. The RBC antibody screening was carried out in a fully automated process with a 3-cell panel (0.8% Surgiscreen RBCs reagents 1, 2, and 3 [Ortho Clinical Diagnostics, Raritan, New Jersey]) in the low-ionic strength saline- (LISS-) IAT. Additionally an enzyme test with 3 enzyme-pretreated (papain) red test cells (ID-DiaCell PI, PII, PIII [BIO-RAD, Hercules, California]) was performed on the ORTHO AutoVue Innova System (Ortho Clinical Diagnostics, Raritan, New Jersey).

2.4. RBC Antibody Identification. If the RBC antibody screening showed a positive result in the LISS-IAT and/or with the enzyme-test (papain), the antibody identification was carried out manually with an 11-cell panel (ID-DiaPanel 1-11 [BIO-RAD, Hercules, California]) in the LISS-IAT and with an enzyme-pretreated (papain) 11-cell panel (ID-DiaPanel-P 1-11 [BIO-RAD, Hercules, California]). If a specific RBC alloantibody was identified, the corresponding blood group antigen was determined to confirm the RBC antibody identification result. The autocontrol was made in the LISS-IAT. Serological reactions were graded from 0 to 4+.

2.5. Data Analysis. Descriptive statistics were performed to analyze the serological ABO and Rh phenotype frequencies and the frequencies and specificities of the RBC alloantibodies.

3. Results

3.1. ABO and Rh D Phenotype Frequencies. Of all patients (n = 2420), 38.18% (924/2420) had blood group O, 44.42% (1075/2420) blood group A, and 12.44% (310/2420) blood group B and 4.96% (120/2420) showed the AB phenotype. All in all 84.42% (2043/2420) were Rh antigen D positive and 15.58% (377/2043) were Rh antigen D negative.

3.2. RBC Antibody Screening Results. In total 4.05% (n = 98) of all patients (n = 2420) showed a positive RBC antibody screening result with the 3-cell panel in the LISS-IAT and/or with the enzyme-pretreated (papain) 3-cell panel. Of them 82.65% were women and 17.35% were men. The median age of patients with a positive RBC antibody result was 42 (range: 17–91) years. In total 95.95% (n = 2322) had a negative test result in the LISS-IAT as well as with the enzyme test.

3.3. RBC Antibody Identification Results. The frequencies and specificities of RBC alloantibodies detected in the LISS-IAT ± enzyme (papain) are illustrated in Table 1: in total, 66.32% (n = 65) of all patients with a positive RBC antibody screening result (n = 98) presented a specific RBC alloantibody identification result. The most common specific RBC alloantibodies were directed against Rhesus (Rh), Lewis (Le), and Kell (K) antigens. Six patients were found with combined specific RBC alloantibodies: three patients had combined anti-D and anti-C, one patient combined anti-D, anti-C, and anti-K, one patient combined anti-E, anti-K, and anti-Fy^a, and one patient had combined anti-c, anti-K, and anti-Fy^a. Eight patients were found with a nonspecific RBC alloantibody identification in the LISS-IAT ± enzyme (papain). The frequencies and specificities of "enzyme-only" detected RBC alloantibodies are shown in Table 2: all in all eleven patients showed a specific RBC alloantibody result with the enzyme test. The identified "enzyme-only" RBC alloantibodies were Rhesus and Lewis system antibodies. Fourteen patients showed a nonspecific RBC alloantibody result with the enzyme test. All specific and nonspecific RBC alloantibody detection results in the LISS-IAT and with the enzyme test are summarized in Table 3.

TABLE 1: Frequencies and specificities of RBC alloantibodies detected in the LISS-IAT ± enzyme (papain) ($n = 73$).

Antibody-specificities	Frequencies	Percent
Anti-D after anti-D prophylaxis	32	32.66
Anti-E	3	3.06
Anti-Le^a	4	4.08
Anti-D	5	5.10
Anti-K	5	5.10
Anti-D and anti-C	3	3.06
Anti-Fy^a	2	2.04
Anti-Kp^a	2	2.04
Anti-M	2	2.04
Anti-C^w	1	1.02
Anti-S	1	1.02
Anti-D, anti-C, and anti-K	1	1.02
Anti-E, anti-K, and anti-Fy^a	1	1.02
Anti-c, anti-K, and anti-Fy^a	1	1.02
Anti-I	1	1.02
Anti-HI	1	1.02
Nonspecific RBC alloantibodies	8	8.17
Total	73	74.49

RBC: red blood cell; Le^a: Lewis^a; K: Kell; Fy^a: Duffy^a; LISS: low-ionic strength saline; IAT: indirect antiglobulin test.

TABLE 2: Frequencies and specificities of "enzyme-only" detected RBC alloantibodies ($n = 25$).

Antibody specificities	Frequencies	Percent
Anti-E	4	4.08
Anti-Le^a	3	3.06
Anti-D after anti-D prophylaxis	3	3.06
Anti-e	1	1.02
Nonspecific RBC alloantibodies	**14**	**14.29**
Total	25	25.51

RBC: red blood cell; Le^a: Lewis^a.

4. Discussion

The ABO and Rh D frequency data of our study population are comparable with the described results in the literature. A study about blood group frequencies in Germany with the data of more than 600,000 donors demonstrated similar results: all in all 41.21% had blood group O, 43.26% blood group A, 10.71% blood group B, and 4.82% blood group AB. 82.71% were Rh D positive and 17.29% were Rh D negative [24].

The RBC antibody screening and the cross-match are used as pretransfusion tests in the daily routine of blood banks and hospitals. Both routine tests are designed to detect agglutinating and hemolyzing erythrocyte antibodies active at 37°C [25]. In this study 4.05% ($n = 98$) of all hospitalized patients ($n = 2420$) showed a positive RBC antibody testing result. Compared to previous studies, blood type alloantibodies have been reported in 0.8% of blood donors, in 1-2% of hospitalized patients, and in 2–9% of patients with a history of blood transfusion [26].

Over the years a lot of distinct blood group antigens have been identified. Carbohydrate antigens (ABO and P/Globo-related system) and protein antigens (Kidd, Duffy, and Rh blood group system) have been described [27]. They can act as functional molecules but also can evoke erythrocyte antibodies [28]. Therefore pretransfusion RBC antibody detection and identification are essential. According to the Austrian Guidelines for Blood Group Serology and Transfusion Medicine (latest version July 2000), the RBC antibody screening must be performed as an IAT with at least two erythrocyte test cells. The completion with an enzyme test is not explicitly postulated. Despite the widespread use of the RBC antibody screening test, differences of opinion exist regarding the use of enzyme-pretreated red test cells [29, 30]. The collected data of the present study illustrate that Rhesus and Lewis system antibodies were identified as the only specificities of "enzyme-only" RBC alloantibodies. These results confirm previous studies, where anti-E and anti-Le^a were found to be the most frequent erythrocyte antibodies active only in the enzyme test [29, 31]. In a retrospective study on blood samples from 10,000 recently transfused patients, the majority of "enzyme-only" antibodies was not clinically significant. Of 19 patients with an "enzyme-only" erythrocyte antibody, who were transfused with antigen-positive RBC units, only one had a delayed hemolytic transfusion reaction [32]. In another work six males with naturally occurring Rh antibodies were investigated. Two subjects with "enzyme-only" Rh antibodies (one anti-E and one anti-D) in papain technique showed a normal survival of incompatible injected RBCs [33]. As far back as 1961 it was considered that Rh antibodies only detectable by an enzyme (papain) method do not play such a clinically significant role in the etiology of hemolytic reactions compared to antibodies detectable by the IAT [20].

In the present study 3.06% ($n = 3$) of all patients with a positive RBC antibody screening result ($n = 98$) showed an "enzyme-only" anti-Le^a in the antibody identification. In general Le antibodies are not considered clinically significant [11]. This is probably because the most of the antibodies in the Lewis system are not active at 37°C [34].

In this study a high number of unwanted positive enzyme reactions were detected. In total 14.29% ($n = 14$) of patients with a positive antibody testing result ($n = 98$) had a nonspecific RBC alloantibody identification result with the enzyme test. These findings confirm the results of other works on this topic. The detection of clinically significant "enzyme-only" erythrocyte antibodies was overshadowed by the high number of nonspecific or clinically insignificant antibodies [29]. Many specialists working on this as a daily routine are convinced that the enzyme test in the RBC antibody screening is not justified because of the high workload in investigating all the initial positive enzyme-method reactions compared with the low number of clinically significant erythrocyte antibodies identified [32].

The limitation of this study is the low number of patients. In a greater study population more "enzyme-only" RBC

TABLE 3: RBC alloantibody detection in the LISS-IAT and with the enzyme test.

$n = 98$	LISS-IAT + enzyme	LISS-IAT	"Enzyme-only"
Specific RBC alloantibodies	60	5	11
Nonspecific RBC alloantibodies	7	1	**14**

RBC: red blood cell; LISS: low-ionic strength-saline; IAT: indirect antiglobulin test.

alloantibodies may be detected and the results of the present study could be substantiated.

5. Conclusions

The data presented in this study demonstrate that Rhesus and Lewis system antibodies were the only specificities of "enzyme-only" detected RBC alloantibodies in patients hospitalized in Austria accompanied by a high number of unwanted nonspecific enzyme reactions. Compared to the existing literature the majority of "enzyme-only" detected RBC antibodies are considered to play a minor part in the etiology of hemolytic transfusion reactions. In clinical practice extra time and additional personnel and labor costs for investigating a high number of unwanted positive enzyme-reactions must be calculated. Based on these facts each hospital "blood-depository" should make its own pragmatic decision whether the enzyme test for routine RBC antibody screening is justified or not in their patient population.

Conflict of Interests

The authors declare that there is no conflict of interests regarding the publication of this paper.

References

[1] R. Owen, "Karl Landsteiner and the first human marker locus," *Genetics*, vol. 155, no. 3, pp. 995–998, 2000.

[2] T. Makarovska-Bojadzieva, M. Blagoevska, P. Kolevski, and S. Kostovska, "Optimal blood grouping and antibody screening for safe transfusion," *Prilozi*, vol. 30, no. 1, pp. 119–128, 2009.

[3] J. P. Aymard, "Karl Landsteiner (1868–1943) and the discovery of blood groups," *Transfusion Clinique Et Biologique*, vol. 19, no. 4-5, pp. 244–248, 2012.

[4] D. R. Branch, "Solving the dilemma of prevention of red cell alloimmunization," *Immunotherapy*, vol. 4, no. 9, pp. 903–905, 2012.

[5] S. Zalpuri, J. J. Zwaginga, and J. G. van der Bom, "Risk Factors for Alloimmunisation after red blood Cell Transfusions (R-FACT): a case cohort study," *British Medical Journal Open*, vol. 2, no. 3, Article ID e001150, 2012.

[6] V. M. Alves, P. R. Martins, S. Soares et al., "Alloimmunization screening after transfusion of red blood cells in a prospective study," *Revista Brasileira De Hematologia e Hemoterapia*, vol. 34, no. 3, pp. 206–211, 2012.

[7] R. de Oliveira Cruz, M. A. Mota, F. M. Conti et al., "Prevalence of erythrocyte alloimmunization in polytransfused patients," *Einstein*, vol. 9, no. 2, pp. 173–178, 2011.

[8] K. M. Byrne, G. S. Booth, J. Y. Lee, and K. R. Ravenell, "The importance of antibody detection and identification in the

chronically transfused patient," *Laboratory Medicine*, vol. 41, no. 5, pp. 261–263, 2010.

[9] C. A. Tormey and G. Stack, "Immunogenicity of blood group antigens: a mathematical model corrected for antibody evanescence with exclusion of naturally occurring and pregnancy-related antibodies," *Blood*, vol. 114, no. 19, pp. 4279–4282, 2009.

[10] S. Pathak, M. Chandrashekhar, and G. R. Whankhede, "Type and screen policy in the blood bank: is AHG cross-match still required? A study at a multispeciality corporate hospital in India," *Asian Journal of Transfusion Science*, vol. 5, no. 2, pp. 153–156, 2011.

[11] M. H. Yazer, "The blood bank "black box" debunked: pretransfusion testing explained," *Canadian Medical Association Journal*, vol. 174, no. 1, pp. 29–32, 2006.

[12] K. A. Downes and I. A. Shulman, "Pretransfusion testing practices in North America, 2005–2010: an analysis of the College of American Pathologists Interlaboratory Comparison Program J-Survey Data, 2005–2010," *Archives of Pathology and Laboratory Medicine*, vol. 136, no. 3, pp. 294–300, 2012.

[13] M. E. Reid, "Transfusion in the age of molecular diagnostics," *Hematology American Society of Hematology Education Program*, pp. 171–177, 2009.

[14] J. Cid, N. Nogués, R. Montero, M. Hurtado, A. Briega, and R. Parra, "Comparison of three microtube column agglutination systems for antibody screening: DG Gel, DiaMed-ID and Ortho BioVue," *Transfusion Medicine*, vol. 16, no. 2, pp. 131–136, 2006.

[15] M. A. Hassan, F. H. Al Gahtani, and A. M. A. Gader, "The frequency of alloantibodies in pregnant and multi-transfused patients—a comparative study between the ID-Micro Typing Gel System and the conventional tube method," *Journal of Applied Hematology*, vol. 2, no. 3, pp. 234–242, 2011.

[16] E. Delaflor-Weiss and V. Chizhevsky, "Implementation of gel testing for antibody screening and identification in a community hospital, a 3-year experience," *Laboratory Medicine*, vol. 36, no. 8, pp. 489–492, 2005.

[17] K. Aho and C. L. Christian, "Studies of incomplete antibodies. 1. Effect of papain on red cells," *Blood*, vol. 27, no. 5, pp. 662–669, 1966.

[18] K. Sagisaka, K. Tokiwa, and N. Yoshioka, "Actions of proteolytic enzymes on agglutinability of M and N blood-group red cells," *Tohoku Journal of Experimental Medicine*, vol. 106, no. 2, pp. 191–197, 1972.

[19] K. Sagisaka and K. Takahashi, "On the agglutinogens of red cells developed with proteolytic enzymes and neuraminidase," *Tohoku Journal of Experimental Medicine*, vol. 120, no. 2, pp. 169–175, 1976.

[20] B. E. Dodd and D. A. Eeles, "Rh antibodies detectable only by enzyme technique," *Immunology*, vol. 4, pp. 337–345, 1961.

[21] F. Gundolf, "Rhesus antibodies demonstrable only by enzyme technique," *Vox Sanguinis*, vol. 24, no. 4, pp. 380–381, 1973.

[22] A. Pereira, R. Mazzara, A. Gelabert, and R. Castillo, "Two-stage papain-indirect antiglobulin test and LISS direct agglutination are not appropriate for pretransfusion screening for unexpected antibodies," *Haematologica*, vol. 76, no. 6, pp. 475–478, 1991.

[23] H. Schennach, C. Gabriel, D. Schönitzer, and B. Blauhut, "Transfusion medicine in Austria," *Transfusion Medicine and Hemotherapy*, vol. 33, no. 5, pp. 364–373, 2006.

[24] F. F. Wagner, D. Kasulke, M. Kerowgan, and W. A. Flegel, "Frequencies of the blood groups ABO, Rhesus, D category VI, Kell, and of clinical relevant high-frequency antigens in South-Western Germany," *Infusionstherapie und Transfusionsmedizin*, vol. 22, no. 5, pp. 285–290, 1995.

[25] S. P. Masouredis, "Pretransfusion tests and compatibility: questions of safety and efficacy," *Blood*, vol. 59, no. 5, pp. 873–875, 1982.

[26] Q. Wang, Q. Yang, Y. Bai, C. Zhang, Y. Diao, and D. Fang, "Frequency of RBC alloantibodies in Chinese surgical patients," *Transfusion Medicine and Hemotherapy*, vol. 39, no. 4, pp. 283–286, 2012.

[27] Y. Lin, K. Pavenski, E. Saidenberg, and D. R. Branch, "Blood group antigens and normal red blood cell physiology: a Canadian blood services research and development symposium," *Transfusion Medicine Reviews*, vol. 23, no. 4, pp. 292–309, 2009.

[28] G. Garratty, M. J. Telen, and L. D. Petz, "Red cell antigens as functional molecules and obstacles to transfusion," *Hematology American Society of Hematology Education Program*, vol. 2002, no. 1, pp. 445–462, 2002.

[29] D. Castellá, J. Cid, M. Panadés, and C. Martín-Vega, "One thousand seventy antibodies detected only by a 2-stage papain test: wanted and unwanted positive reactions," *Immunohematology*, vol. 17, no. 4, pp. 122–124, 2001.

[30] J. Conne, P. Schneider, and J.-D. Tissot, "Role of enzyme-treated cells in RBC antibody screening using the gel test: a study of anti-RH1, -RH2, and -RH3 antibodies," *Journal of Clinical Laboratory Analysis*, vol. 21, no. 2, pp. 61–66, 2007.

[31] M. Pujol, J. M. Sancho, and M. A. Zarco, "The gel enzyme technique in pretransfusion antibody screening," *Haematologica*, vol. 87, no. 10, pp. 1119–1120, 2002.

[32] P. D. Issitt, M. R. Combs, S. J. Bredehoeft et al., "Lack of clinical significance of "enzyme-only" red cell alloantibodies," *Transfusion*, vol. 33, no. 4, pp. 284–293, 1993.

[33] M. Contreras, M. De Silva, P. Teesdale, and P. L. Mollison, "The effect of naturally occurring Rh antibodies on the survival of serologically incompatible red cells," *British Journal of Haematology*, vol. 65, no. 4, pp. 475–478, 1987.

[34] G. Daniels, "ABO, Hh, and Lewis systems," in *Human Blood Groups*, G. Daniels, Ed., pp. 7–98, Blackwell Science, 2002.

15

Assessing Acceptability of Short Message Service Based Interventions towards Becoming Future Voluntary Blood Donors

Sana Saleem,[1] Anum Wasim,[1] Sidra Sabih,[1] Ayisha Farooq Khan,[1] Madiha Hasan Rizvi,[1] Umaima Ayesha Jillani,[1] Mujtaba Jamal Syed,[1] Madiha Mumtaz,[1] Yasmeen Mumtaz,[2] Abdul Moid Shehzad,[1] Om Dawani,[1] Saima Khan,[1] Sheheryar Munir,[1] Nava Asad,[1] and Abdul Nafey Kazi[1]

[1] Dow Medical College, Dow University of Health Sciences, Karachi 74200, Pakistan
[2] Department of Community Medicine, Dow Medical College, Dow University of Health Sciences, Karachi 74200, Pakistan

Correspondence should be addressed to Anum Wasim; anum.wasim5@gmail.com

Academic Editor: Silvano Wendel

All blood bank services, especially those of developing countries, face a major shortfall of blood donations due to lack of voluntary blood donors. Our study aims to evaluate the acceptability of Short Message Service based interventions towards becoming voluntary blood donors among medical university students of Karachi, Pakistan. *Methods.* A total of 350 medical students were approached in medical universities of Karachi, Pakistan, using a nonprobability convenient sampling technique. Data collectors administered a self-made questionnaire to each participant using an interview based format. All data was recorded and analyzed on SPSS 16. *Results.* 350 participants, having a mean age of 21.47 ± 1.36, were included in our study with 30.6% (107/350) being males and 69.4% (243/350) being females. 93.4% (327/350) of participants agreed that donating blood was healthy, but only 26% had donated blood in the past with 79.1% donating voluntarily. 65.7% (230/350) of the participants agreed to take part in Short Message Service based behavioral interventions to become voluntary blood donors with 69.7% (244/350) also agreeing that Short Message Service reminders will promote them to donate blood more often. *Conclusion.* With university students willing to become voluntary blood donors, Pakistani blood banks can carry out Short Message Service based interventions to encourage them to donate blood.

1. Introduction

The continuous major challenge faced by all blood services worldwide is the huge demand-supply gap between blood donors and patients [1]. Although blood donation forms an integral component of medical services, only 92 million blood donations were made to an estimated 234 million major operations performed in 2013 [2]. Developing countries, like Pakistan, experience an even greater crisis, owing to the high incidence of transfusion-requiring medical conditions like high risk obstetrics, thalassemia, trauma, and malaria.

In Pakistan, only 28 people donate blood for every population of 10000 [3]. Replacement donors and paying for donations contribute significantly to Pakistani blood banks that in turn promotes high risk collection of seropositive infectious blood as opposed to the low risk blood products obtained from voluntary donors [4]. In 2012, an estimated 70% donations were replacement or paid for donations with 50% cases receiving unscreened blood transfusions [5].

Recruitment of low risk voluntary blood donors is a primary solution of replenishing this shortfall in blood banks [6]. University student populations, medical university students in particular, are considered the best candidates to become voluntary blood donors. Nevertheless, experience at blood banks suggests that not all university students voluntarily donate blood on a regular basis [7]. The literature reveals misconceptions, lack of knowledge (even in medical students), and fear as the primary factors preventing students from becoming voluntary blood donors [8]. In this rapid age of progress, a more novel approach is needed for a developing country like Pakistan.

With more than 5 billion worldwide mobile phone subscribers [9], mobile phone technology is rapidly progressing in the field of medicine especially for Short Message Service based interventions. In the last few years, Short Message Service (SMS) based interventions have displayed significant results for diseases like diabetes mellitus, HIV, and tuberculosis in both developed and developing countries [10, 11]. This form of intervention has proven to be cheap, accessible, and an easy way of communication [12].

Mobile phone use has risen remarkably over the last decade in Pakistan. Since 2004, the number of mobile phones in use in the country has increased from 5 million to 130 million, with almost every household in the country now having at least one mobile phone [13]. Even a normal SMS costs less than US$0.01 to send, and rates are even lower for computerized SMS packages.

Keeping our current study domain in mind, which has had a limited assessment in this regard in the past, we aim to assess the acceptability of SMS based interventions towards becoming future voluntary blood donors among medical university students of Karachi, Pakistan, so that a foundation may be laid in solving the solution of shortfall in a low income country like Pakistan. The secondary aim was to sensitize the medical student population regarding donating blood.

2. Methodology

2.1. Ethics Statement. The study has been approved by the Ethical Review Board of Dow University of Health Sciences. Each participant gave a written informed consent and all their information was kept confidential.

2.2. Sample Size. Using an estimated response distribution of 50%, as in previous studies [7, 14] conducted in other countries and a confidence interval of 95%, the sample size of this study was calculated to be a total of 350 medical students. A total of 432 participants were approached to participate in our study. 54 students were excluded for not meeting the respective inclusion criteria while 28 students declined to participate in the study.

2.3. Data Collection Process. The study was conducted amongst the two largest public sector medical universities of Karachi: Dow Medical College and Jinnah-Sindh Medical University from September 1, 2013, to September 30, 2013. Selection of these universities was based on the criteria of highest number of medical students studying in a single medical university in Karachi.

Coauthors of this study, who were also the data collectors, approached the participants at the study site. Limited availability of clinical years due to ward rotations and distributed schedules of nonclinical years made us choose nonprobability convenient sampling technique for this study. Each participant was initially assessed for eligibility criteria: participant should be a medical student currently enrolled in a 5-year

MBBS program at his/her university with an age of 18 or above and should not be a registered voluntary blood donor. Any participant that failed to meet all three criteria was excluded from the study.

Data collectors informed each participant of the study topic and its implications. Participants agreeing to take part gave a written informed consent. Data collectors then administered the questionnaire to each participant using an interview based format. Each data collector verbally read out close ended questions from the questionnaire to the participants in a private and secluded place and recorded their answer on the questionnaire. An average of 5–10 mins was taken by a data collector to interview one participant. At the end, each participant was thanked and assured of complete confidentiality.

2.4. Questionnaire. Using template questions of Giri and Phalke's [7] questionnaire, we modified and designed a self-made questionnaire based on Pakistani blood bank settings for our study. The questionnaire was divided into four different sections.

(i) *General Blood Donation Knowledge.* This section assessed the familiarity of medical students regarding blood donations and working of blood banks in Pakistan.

(ii) *Personal Blood Donation Attitude/Practices.* This section assessed personal approach of each medical student regarding previously donated blood, reasons of donating blood/not donating blood, fear of donating blood, and whether they would like to donate blood anytime in the future.

(iii) *Implication of Being a Volunteer Blood Donor.* This section assessed the implications of medical students on becoming volunteer blood donors in Pakistan.

(iv) *Short Message Service Intervention.* This section evaluated the baseline characteristics of Short Message Service and acceptability of participants towards any Short Message Service interventional studies to become voluntary blood donors in the future.

Close ended questions comprised the majority and important part of the questionnaire with multiple choice answers (yes, no, and maybe).

2.5. Statistical Analysis. All the data was recorded in a structured compilation sheet and analyzed through application of statistical tools of analysis. A descriptive statistical analysis was carried out on SPSS 16 software with mean, mode, and standard deviations calculated.

3. Results

350 participants, having a mean age of 21.47 ± 1.36, were included in our study with 30.6% (107/350) being males and 69.4% (243/350) being females.

The first component of our questionnaire dealt with knowledge of Pakistani blood bank working and blood donations (Table 1). 95.1% (333/350) participants were familiar

TABLE 1: Knowledge of Pakistani blood banks and blood donations.

Question	Correct answer, n (%)	Wrong answer, n (%)	Did not know, n (%)
Weight criterion permitted in Pakistan	219 (62.6)	93 (26.6)	38 (10.8)
Compatibility of blood Transfusions	333 (95.1)	17 (4.1)	—
Screening by blood banks	316 (90.3)	34 (9.7)	—
Amount of donated blood permitted in Pakistan	129 (36.9)	95 (27.2)	126 (36)
Maximum components from a single donation	149 (42.6)	140 (40)	61 (17.4)
Number of days for discarding unutilized blood products in Pakistan	94 (26.9)	230 (65.7)	26 (7.4)
Time duration to redonate blood in Pakistan	220 (62.9)	110 (31.4)	20 (5.7)
Type of blood component commonly utilized in Pakistan	225 (64.3)	107 (30.5)	18 (5.2)

about the compatibility of different blood transfusions while 90.3% (316/350) participants were aware of screening by blood banks. 62.9% (220/350) participants knew the right time permitted to redonate blood in Pakistan whereas 62.6% (219/350) participants knew that 50 kg was the borderline weight criterion for donating blood in Pakistan. Only 36.9% (129/350) participants knew that 450 mL blood is donated by a volunteer in Pakistan while 36% (126/350) participants did not have any idea. Similarly, knowledge of discarding unutilized blood products was low as well with 38.9% (136/350) participants having no clue and 34.2% (230/350) giving a wrong answer.

Our second component dealt with attitude and personal practices among the participants regarding donating blood. 93.4% (327/350) participants agreed that donating blood was healthy. A large number of the participants, 74% (259/350), had never donated blood in their life. Assessment of reasons for not donating blood found that 47.6% (123/259) did not fit blood donation criteria followed by 24.7% (64/259) who did not feel like donating. The rest of the participants never thought of donating.

Genderwise, 206/243 (84.8%) females did not donate blood in comparison to 53/107 (49.5%) males. The majority of the females, 53.3% (110/206), did not donate blood as they did not completely fit the blood donation criteria while 52.8% (28/53) of the males did not donate blood as they did not feel like donating. However, 60% (155/259) of the participants agreed to become voluntary blood donors through any sort of intervention.

Only 26% (91/350) participants were first time donors. Assessment of reasons among the first time donors found that 79.1% (72/91) had donated as replacement donors with the rest of them (19/91) as paid for donors. Furthermore, 87.9% (80/91) of these participants agreed to become regular voluntary blood donors if given an initiative, reminder, or boost.

Fear of donating blood was kept as a separate entity in our study. 68.6% (240/350) participants had no fear of donating blood while 31.4% (110/350) did have a fear. Evaluation of the reasons for fear among these 110 participants found that 36.36% (40/110) of the participants had a fear of needle prick followed by 33.6% (37/103) participants fearing that they would feel weak.

Genderwise, 71% (78/110) of the females had a fear of donating blood in comparison to 29% (32/110) of the males. Needle prick was the major fear factor for 38.4% (30/78)

TABLE 2: Implications of knowing and becoming a voluntary blood donor.

Implications	Yes n (%)	No n (%)
Definition of voluntary blood donor	329 (94)	21 (6)
Asking family relatives/replacement donors to donate blood	317 (90.6)	33 (9.4)
Blood banks pay voluntary blood donors in Pakistan	265 (75.7)	85 (24.3)
Incentives should be given to voluntary blood donors in Pakistan	187 (53.4)	163 (46.6)
Maintaining a registry by blood banks of voluntary blood donors	328 (96.6)	12 (3.4)

females not donating blood. 31.25% (10/32) of the males had a fear of needle prick with 31.25% (10/32) males also having a fear of feeling weak after donating. However, 88.3% (91/110) participants agreed to take part in an intervention to help remove the fear and become voluntary blood donors.

The third component of our study dealt with implications of knowing and becoming a voluntary blood donor in Pakistan (Table 2).

The last and most important component of our study dealt with acceptability and baseline characteristics in taking part in Short Message Service based interventions. Among baseline characteristics, 98.9% (346/350) participants had a cell phone and 96.9% (339/350) were comfortable using SMS (Table 3).

65.7% (230/350) of the total participants agreed to take part in SMS based behavioral interventions to become voluntary blood donors. The intervention could be related to removal of fear, promoting knowledge, or any other reason that may help the individual to donate blood voluntarily. 69.7% (244/350) of the participants gave a desirable answer that SMS reminders can remind and encourage them to donate blood more often. However, 40% (140/350) of the participants wanted an incentive (cash) to take part in such interventions to become future voluntary blood donors (Table 4).

4. Discussion

Over the last few decades, knowledge, attitudes, and decision making practices with regard to voluntary blood donation

TABLE 3: Baseline characteristics of participants for Short Message Service intervention.

Question	Answer (n)
Having a cell phone	(i) Yes = 346 (ii) No = 4 Total = **350**
Comfortable using SMS	(i) Yes = 339 (ii) No = 11 Total = **350**
Time of day comfortable receiving SMS	(i) Morning = 27 (ii) Afternoon = 32 (iii) Evening = 69 (iv) Night = 42 (v) Anytime = 180 Total = **350**
Language you wish to receive SMS	(i) English = 228 (ii) Urdu = 30 (iii) Roman Urdu = 92 Total = **350**

TABLE 4: Acceptability of taking part in SMS based interventions.

	Yes n (%)	No n (%)
Behavioral intervention	230 (65.7)	120 (34.3)
Blood donation reminder intervention	244 (69.7)	106 (30.3)
Want an incentive to take part	140 (40)	210 (60)

have been assessed in order to develop a better understanding of the process, so that donation efficiency, safety, retention, collection numbers, and donor pool diversity may be effectively regulated. In our current setup, results of our study act as pivotal tool in bringing about further improvements in future blood donation practices.

While knowledge of blood bank working and practices is not a major determinant in donor motivation [15], knowledge of donating blood among donors is an essential aspect for donor recruitment, especially volunteer donors [16]. The literature reveals that medical students are justifiably expected to have better knowledge of both blood donations and blood banks than other groups in society [15]. Our study reported medical students having an overall mixed approach on both aspects. Parts like screening and blood group compatibility had better results while amount of blood donated and discarding blood products showed low results. Overall, the results were below par in comparison to studies conducted in Greece and India [17, 18] but conformed more towards Alam and El Din Masalmeh's study in Saudi Arabia [19]. It is, however, important to note that all three aforementioned studies were done amongst the general population. Even Sabu et al.'s study on Indian medical students concluded much better results [20]. Such poor knowledge among Pakistani medical students acts as a major hindrance for voluntary blood donation.

93.4% of the participants deemed blood donation to be a healthy and positive practice, but only 26% students had actually ever donated blood. 15.2% of the Pakistani medical students in Siddiqui et al.'s study and 23% of the Pakistani

medical students in Khan et al.'s study reported the same practice [14, 21]. Almost all medical students in both studies were also aware that donating blood was healthy. Similar studies conducted upon university students of other developing countries like Thailand, Iran, and India have also revealed similarly low donor percentages [1, 20, 22]. Shah et al.'s decade old behavioral study on Dhaka University students showed corresponding outcomes to our study as well [23]. This goes on to prove that while technology is soaring sky high with each passing day, behavioral patterns continue to remain stagnated, therefore highlighting a dire need for effective and motivational donor recruitment programs.

Careful assessment of factors which hinder a process is a key player in reaching a solution and formed a substantial portion of our study results. Among the nondonor respondents, the majority did not fit the blood donation criteria, comprising mostly females. The ratio of female students studying in Pakistani Medical Universities is very high as compared to male students. A similar finding was suggested by Hosain et al. [24]. Male participants, who did not donate, admitted that they did not feel like donating, reflecting a clear sense of nonchalance and lack of stimulation as compared to their female counterparts who wanted to donate but were not eligible to do so. These factors exhibit a high likeability to previous studies in Pakistan and other developing countries [21, 25, 26]. However, one South Indian study showed no statistical difference between gender and attitude toward donating blood [20].

The literature review has also explicitly unveiled fear as a colossal reason which hinders all types of potential donors from donating blood. Out of the 31.4% respondents who nurtured a fear, the majority hailed from amidst the female gender. Reasons of fear elicited were risk of catching infection and weakness after donating. However, fear of needle prick was the most popular response, comparable to Siddiqui et al.' study [14] as well as other studies on medical students [20, 25]. Much of this fear is reported to have escalated ever since HIV took over the global health scene by storm, sowing the seeds for apprehension among the already reluctant populace.

But despite low percentages reported in knowledge, attitude, and practices of our study and other studies in Pakistan, Siddiqui et al. suggested that medical students in Pakistan still comprise the major portion of regular voluntary donors and are more likely to be driven by altruism and humanitarian causes as compared to other groups in the donor pool [14]. This is clearly true, as 60% of nondonor respondents and 87.9% of first time donors in our study were willing to become regular voluntary blood donors through an intervention. Such health interventions for Pakistan will depend on accessibility, resourcefulness, cost, and time frame.

The dramatic rise of cellphone and SMS usage in Pakistan can be a solution to this problem. Baseline information of mobile phones in our study found that 98.9% participants had a cell phone and 96.9% were comfortable using SMS. These baseline results correlate with the information released by the Pakistan Telecommunication Authority (PTA). To date, almost every individual in Pakistan has at least one cellphone [13]. Furthermore, in 2011, an average of 250 daily texts was sent by an individual in Pakistan [13]. Such statistics prove that mobile phone usage in Pakistan has penetrated all levels of society, especially the lower class. A foundation to potentiate many other different types of SMS based health interventions in Pakistan can be based on this data.

A behavioral intervention is defined as improving or modifying a behavior for a positive impact. In our study, SMS behavioral interventions would aim at helping remove fear or improving knowledge by removing any taboo or misconception via SMS. 65.7% of the participants agreed to be part of such SMS based behavioral interventions indicating a positive attitude. Gombachika and Monawe's study among the general population of Malawi also indicated a positive attitude towards SMS based behavioral interventions [27]. Low lying, cheap, and accessible technology of mobile phones can easily be used by developing countries like Pakistan and Malawi to initiate SMS based interventions in improving blood donations.

SMS reminders for blood donation are also currently in use in many blood banks of developing countries including India [28]. 69.7% respondents of our study were affirmative in receiving SMS blood donation reminders. Fung et al.'s study stated better attendance rates amongst American donors who received SMS reminders, hence proving the effectiveness of SMS reminders [29]. SMS reminders can tackle the "nobody told me to donate" respondents and first time donors by continuous encouragement to them to donate. Blood banks can be made responsible for sending tailored SMS to the people and in turn use this data in developing a registry of voluntary blood donors that currently does not exist in Pakistan.

There are several limitations to our study. First of all, our study was limited to only a certain population that could read SMS. SMS based interventions will only work among those who can read SMS. This will rule out a large major portion of the population that is illiterate. Secondly, these SMS based interventions may become gender biased towards males. Females in Pakistan mostly do not donate blood due to blood donation criteria that cannot be changed by an intervention.

5. Conclusion

There is still major workup needed to create more awareness about blood donation among medical students keeping in mind their future professional link to it. We recommend inclusion of such awareness programs as part of curriculum of medical students. However, pertaining to attitude and practices, there are positive outcomes with high acceptability among medical students to take part in SMS based interventions to become voluntary blood donors. If proper authorities, especially blood banks, work on these interventions, a larger pool of voluntary blood donors in Pakistan can be built.

Conflict of Interests

The authors declare that there is no conflict of interests regarding the publication of this paper.

References

[1] H. Safizadeh, N. Pourdamghan, and B. Mohamadi, "University students awareness and attitude towards blood donation in Kerman City," *Iranian Journal of Blood and Cancer*, vol. 1, no. 3, pp. 107–110, 2009.

[2] WHO, *Towards 100% Voluntary Blood Donation: A Global Framework for Action*, WHO, 2013.

[3] "Pakistan suffering from lack of blood donors: seminar told," http://www.dawn.com/news/1011774/pakistan-suffering-from-lack-of-blood-donors-seminar-told.

[4] H. Bönig, M. Schmidt, K. Hourfar, J. Schüttrumpf, and E. Seifried, "Sufficient blood, safe blood: can we have both?" *BMC Medicine*, vol. 10, article 29, 2012.

[5] "70% blood donations in Pakistan are either replacement or paid for," http://www.thenews.com.pk/Todays-News-2-114368-70pc-of-blood-donations-in-Pakistan–are-either-replacement-or-paid-for.

[6] B. N. Sojka and P. Sojka, "The blood-donation experience: perceived physical, psychological and social impact of blood donation on the donor," *Vox Sanguinis*, vol. 84, no. 2, pp. 120–128, 2003.

[7] P. A. Giri and D. B. Phalke, "Knowledge and attitude about blood donation amongst undergraduate students of pravara institute of medical sciences deemed university of central India," *Annals of Tropical Medicine and Public Health*, vol. 5, no. 6, pp. 569–573, 2012.

[8] N. Zaller, K. E. Nelson, P. Ness, G. Wen, X. Bai, and H. Shan, "Knowledge, attitude and practice survey regarding blood donation in a Northwestern Chinese city," *Transfusion Medicine*, vol. 15, no. 4, pp. 277–286, 2005.

[9] Z. Awan, "Do mobile phones cause tumors?" *Journal of Pakistan Medical Students*, vol. 2, no. 2, pp. 64–67, 2012.

[10] M. Vervloet, L. van Dijk, J. Santen-Reestman, B. van Vlijmen, M. L. Bouvy, and D. H. de Bakker, "Improving medication adherence in diabetes type 2 patients through real time medication monitoring: a randomised controlled trial to evaluate the effect of monitoring patients' medication use combined with short message service (SMS) reminders," *BMC Health Services Research*, vol. 11, article 5, 2011.

[11] C. Pop-Eleches, H. Thirumurthy, J. P. Habyarimana et al., "Mobile phone technologies improve adherence to antiretroviral treatment in a resource-limited setting: a randomized controlled trial of text message reminders," *AIDS*, vol. 25, no. 6, pp. 825–834, 2011.

[12] G. Eysenbach, "CONSORT-EHEALTH: improving and standardizing evaluation reports of Web-based and mobile health interventions," *Journal of Medical Internet Research*, vol. 13, no. 4, article e126, 2011.

[13] "Pakistan Telecommunication authority," http://www.pta.gov.pk/index.php?option=com_content&view=article&id=269:telecom-indicators&catid=124:industry-report&Itemid=599.

[14] U. F. Siddiqui, A. Yasmeen, N. Hina, and S. N. Alam, "Who donates more; medical or non-medical Students?" *Journal of the Dow University of Health Sciences*, vol. 6, no. 1, pp. 17–21, 2012.

[15] P. London and B. M. Hemphill, "The motivations of blood donors." *Transfusion*, vol. 5, no. 6, pp. 559–568, 1965.

[16] L. Kasraian and M. Maghsudlu, "Blood donors' attitudes towards incentives: influence on motivation to donate," *Blood Transfusion*, vol. 10, no. 2, pp. 186–190, 2012.

[17] O. Marantidou, L. Loukopoulou, E. Zervou et al., "Factors that motivate and hinder blood donation in Greece," *Transfusion Medicine*, vol. 17, no. 6, pp. 443–450, 2007.

[18] N. Shenga, R. Pal, and S. Sengupta, "Behavior disparities towards blood donation in Sikkim, India," *Asian Journal of Transfusion Science*, vol. 2, no. 2, pp. 56–60, 2008.

[19] M. Alam and B. El Din Masalmeh, "Knowledge, attitudes and practices regarding blood donation among the Saudi population," *Saudi Medical Journal*, vol. 25, no. 3, pp. 318–321, 2004.

[20] K. Sabu, A. Remya, V. S. Binu, and R. Vivek, "Knowledge, attitude and practice on blood donation among health science students in a University campus, South India," *Online Journal of Health and Allied Sciences*, vol. 10, no. 2, article 6, 2011.

[21] "Blood Donation among medical students: Knowledge, Attitude and Practices," http://www.researchgate.net/publication/224982224_Blood_Donation_among_Medical_Students_Knowledge_Attitude_and_Practices.

[22] V. Wiwanitkit, "Knowledge about blood donation among a sample of Thai university students," *Vox Sanguinis*, vol. 83, no. 2, pp. 97–99, 2002.

[23] M. Shah, S. Hasan, S. Malik, and C. T. Sreeramareddy, "Perceived stress, sources and severity of stress among medical undergraduates in a Pakistani medical school," *BMC Medical Education*, vol. 10, no. 1, article 2, 2010.

[24] G. M. Hosain, M. Anisuzzaman, and A. Begum, "Knowledge and attitude towards voluntary blood donation among Dhaka University students in Bangladesh," *East African Medical Journal*, vol. 74, no. 9, pp. 549–553, 1997.

[25] A. Agrawal, A. K. Tiwari, A. Ahuja, and R. Kalra, "Knowledge, attitude and practices of people towards voluntary blood donation in Uttarakhand," *Asian Journal of Transfusion Science*, vol. 7, no. 1, pp. 59–62, 2013.

[26] S. Uma, R. Arun, and P. Arumugam, "The knowledge, attitude and practice towards blood donation among voluntary blood donors in Chennai, India," *Journal of Clinical and Diagnostic Research*, vol. 7, no. 6, pp. 1043–1046, 2013.

[27] H. Gombachika and M. Monawe, "Correlation analysis of attitudes towards SMS technology and blood donation behaviour in Malawi," in *Proceedings of the 3rd International ICST Conference (AFRICOMM '11)*, pp. 239–247, 2011.

[28] "Donate, receive blood via SMS," http://articles.timesofindia.indiatimes.com/2011-06-13/pune/29652354_1_blood-donors-voluntary-donors-blood-banks.

[29] M. K. Fung, B. Briggs, and A. Frascoia, "The effects of text message reminder on blood donor show rate," *Transfusion*, vol. 49, Abstract SP34, p. 65A, 2009.

16

Prevalence and Incidence of Syphilis among Volunteer Blood Donors in Israel

Leibovici Vera,[1] Donchin Milka,[2] Strauss-Liviatan Nurith,[3] and Shinar Eilat[4]

[1] *Department of Dermatology, Hadassah-Hebrew University Hospital, P.O. Box 12018, Jersalem, Israel*
[2] *Brown School of Public Health, Hadassah University Hospital, Jersalem, Israel*
[3] *Private Practice, P.O. Box 84027, 90805 Mevaseret Zion, Israel*
[4] *Magen David Adom National Blood Services, 52621 Ramat Gan, Israel*

Correspondence should be addressed to Leibovici Vera; vleibovici@hadassah.org.il

Academic Editor: Rajendra Chaudhary

Data of 1,290,222 volunteer blood donors, in a 5-year period, was analyzed for prevalence and incidence of syphilis. Subsequent testing of donations positive in *Treponema pallidum* hemagglutination assay included Venereal Disease Research Laboratory and fluorescent Treponemal antibody absorption. Stepwise logistic regression model was used to identify positive syphilis serology. Prevalence of syphilis was 47 : 100,000, similar in men and women and increased significantly with age ($P < 0.001$). Native Israelis had the lowest prevalence rate of syphilis (21 : 100,000), while a significantly higher prevalence was found among immigrants from Africa, Eastern Europe, and South America (odds ratios of 19.0, 10.8, and 7.3, resp., $P < 0.001$ for each). About 33.2% of the seropositive donors had evidence of recent infection, and 66.8% had past infections. Incidence rate reached 8 : 100,000 person-years. Coinfection with HIV, HCV, and HBV was calculated as 8%, 1.88%, and 0.37% for positive donations, respectively. The data support the need to continue screening blood donors in Israel for syphilis and employ preventive measures to populations at risk, in order to improve public health, blood safety, and quality. A subsequent study to assess blood donors' knowledge, attitude, and behavior is planned. In times of global migration this information may be useful to blood services worldwide.

1. Introduction

Syphilis is a sexually transmitted disease (STD) caused by *Treponema pallidum*, which can also be transmitted via accidental direct inoculation, transplacenta during pregnancy, and, rarely, via blood transfusion [1, 2].

Although the value of routine serologic screening of blood donors for syphilis has been a question in debate for years [3–5], and refrigerated blood components are less infective for syphilis, transmissions through blood components still occur [6]. Therefore, standard operating procedures of blood establishments worldwide include demands/recommendations for such screening [7, 8]. New draft guidance for screening, testing, and management of blood donors and components was recently distributed by the FDA [9].

In many parts of the world, the incidence and prevalence of syphilis still remain high in both volunteer and family/replacement blood donors [10–15]. There are numerous reports in high-risk groups in the literature, both from developed and developing countries, indicating rising prevalence and incidence of syphilis [16–20].

In Israel, screening tests for syphilis are conducted in community STD clinics for the general and high-risk populations, by the National Blood Services on each blood unit donated (all collected from volunteer blood donors), and also in all pregnant women. Confirmatory tests for all positive samples are performed exclusively by the Central National Reference Laboratory for Venereal Diseases of the Ministry of Health (MOH), thus forming a national registry for surveillance and followup.

Data reported by the Israeli MOH to the WHO regional office in Europe showed that the incidence of syphilis in the general population in Israel was 2.52, 5.8, and a low 0.7 per 100,000 in 1996, 2001, and 2005, respectively [21]. Although the incidence of syphilis in Israel in the general population in 2005 was rather low, further reports between 2004 and 2009

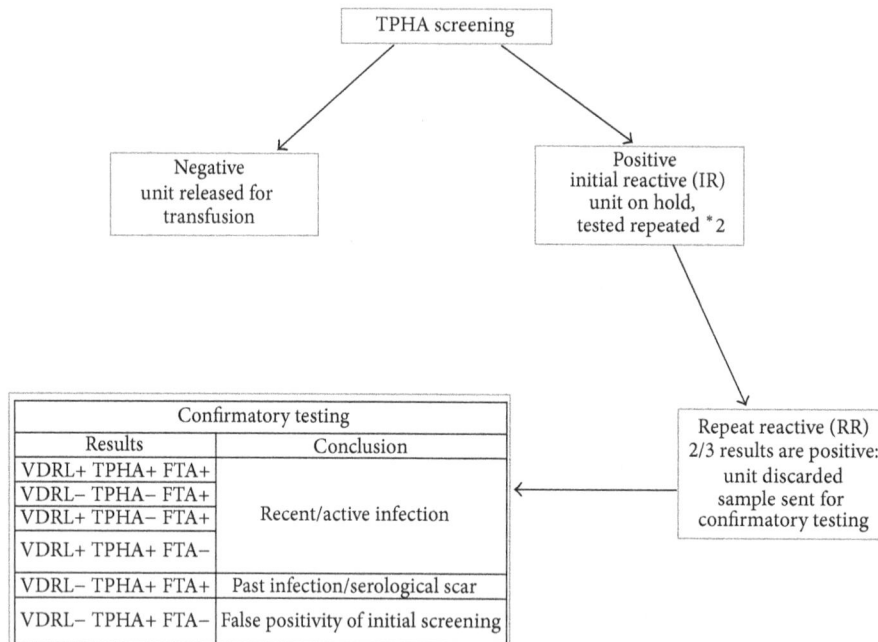

FIGURE 1: Algorithm for syphilis screening and confirmatory testing.

in people with high-risk sexual behavior show an increase of the prevalence and incidence of syphilis in this specific group [22–25]. We studied the prevalence and incidence of syphilis and coinfection with other transfusion-transmitted diseases in volunteer blood donors of the Israeli National Magen David Adom Blood Services (MDABS) during 2005–2009 to assess the determinants of this sexually transmitted disease in this selected population.

2. Materials and Methods

2.1. Study Population. All blood donors in Israel are non-remunerated volunteers. Units are collected throughout the country in mobile vehicles or in fixed-site donor rooms. Before donation each potential donor fills a detailed health history questionnaire, which includes data regarding age, gender, country of birth, and year of immigration (if applicable), and questions concerning the donor's general health, lifestyle and risk behavior, followed by a short private interview, blood pressure and hemoglobin determination, and physical examination. Donors may be disqualified and deferred from donating based on their written and verbal answers or on previous information in the MDABS database. Relevant deferral criteria include, among others, permanent deferral for known HIV or hepatitis, by past testing or self-report, men who have had sex with men (MSM) since 1977, and people who have been given money for sex (sex workers). A 12-month temporary deferral includes donors who were treated for syphilis or gonorrhea within the previous year and those who had sex with people mentioned above [7]. The study was carried out using the computerized database of MDA Blood Services donors' records for the period 2005–2009.

2.2. Laboratory Tests

2.2.1. Screening for Syphilis (see Figure 1). Tests were done using a specific serological *Treponema Pallidum* hemagglutination assay (TPHA) of Biokit-Syphagen TPHA autoindirect hemagglutination test (Biokit, Barcelona, Spain), performed on Olympus PK 7200 blood-typing equipment (Olympus, Japan). Each initial reactive sample was further tested in duplicate, according to the manufacturer's instructions. If two out of three results were positive (Repeat Reactive), the unit was discarded and the sample was sent to the National Reference Laboratory for Venereal Diseases of the Israeli Ministry of Health for serological confirmation testing using a different TPHA hemagglutination assay, the nonspecific treponemal assay Venereal Disease Research Laboratory (VDRL), using BD VDRL Antigen (Becton Dickinson, USA), and fluorescent Treponemal absorption test (FTA-ABS) with Trepo-Spot IF, Fluoline H (Biomerieux France).

According to the confirmatory results donors were defined as

(a) "Recent/Active Infection": if confirmatory results were one of the following: VDRL+ TPHA+ FTA+; VDRL− TPHA− FTA+; VDRL+ TPHA− FTA+ or VDRL+ TPHA+ FTA−, the donors have not been treated and therefore may be infectious [26];

(b) "Past Infection/Serological Scar": if confirmatory results were VDRL− TPHA+ FTA+

The test was defined as false positive when VDRL− TPHA+ and FTA−.

Prevalence was defined as the number of TPHA positive donors in the total donors' population. *Incidence* was defined as the number of new TPHA positive donors in the total donors' population. *Seroconversion* was defined when the

TABLE 1: Prevalence (%) of seropositive donors by gender, age, country of birth, and year of immigration.

Variable	Number of donations	Number of donors	Number of seropositives	Prevalence (%)	95% C.I. of prevalence
Total	1,290,222	606,549	283	0.0467	(0.0415, 0.0524)
Gender					
Men	945,653	417,475	189	0.0453	(0.0393, 0.0522)
Women	344,569	189,074	94	0.0497	(0.0406, 0.0608)
Age					
≤24	440,712	207,203	24	0.0116	(0.0078, 0.0172)
25–34	357,888	170,781	74	0.0433	0.0345, 0.0544
35–44	217,965	107,251	81	0.0755	(0.0608, 0.0938)
≥45	273,657	121,314	104	0.0857	(0.0708, 0.1039)
Country of origin					
Israel	1,022,071	474,140	101	0.0213	(0.0175, 0.0259)
Asia	29,423	14,580	17	0.1166	(0.0728, 0.1867)
Africa	9,921	5,047	9	0.1783	(0.0938, 0.3386)
USSR and Eastern Europe	141,894	70,766	136	0.1922	(0.1625, 0.2273)
Western Europe North America and Oceania	66,106	32,370	11	0.0340	(0.0190, 0.0608)
South America	19,159	8,863	9	0.1015	(0.0534, 0.1929)
Unknown	1,648	783	0		
Time of immigration					
Israeli born	1,022,071	474,140	101	0.0213	(0.0175, 0.0259)
<1990	109,483	47,774	39	0.0816	0.0597, 0.1116
≥1990	142,292	72,188	136	0.1884	(0.1593, 0.2228)
Unknown	16,376	12,447	7	0.0562	(0.0272, 0.1161)

current donation from a previously seronegative repeat donor gave a seropositive confirmed reaction.

2.2.2. Screening for Other Transfusion Transmitted Viruses. Tests were performed at MDABS laboratories using chemiluminescentimmunoassay for human immunodeficiency virus (HIV), hepatitis B (HBV), hepatitis C (HCV), and human T-lymphotropic virus (HTLV) (Prism, Abbott laboratories, USA), and Individual Unit Nucleic Acid Testing (ID-NAT) for HIV, HBV, and HCV using Procleix Ultrio (Novartis, USA).

2.3. Statistical Analyses. Seroprevalence was defined as the proportion of donors serologically confirmed as positives from the total number of donors and was given with 95% confidence intervals.

The seroconversion rate per 100,000 person-years was calculated by the number of donors who seroconverted, divided by the total number of person-years between consecutive donations, multiplied by 100,000.

Proportion comparisons were performed with the normal approximation. The chi-square test was used to test the association between categorical variables.

Two models of stepwise logistic regression were used to investigate which variables are associated with total seropositivity (Yes/No) and with recent infection (Yes/No).

We estimated the models with the following explanatory variables: age, country of birth (grouped into Israeli-born, East Europe, and former USSR countries, West Europe, North America, and Oceania, Africa, Asia, and South America), year of immigration (equals 1 for immigration year ≥ 1990 and 0 before 1990), and the 2-way interactions between immigration year and country group. Country group was a categorical variable, with Israel as the reference category to each of the other five country groups. We used the forward conditional method for variable selection. The final models are presented. *P* values are given for the significant variables, and estimates of the odds ratios with their corresponding 95% confidence intervals are given.

3. Results

Data for analysis included a total of 1,290,222 valid blood donations, collected from 605,549 donors, with an average of 2.1 units/donor (range 1–57). About 69% of the donors were men and 31% were women. Median age was 29, ranging from 17 to 70 years. Mean age of the donors was 33 ± 12.4 years. About 79% of the blood donors were born in Israel, and 21% had emigrated from different countries (Table 1).

Out of the 605,549 volunteers who donated blood in 2005–2009, 283 were seropositive, indicating a prevalence of 47 per 100,000. Prevalence rates of all the syphilis seropositive

TABLE 2: Distribution of donors with recent versus past syphilis by country of origin, age, and time of immigration.

	Active infection	Past infection	Total
Country of origin			
Total	**94 (100%)**	**189 (100%)**	**283 (100%)**
Israel	36 (38.3%)	65 (34.4%)	**101 (35.7%)**
Asia	8 (8.5%)	9 (4.8%)	**17 (6.0%)**
Africa	4 (4.3%)	5 (2.6%)	**9 (3.2%)**
USSR and Eastern Europe	39 (41.5%)	97 (51.3%)	**136 (48.1%)**
Western Europe North America and Oceania	4 (4.3%)	7 (3.7%)	**11 (3.9%)**
South America	3 (3.2%)	6 (3.2%)	**9 (3.2%)**
Age (years)			
≤24	9 (9.6%)	15 (7.9%)	**24 (8.5%)**
25–34	23 (24.5%)	51 (27.0%)	**74 (26.1%)**
35–44	28 (29.8%)	53 (28.0%)	**81 (28.6%)**
≥45	34 (36.2%)	70 (37.0%)	**104 (36.7%)**
Year of immigration			
<1990	15 (16.1%)	24 (13.1%)	**39 (14.1%)**
≥1990	42 (45.2%)	94 (51.4%)	**136 (49.3%)**
Israeli born	36 (38.7%)	65 (35.5%)	**101 (36.6%)**

donors (with both recent and past infection) analyzed by gender, age, country of origin, and time of immigration to Israel are depicted in Table 1.

Men and women had similar prevalence rates of syphilis of 45 and 49 per 100,000, respectively. There was a significant increase ($P < 0.001$) in the prevalence rate of syphilis with age: donors age 45 years and older, who donated about one-fifth of the total number of units, comprised 36.7% of the seropositives. Prevalence rates were 7.4, 6.5, and 3.7 times higher in donors age 45 or older, 35–44, and 25–35, respectively, compared to ≤24 years.

When analyzed by country of origin, the highest rates of seropositivity were detected in donors born in Eastern Europe and Africa (192 per 100,000 and 178 per 100,000, resp.), when compared to native Israeli.

Ninety-four of the 283 seropositive donors (33%) were diagnosed as Recent Infections by the National Reference Laboratory for Venereal Diseases, and 189/283 (67%) were defined as Past Infection/Serological Scars. The distribution of seropositives between donors defined as recent or past infections was similar between the two groups (Table 2) including following a review of the donors' history and questionnaires.

The logistic regression model (Table 3) enables identification of the marginal contribution of the above determinants to the risk of seropositivity, both total and recent infection.

Age increased the risk of syphilis in the given population of blood donors (controlling for the other variables in the model). Every additional year of age adds 6% to the risk of either total seropositivity or recent infection (odds ratio = 1.06, $P < 0.001$). The interaction of immigration year (above and below 1990) and country of birth group was also significant. More specifically, new immigrants (immigration year

≥ 1990) from Africa, Eastern Europe, and South America had a significantly higher risk for syphilis (with odds ratios of 19.0, 10.8, and 7.3, resp., $P < 0.001$ for each) compared to the risk of Israeli-born donors and those who immigrated before 1990. Similar results are presented for the recent infection model.

Seroconversion was found in 51 donors, giving an incidence rate of 8 per 100,000 person-years. No significant differences were found when compared to the other seropositive donors, by the studied parameters.

Incidence by year is given in Figure 2.

Coinfection of seropositivity for syphilis with other transfusion-transmitted diseases was found: two out of 25 HIV-positive donors were seropositive for syphilis (8%), compared to 0.046% among the HIV-negative blood donors ($P < 0.001$). In addition, 0.37% and 1.88% of the seropositive donors for hepatitis B and C, respectively, were positive for syphilis, compared with 0.046 and 0.045% among the negative donors for these two hepatitis viruses ($P < 0.001$ for each test).

4. Discussion

Previous studies of the prevalence of syphilis in Israel mostly took place among people with high-risk sexual behavior, such as MSM or sex workers. Only in one study, reported in 2005 and conducted in a limited region, a low incidence of 0.7 cases of syphilis in 100,000 people was found [21].

The volunteer blood donors are considered a selective population, since they are prescreened for previous diseases and sexual behavior, both by the detailed questionnaire and during a discrete personal interview before donation. However, since blood donation is performed by all citizens,

TABLE 3: Odds ratio (OR) of the determinants of seropositivity for syphilis, total and recent infection—logistic regression models.

Variable	Total seropositivity						Recent infection					
	B-Coefficient in model	Standard error	Sig.	OR	95% C.I. for OR Lower	Upper	B-Coefficient in model	Standard error	Sig.	OR	95% C.I. for OR Lower	Upper
Age	0.055	0.004	<0.0001	1.06	1.047	1.065	0.054	0.008	<0.0001	1.06	1.040	1.072
Immigration Year 1990* Country Group			<0.0001						<0.0001			
Imm. Year 1990 by Country Group (Asia)	1.286	1.004	0.2004	3.62	0.505	25.906	2.295	1.011	0.0231	9.92	1.368	71.928
Imm. Year 1990 by Country Group (Africa)	2.944	0.419	<0.0001	19.00	8.360	43.168	3.256	0.596	<0.0001	25.94	8.068	83.412
Imm. Year 1990 by Country Group (Eastern Europe)	2.381	0.127	<0.0001	10.82	8.442	13.870	2.101	0.226	<0.0001	8.17	5.244	12.731
Imm. Year 1990 by Country Group (Western Europe)	−0.711	1.004	0.4789	0.49	0.069	3.514	0.297	1.011	0.7687	1.35	0.186	9.757
Imm. Year 1990 by Country Group (South America)	1.991	0.456	<0.0001	7.32	2.994	17.912	2.487	0.596	<0.0001	12.02	3.738	38.677

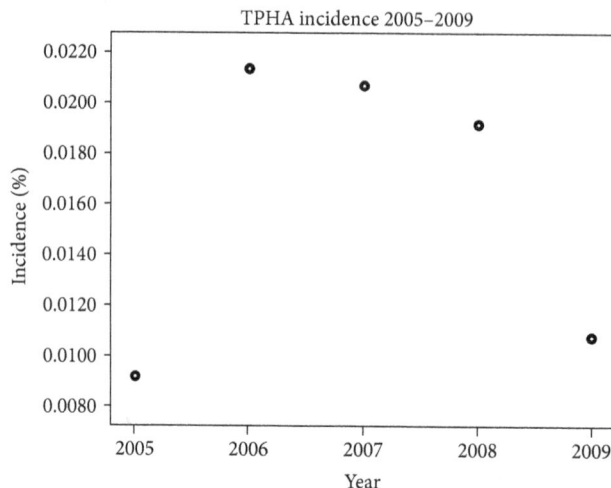

FIGURE 2: Incidence of TPHA seropositivity during the study period.

it could provide an updated picture about incidence and prevalence of syphilis in this population.

Data obtained during the period 2005–2009 show a prevalence of 47 per 100,000, of which 33% were diagnosed as recently infected and 67% were defined as past infection/ "serological scars." In addition, an incidence of 8 per 100,000 person-years was detected, which is an 11.4-fold increase since 2005.

Three major variables in our study had statistically significant impact on the risk of seropositivity (either for the entire group or for recent infection): age of the donors, their country of origin, and the time of immigration to Israel.

Age. The prevalence rates of syphilis increased with age.

Donors. The 35–44 year age group and those older than 45 years had a 6.5-fold and 7.4-fold higher prevalence of syphilis, respectively, when compared to the younger donors (aged 24 years or less). This is in agreement with others with similar findings among blood donors (18) or who described an increase of primary and secondary syphilis in older adults in the USA [27, 28].

Country of Origin and Oime of Immigration. Israel is a country that absorbs Jewish immigrants from all over the world. In particular, from 1990 to 2001 more than 900,000 immigrants came to the country (13% of the total Israeli population), mostly from the former Soviet Union and from Africa [29].

Our study revealed that the new immigrants from Africa and from Eastern Europe who arrived in Israel after 1990 had a 19-fold and 10.8-fold (resp.) higher risk for syphilis seropositivity than donors born in Israel. The findings were similar to the prevalence in their countries of origin, as reported by the Israeli MOH [30] and the 2001 WHO European Health database [21]. These results are in accordance with the high incidence of syphilis in the former communist countries of Eastern Europe, with rates of 262, 245, and 150 cases per 100,000 in the Russian Federation, Kazakhstan and Ukraine, respectively [21], and with data published from Africa in 2001, with infection rates of 1000, 300–400, and 100–200 cases per 100,000 found in Zambia, Kenya, and Benin, respectively [31].

The study also depicted an association between syphilis and other transfusion-transmitted diseases such as HIV, hepatitis B, and C, when compared to the donor population that was seronegative for syphilis, and it concurred with our previous observations of higher prevalence of hepatitis C among blood donors who immigrated to Israel from the former USSR [32].

It is worth mentioning that about 62% of the units were donated by native Israelis, with the lowest risk for recent infection, thus contributing to the safety of the national inventory.

In view of the ongoing discussion regarding the recent FDA's draft Recommendation for Screening, Testing and Management of Blood Donors, and Blood Components Based on Screening Tests for Syphilis [9], our findings demonstrate that screening for syphilis may still retain certain value in Israel and should be considered in some other regions in the world, depending on their blood donors' epidemiology data.

Given the high prevalence of syphilis in Israel allied with active immigration, special attention should be invested in targeting preventive measures to the blood donor populations and populations at risk. A future study is planned to assess the knowledge, attitude, and behavior of the volunteer blood donors' population. These measures will most probably improve public health and increase blood safety and quality.

In times of global migration the reported information may be useful to blood services worldwide.

Conflict of Interests

The authors declare that there is no conflict of interests regarding the publication of this paper.

Acknowledgments

The authors express our gratitude to Mrs. Becky Rubin for preparing the data set and to Dr. Veronica Gendelman, from MDA Blood Services.

References

[1] E. Van Dyck, R. Musonda, L. Zekeng et al., "Study Group on Heterogeneity of HIV Epidemics in Zeltser R, Kurban AK. Syphilis," *Clinics in Dermatology*, vol. 22, pp. 461–468, 2004.

[2] C. Gardella, A. A. Marfin, R. H. Kahn, E. Swint, and L. E. Markowitz, "Persons with early syphilis identified through blood or plasma donation screening in the United States," *Journal of Infectious Diseases*, vol. 185, no. 4, pp. 545–549, 2002.

[3] J. Case, "Serologic test for syphilis: a discredited surrogate test for HIV infection," *Transfusion*, vol. 38, no. 2, p. 218, 1998.

[4] S. Orton, "Syphilis and blood donors: what we know, what we do not know, and what we need to know," *Transfusion Medicine Reviews*, vol. 15, no. 4, pp. 282–291, 2001.

[5] L. M. Katz, "A test that won't die: the serologic test for syphilis," *Transfusion*, vol. 49, no. 4, pp. 617–619, 2009.

[6] S. Attaullah, S. Khan, and J. Khan, "Trend of transfusion transmitted infections frequency in blood donors: provide a road map for its prevention and control," *Journal of Translational Medicine*, vol. 10, no. 1, article 20, 2012.

[7] *Standards for Blood Banks and Transfusion Services*, AABB, 28th edition, 2012.

[8] Guide for the Preparation: Recommendation for Screening, *Testing and Management of Blood Donors and Blood Components Based on Screening Tests for Syphilis*, European Directorate for the Quality of Medicines and Healthcare, 16th edition, 2011.

[9] Guidance for the Industry: Recommendation for Screening, *Testing and Management of Blood Donors and Blood Components Based on Screening Tests For Syphilis*, FDA, CBER, 2013.

[10] M. L. K. Mogtomo, S. L. Fomekong, H. F. Kuate, and A. N. Ngane, "Screening of infectious microorganisms in blood banks in Douala (1995-2004)," *Cahiers Sante*, vol. 19, no. 1, pp. 1–8, 2009.

[11] S. Zou, E. P. Notari, C. T. Fang, S. L. Stramer, and R. Y. Dodd, "Current value of serologic test for syphilis as a surrogate marker for blood-borne viral infections among blood donors in the United States," *Transfusion*, vol. 49, no. 4, pp. 655–661, 2009.

[12] J. Liu, Y. Huang, J. Wang et al., "The increasing prevalence of serologic markers for syphilis among Chinese blood donors in 2008 through 2010 during a syphilis epidemic," *Transfusion*, vol. 52, pp. 1741–1749, 2012.

[13] Z. H. Ji, C. Y. Li, Y. G. Lv et al., "The prevalence and trends of transfusion-transmissible infectious pathogens among first-time, voluntary blood donors in Xi'an, China between 1999 and 2009," *International Journal of Infectious Diseases*, vol. 17, pp. 259–262, 2013.

[14] J. J. Noubiap, W. Y. Joko, J. R. Nansseu, U. G. Tene, and C. Siaka, "Sero-epidemiology of human immunodeficiency virus, hepatitis B and C viruses, and syphilis infections among first-time blood donors in Edéa, Cameroon," *International Journal of Infectious Diseases*, vol. 17, no. 10, pp. e832–e837, 2013.

[15] S. L. Gottlieb, V. Pope, M. R. Sternberg et al., "Prevalence of syphilis seroreactivity in the United States: Data from the National Health and Nutrition Examination Surveys (NHANES) 2001-2004," *Sexually Transmitted Diseases*, vol. 35, no. 5, pp. 507–511, 2008.

[16] *Department of Health and Human Services Cf DCaP National Center For HIV, STD and TB Prevention*, Division of STD Prevention, 2005.

[17] P. Pathela, S. L. Braunstein, J. A. Schillinger, C. Shepard, M. Sweeney, and S. Blank, "Men who have sex with men have a 140-fold higher risk for newly diagnosed HIV and syphilis compared with heterosexual men in New York City," *Journal of Acquired Immune Deficiency Syndromes*, vol. 58, no. 4, pp. 408–416, 2011.

[18] K. Salado-Rasmussen, T. L. Katzenstein, J. Gerstoft et al., "Risk of HIV or second syphilis infection in Danish men with newly acquired syphilis in the period 2000—2010," *Sexually Transmitted Infections*, vol. 89, no. 5, pp. 372–376.

[19] E. Muldoon and F. Mulcahy, "Syphilis resurgence in Dublin, Ireland," *International Journal of STD and AIDS*, vol. 22, no. 9, pp. 493–497, 2011.

[20] C. Hao, H. Yan, H. Yang et al., "The incidence of syphilis, HIV and HCV and associated factors in a cohort of men who have sex with men in Nanjing, China," *Sexually Transmitted Infections*, vol. 87, no. 3, pp. 199–201, 2011.

[21] *WHO Meeting on Prospects For the Public Health Approach To the Prevention and Care of Sexually Transmitted Infections in Countries of Eastern Europe and Central Asia*, WHO European Health for All Database, 2001.

[22] E. Hefer, L. Rubin, I. Volovik, and S. Rishpon, "Sexually transmitted disease morbidity trends in the Haifa District during 2001-2004," *Harefuah*, vol. 146, no. 6, pp. 425–428, 2007.

[23] H. Joffe, E. Bamberger, S. Nurkin et al., "Sexually transmitted diseases amon patients with human immunodeficiency virus in Northern Israel," *Israel Medical Association Journal*, vol. 8, no. 5, pp. 333–336, 2006.

[24] Y. Linhart, T. Shohat, Z. Amitai et al., "Sexually transmitted infections among brothel-based sex workers in Tel-Aviv area, Israel: high prevalence of pharyngeal gonorrhoea," *International Journal of STD and AIDS*, vol. 19, no. 10, pp. 656–659, 2008.

[25] T. Brosh-Nissimov, Z. Mor, E. Avramovich et al., "Syphilis outbreak among men who have sex with men, Tel Aviv, Israel, 2008-2009," *Israel Medical Association Journal*, vol. 14, no. 3, pp. 152–156, 2012.

[26] S. Nesteroff, *RCPA Serology*, QAP, Serology, 2004.

[27] L. A. Jeffers and M. C. DiBartolo, "Raising health care provider awareness of sexually transmitted disease in patients over age 50," *Medsurg Nursing*, vol. 20, no. 6, pp. 285–290, 2011.

[28] J. Holden and L. Trachtman, "Increase in primary and secondary syphilis cases in older adults in Louisiana," *The Journal of the Louisiana State Medical Society*, vol. 163, no. 6, pp. 308–311, 2011.

[29] The Israeli Central Bureau of Statistics, *Immigrant Population From the Former USSR*, Demographic Trends, 2001.

[30] *Notifiable Infectious Diseases in Israel- 60 Years of Surveillance (1951-2010), Center For Disease Control (ICDC) and the Division of Epidemiology*, Public Health Services, The Israeli MOH, 2012.

[31] A. Buvé, H. A. Weiss, M. Laga et al., "The epidemiology of gonorrhoea, chlamydial infection and syphilis in four African cities," *AIDS*, vol. 15, no. 4, pp. S79–S88, 2001.

[32] H. Kerzman, M. S. Green, and E. Shinar, "Risk factors for hepatitis C virus infection among blood donors in Israel: a case-control study between native Israelis and immigrants from the former Soviet Union," *Transfusion*, vol. 47, no. 7, pp. 1189–1196, 2007.

17

Factors Associated with Intention to Donate Blood: Sociodemographic and Past Experience Variables

Pule Ishmael Pule, Boitshwarelo Rachaba, Mgaywa Gilbert Mjungu Damas Magafu, and Dereje Habte

Faculty of Medicine, University of Botswana, Private Bag 00713, Gaborone, Botswana

Correspondence should be addressed to Dereje Habte; derejehabte@yahoo.com

Academic Editor: Rajendra Chaudhary

Background and Objectives. This study was conducted to assess the level of intention of the general public towards blood donation and the factors associated with it. *Methods*. A descriptive cross-sectional study was conducted in South-East Botswana amongst participants aged 21–65 years. An interviewer-administered questionnaire was completed for 384 participants. *Results*. Of the 384 participants, 104 (27.1%) reported that they had donated blood in the past and 269 (70.1%) stated that they were willing to donate blood in the future. Thirteen out of the 104 past donors (12.5%) reported that they had donated blood in the 12 months preceding the survey and only 10 (9.6%) participants reported that they have been regular donors. In the backward logistic regression analysis, the variables that remained significant predictors of the intention to donate blood were secondary education (adjusted odds ratio (AOR) (95% confidence interval (CI)): 2.92 (1.48, 5.77)), tertiary education (AOR (95% CI): 3.83 (1.52, 9.62)), and knowing a family member who had ever donated blood (AOR (95% CI): 2.84 (1.58, 5.12)). *Conclusion*. Being informed about blood transfusion and its life-saving benefits through either the education system or the experience made people more likely to intend to donate blood. Evidence-based interventions to retain blood donors as regular donors are recommended.

1. Introduction

Blood transfusion is becoming a crucial component in the management of patients presenting with accident injuries, surgical conditions, malignancies, pregnancy complications, and other medical conditions [1, 2]. In high income countries, the major indications for transfusion include sophisticated medical and surgical procedures, malignancies, and trauma. Pregnancy complications and childhood anemia are the conditions that largely need blood transfusion in middle and low income countries. More than one-quarter of maternal deaths could be averted by having access to safe blood [2–4].

WHO estimates that at least 1% of the population needs to donate blood to meet the minimum requirement of blood for a country [1]. Globally, 70 countries have a blood donation level less than the optimal level of 10/1000 population [1]. The African continent managed to collect blood to satisfy only 41% of the demand in 2006 [5, 6]. The gap between supply and demand for blood is wider in developing and transitional countries than in developed counterparts [1, 2]. According to Botswana National Blood Transfusion Services (NBTS), the country needs 36,000 units of blood annually. Records show that 23,275 units of blood were collected in the year 2009 followed by a reduction to 20,401 units collected in 2010 and 16,562 units collected in 2011 (unpublished report by Botswana NBTS, 2012).

Altruism, social responsibility, peer influence, access to health communication, and knowledge about importance of blood donation are mentioned as some of the factors that motivate individuals to donate blood [7–12]. Transmission of values to generations among family members practicing donation and the influence of active blood donors on others are also noted [12, 13]. The retention of blood donors as regular donors is critical to ensure regular supply of blood which is influenced by a range of factors, namely, demographic, psychosocial, altruism, social obligation, prior donation frequency, satisfaction with the last donation experience, and behavioral factors [14–18].

Studies have demonstrated that the intention to donate blood predicts the practice of blood donation [18, 19]. Demographic, knowledge status, and behavioral factors are shown to determine individuals' intention to donate blood [20–22]. Hence, it is worthwhile to study the intention of community members for blood donation in Botswana to understand the situation and come up with evidence-based interventions. This study was conducted to assess the level of intention of the general public in South-East Botswana towards blood donation and the factors associated with the intention.

2. Methods

2.1. Study Site and Study Population. A descriptive cross-sectional study was conducted in Kweneng district in South-East Botswana. The population of the district was estimated to be 304,674 with a density of 6.4 people per square kilometer [23]. The study participants were recruited from Molepolole village which is the capital of Kweneng district with a population of 67,598 [23]. The study was conducted amongst members in the selected households in Molepolole. They were aged 21–65 years irrespective of gender.

2.2. Sample Size and Sampling. Epi-Info software version 3.5.3 (US CDC, Atlanta, Georgia) was utilized to compute the sample size. The proportion of the intention to donate blood was assumed to be 50% to attain the maximum sample size. With a margin of error of 5% at 5% level of significance, a sample size of 384 was determined. EPI-random walk method [24] was used to select the households. The starting point was selected at Kgosing, the office for local leaders (at the center of the village). A bottle was spun and households along the direction of the bottle top were included in the data collection. One eligible member in each selected household was interviewed until reaching the required sample size. If there were more than one eligible person in the selected household, only one randomly selected participant was included using lottery method.

2.3. Data Collection and Analysis. A questionnaire was developed in English after a thorough literature review to include the relevant variables. It was then pilot tested and validated. Two enumerators trained on the questionnaire collected the data. The principal investigators were involved in the supervision of the data collection. Data were collected between August 27 and September 21, 2012. In this study, a regular blood donor was a person who voluntarily donated blood routinely, that is, 2–4 times a year [1].

Data were entered using Epi-Info software version 3.5.3 and exported to SPSS version 20 (IBM, NY, USA) for analysis. Frequency, percentage, and mean were computed to describe the findings. The crude and adjusted odds ratio (COR/AOR) and 95% confidence intervals (CI) were analyzed to explore associations. Backward logistic regression analysis was employed to control the effect of confounding variables. P values less than 0.05 were considered statistically significant.

TABLE 1: Background characteristics of study participants.

Characteristic	Frequency ($n = 384$)	Percentage
Age in years		
21–30	187	48.7
31–40	105	27.3
41–50	47	12.2
51 and above	45	11.7
Gender		
Male	156	40.6
Female	228	59.4
Education level		
No formal education	44	11.5
Primary	56	14.6
Secondary	229	59.6
Tertiary	55	14.3
Marital status		
Married	67	17.4
Single	311	81.0
Widowed	2	0.5
Divorced	2	0.5
No response	2	0.5
Religion		
Christianity	308	80.2
Botswana traditional religion	6	1.6
Atheism	7	1.8
Rastafarian	1	0.3
No religion	58	15.1
No response	4	1

2.4. Ethical Issues. Ethical approval was secured from the Institutional Review Boards of the University of Botswana and the Ministry of Health Research Unit of Botswana. The District Health Management Team and the local administrators granted permission to conduct the research. Signed consent was obtained from all participants before the conduct of the interview. No personal identifying details were recorded on the questionnaire.

3. Results

A total of 384 participants were included in the study with female to male ratio of 1.46. Three-fourths of the participants were in the age range of 21–40 years and 73.9% had educational level of secondary school and above. Married and singles accounted for 17.4% and 81% of the sample, respectively. The vast majority (80.2%) were followers of Christianity while 15.1% were not followers of any religion (Table 1). The younger the age of the study participants, the better their educational achievement ($P = 0.00$).

Over four-fifths of the study participants (327) had heard about blood donation in the past of which 104 (31.8%) have ever donated blood. The major sources of information on blood donation were school (35.8%), health facilities (26.6%), and the media (30.6%). Most participants knew at least one condition that may need blood transfusion as

TABLE 2: Participants' knowledge and practice of blood donation.

Characteristic	Frequency	Percentage
Ever heard about blood donation ($n = 384$)		
Yes	327	85.2
No	57	14.8
Source of information ($n = 327$)[a]		
School	117	35.8
Health facilities	87	26.6
Media	100	30.6
Blood transfusion center	6	1.8
Red cross	5	1.5
Blood donation campaign	6	1.8
Work place	11	3.4
Family or friends	14	4.3
Public service centers (offices, kgotla, church, and mall)	9	2.8
Knows a health condition that requires blood transfusion ($n = 384$)		
Yes	295	76.8
No	89	23.2
Knowledge on blood donation by gender ($n = 384$)		
Males and females can donate	350	91.1
Only males can donate	34	8.9
Number of possible donations in one year ($n = 384$)		
One	21	5.5
Two	54	14.1
Three	36	9.4
Four	4	1.0
No idea	269	70.1
Ever donated blood ($n = 384$)		
Yes	104	27.1
No	280	72.9
Donated blood in the past 12 months ($n = 104$)		
Yes	13	12.5
No	91	87.5
Status of blood donation ($n = 104$)		
Regular donor	10	9.6
Nonregular donor	94	90.4
Willingness to donate blood in the future ($n = 384$)		
Yes	269	70.1
No	115	29.9

[a]% exceeded 100% as some participants had more than one response.

a treatment. Of the 384 participants, 104 (27.1%) reported that they had donated blood in the past and 269 (70.1%) stated that they were willing to donate blood in the future. Thirteen out of the 104 past donors (12.5%) reported that they had donated blood in the 12 months preceding the survey and only 10 participants (9.6%) reported that they had been regular donors (Table 2). The reasons for blood donation among donors were largely individual initiative (73%) and organizational initiative (20%) (Figure 1). Among the participants who never donated blood, lack of knowledge, absence of opportunities, medical reasons, lack of interest, and fear were among the reasons listed for not donating blood (Figure 2).

Only 31% reported that they came across a close family member who had ever donated blood. Similarly, 26.8%

reported that they knew a friend who had donated blood in the past. Participants whose close family member had ever needed blood transfusion in the past constituted 116 (30.2%), of which 97 (83.6%) managed to receive the transfusion. Unavailability of blood, cultural reasons, and patient death were amongst the reasons for the patients' failure to receive blood transfusion (Table 3).

Table 4 shows the COR and AOR for the different exposure variables versus willingness to donate blood. A backward logistic regression analysis was made to compute AORs and only two variables were retained in the final regression model. In the bivariate analysis, younger age group and secondary and tertiary educational levels were amongst the sociodemographic variables that showed significantly increased willingness as compared to the reference groups.

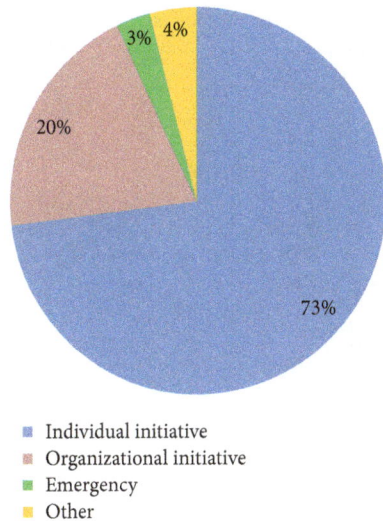

Figure 1: Reasons for blood donation among donors ($n = 104$).

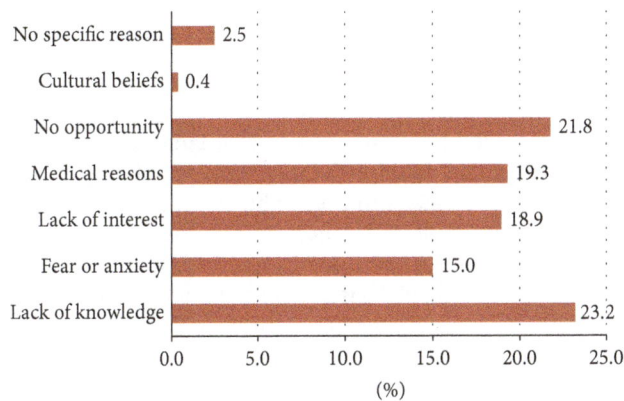

Figure 2: Reasons for not donating blood among nondonors.

Other exposure measures that showed significantly increased association in the bivariate analysis included prior history of blood donation (COR (95% CI): 1.99 (1.17, 3.43)), knowing a family member who ever donated blood (COR (95% CI): 3.52 (1.99, 6.23)), and knowing a friend who ever donated blood (COR (95% CI): 3.24 (1.78, 5.90)). In the backward logistic regression analysis, the variables that remained significant predictors of willingness to donate blood were secondary education (AOR (95% CI): 2.92 (1.48, 5.77)), tertiary education (AOR (95% CI): 3.83 (1.52, 9.62)), and knowing a family member who had ever donated blood (AOR (95% CI): 2.84 (1.58, 5.12)).

4. Discussion

This study was a community-based study representing one of the urban villages in Botswana. Findings from a community-based study are more representative of the general public's intention to donate blood than findings from a facility-based study. The study population was homogeneous in terms of marital status, religion, and residence of participants whereby the large majority were single, Christians, and urban residents. Such homogeneity is thought to act as a self-control mechanism for potential confounding that may be caused by certain variables. The Botswana Demographic Survey also demonstrated a similar distribution in relation to gender, marital status, and religion [25]. Hence, the study should be considered to have acceptable representation of the population studied.

The main finding of this study is that better educational background and exposure to past donors were the predictors of intention to donate blood. Both younger age group and better educational status were factors that were significantly associated with the intention to donate blood in the bivariate analysis. However, only the latter turned out to be statistically significant in the multivariable analysis. The result demonstrated that the educational status of younger participants was better than that of their older counterparts. Hence the higher willingness to donate blood among the younger age groups may be attributed to the direct effect of the better educational background of the younger age groups rather than to their age. Individuals who reported that they had donated blood in the past and who reported that they knew someone who had ever donated blood were more likely to intend to donate blood in the future, results which are in conformity with studies done in different settings [12, 13, 20, 21]. In contrast, another study reported that blood drive organizers and/or recruiters were more important than family and/or peers in encouraging donors [11]. It is likely that witnessing blood donors without any complication following the procedure improves the confidence and disproves misconceptions among community members. The influence of family and other active blood donors on their contacts is also demonstrated in previous studies [12, 13]. Programs need to consider close family members and friends who donated blood in the past as change agents in community blood donation mobilization efforts.

A total of 327 study participants reported that they have heard about blood donation of which 104 (31.8%) have ever donated blood. A significant proportion of participants had heard about blood donation which was not reflected in relation to the practice of blood donation in the past. It shows that information alone is not sufficient and behavior change communication approach needs to be employed to guarantee blood donation practice. Blood transfusion centers, the Red Cross Society, and blood donation campaigns were cited as sources of information by few participants. Moreover, public service centers like offices, kgotlas (local leaders' institutions), and churches were cited as information sources by the minority. It is quite important to diversify health education efforts by including such centers in order to bring about the desired behavior change especially through the involvement of community and religious leaders. Religious leaders were demonstrated to have an influential role in studies done among African Americans and the Middle East [26–28].

TABLE 3: Past experiences of blood donation and transfusion among close contacts.

Characteristic	Frequency	Percentage
Knows a close family member who donated blood ($n = 384$)		
Yes	119	31.0%
No	265	69.0%
Knows a friend who donated blood ($n = 384$)		
Yes	103	26.8%
No	281	73.2%
Close family member ever needed blood transfusion ($n = 384$)		
Yes	116	30.2%
No	268	69.8%
Close family member ever got blood transfusion ($n = 116$)		
Yes	97	83.6%
No	19	16.4%
Reason for no blood transfusion ($n = 19$)		
Unavailability of blood	6	31.6%
Cultural reasons	2	10.5%
Patient died soon	5	26.3%
No response	6	31.6%

Over a quarter of the participants reported that they have ever donated blood which is a good proportion if they were retained as regular blood donors. The level of those who had ever donated blood from one study in India ranged from 7.7% to 12.7% [29, 30] whereas two-thirds of the participants reported that they have ever donated blood in studies done in the Middle East and USA [28, 31]. In the current study, only 12.5% of the participants who mentioned that they have ever donated blood reported that they have donated the blood in the 12 months preceding the survey. There is a significant gap in that those who reported to have ever donated blood were not retained to be regular donors. Studies have demonstrated that higher prior donation frequency was a predictor for donor return [18, 19]. Once individuals come for blood donation to the centers, a mechanism to retain them as regular blood donors needs to be devised. WHO and the International Federation of Red Cross and Red Crescent Societies recommend establishing a database of loyal and regular donors as a means of having access to a safe blood supply. This includes having a mechanism for routinely recalling donors so that they can donate every 3-4 months [1].

Intention to donate in the future was reported by more than two-thirds of the participants. Willingness is the starting point for behavior change as was demonstrated by a study done among new and experienced blood donors [18]. It is an indication that the opportunity still exists in terms of intention despite the low level of past practice of donation. However, it is worth noting that not all intending people can be eligible for blood donation in a setting like Botswana with a national HIV prevalence of 16.9%. The HIV prevalence in the age range 30–49 years was reported to be higher than the national average estimate (range: 33.9%–43.7%)

[32]. Hence, there is a need to have a larger pool of volunteers to compensate for the potential ineligibility despite individuals' willingness to donate blood. The reasons given for not donating blood in the past are diverse and future interventions need to take into account such factors. In-depth investigation on those factors is of paramount importance to clearly understand the root causes and come up with evidence-based interventions.

It is worth noting the following limitations of this study. We used nonprobability sampling and the presence of sampling bias cannot be ruled out. The sample might not be fully representative of the rural population as the study was conducted in a semiurban setting. The intention to donate blood reported during data collection may not necessarily be genuine, which is one of the limitations of reported responses. This study did not explore the reasons why one-time donors ended up donating only once. Could it be that they had a bad experience at their first donation? Future research studies should explore the reasons why some donors donate blood only once.

5. Conclusion

Being informed about blood transfusion and its life-saving benefits through either the education system or the life experiences had made people more likely to intend to donate blood. The intention for future blood donation far outweighs past practice of blood donation. The high level of willingness to donate blood needs to be considered as an opportunity for future community mobilization initiatives. Health programs need to target behavior change using diverse approaches including the use of current blood donors and local leaders as change agents. Evidence-based interventions

TABLE 4: Factors associated with the intention to donate blood in the future.

Factor	Willing to donate blood		Crude odds ratio (95% CI)	Adjusted odds ratio (95% CI)
	Yes	No		
Age in years				
21–30	151	36	4.39 (2.20, 8.73)**	
31–40	70	35	2.09 (1.03, 4.26)*	
41–50	26	21	1.29 (0.57, 2.94)	
51 and above	22	23	Reference	
Gender				
Male	112	44	Reference	
Female	157	71	0.87 (0.56, 1.36)	
Education level				
No formal education	22	22	Reference	Reference
Primary	25	31	0.81 (0.37, 1.78)	0.81 (0.36, 1.82)
Secondary	177	52	3.40 (1.75, 6.63)**	2.92 (1.48, 5.77)**
Tertiary	45	10	4.50 (1.82, 11.12)**	3.83 (1.52, 9.62)**
Ever heard about blood donation				
Yes	235	92	1.73 (0.97, 3.09)	
No	34	23	Reference	
Knows a health condition that requires blood transfusion				
Yes	210	85	1.26 (0.76, 2.09)	
No	59	30	Reference	
Ever donated blood				
Yes	83	21	1.99 (1.17, 3.43)*	
No	186	94	Reference	
Knows a close family member who donated blood				
Yes	102	17	3.52 (1.99, 6.23)**	2.84 (1.58, 5.12)**
No	167	98	Reference	Reference
Knows a friend who donated blood				
Yes	88	15	3.24 (1.78, 5.90)**	
No	181	100	Reference	
Close family member ever needed blood transfusion				
Yes	86	30	1.33 (0.82, 2.17)	
No	183	85	Reference	

*P value less than 0.05; **P value less than 0.01.

to retain blood donors as regular donors are of paramount importance. Further studies to understand the root causes among nondonors as well as the reasons behind failure to retain regular blood donors are recommended.

Conflict of Interests

The authors declare that there is no conflict of interests regarding the publication of this paper.

Acknowledgment

The authors would like to acknowledge the study participants for their valuable time.

References

[1] "Towards 100% voluntary blood donation: a global framework for action," WHO/International Federation of Red Cross and Red Crescent Societies, http://www.who.int/bloodsafety/publications/9789241599696_eng.pdf.

[2] World Health Organization, "Blood safety and availability," WHO Fact Sheet no. 279, World Health Organization, 2014.

[3] T. D. Haile, G. Richard, M. Colin, and T. Amardeep, "Surgery," in Disease Control Priorities in Developing Countries, D. T. Jameson, J. G. Breman, A. R. Measham et al., Eds., World Bank/Oxford University Press, Washington, DC, USA, 2nd edition, 2006.

[4] T. G. Weiser, S. E. Regenbogen, K. D. Thompson et al., "An estimation of the global volume of surgery: a modelling strategy

based on available data," *The Lancet*, vol. 372, no. 9633, pp. 139–144, 2008.

[5] WHO, *WHO Blood Safety Indicators in 2007*, World Health Organization, 2009.

[6] J. B. Tapko, P. Mainuka, and A. J. Diarra-Nama, *Status of Blood Safety in the WHO African Region: Report of the 2006 Survey*, World Health Organization Regional Office for Africa, Brazzaville, Congo, 2009.

[7] N. Zaller, K. E. Nelson, P. Ness, G. Wen, X. Bai, and H. Shan, "Knowledge, attitude and practice survey regarding blood donation in a Northwestern Chinese city," *Transfusion Medicine*, vol. 15, no. 4, pp. 277–286, 2005.

[8] E. Ferguson, K. Farrell, and C. Lawrence, "Blood donation is an act of benevolence rather than altruism," *Health Psychology*, vol. 27, no. 3, pp. 327–336, 2008.

[9] W. R. Steele, G. B. Schreiber, A. Guiltinan et al., "The role of altruistic behavior, empathetic concern, and social responsibility motivation in blood donation behavior," *Transfusion*, vol. 48, no. 1, pp. 43–54, 2008.

[10] B. N. Sojka and P. Sojka, "The blood donation experience: self-reported motives and obstacles for donating blood," *Vox Sanguinis*, vol. 94, no. 1, pp. 56–63, 2008.

[11] S. A. Glynn, S. H. Kleinman, G. B. Schreiber et al., "Motivations to donate blood: demographic comparisons.," *Transfusion*, vol. 42, no. 2, pp. 216–225, 2002.

[12] A. H. Misje, V. Bosnes, O. Gåsdal, and H. E. Heier, "Motivation, recruitment and retention of voluntary non-remunerated blood donors: a survey-based questionnaire study," *Vox Sanguinis*, vol. 89, no. 4, pp. 236–244, 2005.

[13] A. Quéniart, "Blood donation within the family: the transmission of values and practices," *Transfusion*, vol. 53, no. 5, pp. 151S–156S, 2013.

[14] A. H. Misje, V. Bosnes, and H. E. Heier, "Recruiting and retaining young people as voluntary blood donors," *Vox Sanguinis*, vol. 94, no. 2, pp. 119–124, 2008.

[15] B. M. Masser, K. M. White, M. K. Hyde, and D. J. Terry, "The psychology of blood donation: current research and future directions," *Transfusion Medicine Reviews*, vol. 22, no. 3, pp. 215–233, 2008.

[16] A. H. Misje, V. Bosnes, and H. E. Heier, "Gender differences in presentation rates, deferrals and return behaviour among Norwegian blood donors," *Vox Sanguinis*, vol. 98, no. 3, part 1, pp. e241–e248, 2010.

[17] M. Germain, S. A. Glynn, G. B. Schreiber et al., "Determinants of return behavior: a comparison of current and lapsed donors," *Transfusion*, vol. 47, no. 10, pp. 1862–1870, 2007.

[18] G. Godin, M. Conner, P. Sheeran, A. Bélanger-Gravel, and M. Germain, "Determinants of repeated blood donation among new and experienced blood donors," *Transfusion*, vol. 47, no. 9, pp. 1607–1615, 2007.

[19] K. S. Schlumpf, S. A. Glynn, G. B. Schreiber et al., "Factors influencing donor return," *Transfusion*, vol. 48, no. 2, pp. 264–272, 2008.

[20] D. K. Tscheulin and J. Lindenmeier, "The willingness to donate blood: an empirical analysis of socio-demographic and motivation-related determinants," *Health Services Management Research*, vol. 18, no. 3, pp. 165–174, 2005.

[21] G. Godin, P. Sheeran, M. Conner et al., "Factors explaining the intention to give blood among the general population," *Vox Sanguinis*, vol. 89, no. 3, pp. 140–149, 2005.

[22] M. J. Polonsky, A. M. N. Renzaho, A. S. Ferdous, and Z. McQuilten, "African culturally and linguistically diverse communities' blood donation intentions in Australia: integrating knowledge into the theory of planned behavior," *Transfusion*, vol. 53, no. 7, pp. 1475–1486, 2013.

[23] *Population and Housing Census, Preliminary Results Brief*, Botswana Central Statistics Office, 2011.

[24] P. Milligan, A. Njie, and S. Bennett, "Comparison of two cluster sampling methods for health surveys in developing countries," *International Journal of Epidemiology*, vol. 33, no. 3, pp. 469–476, 2004.

[25] *The 2006 Botswana Demographic Survey*, Botswana Central Statistics Office, 2006.

[26] B. Grossman, A. R. Watkins, F. Fleming, and M. R. DeBaun, "Barriers and motivators to blood and cord blood donations in young African-American women," *American Journal of Hematology*, vol. 78, no. 3, pp. 198–202, 2005.

[27] M. Alam and B. El Din Masalmeh, "Knowledge, attitudes and practices regarding blood donation among the Saudi population," *Saudi Medical Journal*, vol. 25, no. 3, pp. 318–321, 2004.

[28] B. H. Abderrahman and M. Y. N. Saleh, "Investigating knowledge and attitudes of blood donors and barriers concerning blood donation in Jordan," *Procedia—Social and Behavioral Sciences*, vol. 116, pp. 2146–2154, 2014.

[29] N. Shenga, R. Pal, and S. Sengupta, "Behavior disparities towards blood donation in Sikkim, India," *Asian Journal of Transfusion Sciences*, vol. 2, no. 2, pp. 56–60, 2008.

[30] B. Singh, R. Pandey, N. Dsouza et al., "Knowledge, attitudes and socio-demographic factors differentiating blood donors from non-donors in an urban slum of Delhi," *Indian Journal of Community Medicine*, vol. 27, no. 3, p. 118, 2002.

[31] L. E. Boulware, L. E. Ratner, P. M. Ness et al., "The contribution of sociodemographic, medical, and attitudinal factors to blood donation among the general public.," *Transfusion*, vol. 42, no. 6, pp. 669–678, 2002.

[32] *Preliminary Results Botswana AIDS Impact Survey IV*, Botswana Central Statistics Office, 2013.

18

Mapping Rare Erythrocyte Phenotypes in Morocco: A Tool to Overcome Transfusion Challenges

A. Benahadi,[1,2] **S. Boulahdid,**[1,2] **B. Adouani,**[1,2] **A. Laouina,**[1,2] **A. Mokhtari,**[2] **A. Soulaymani,**[2] **K. Hajjout,**[1] **M. Benajiba,**[1] **and R. Alami**[1]

[1] Centre National de Transfusion Sanguine, Rue Lamfadal Charkaoui, Madinat Al Irfane, BP 180, Rabat, Morocco
[2] Laboratoire de Génétique et de Biométrie, Faculté des Sciences, University Ibn Tofaïl, Kenitra, Morocco

Correspondence should be addressed to R. Alami; raoufalami@yahoo.com

Academic Editor: Arturo Pereira

The aim of this research is to search for the distribution of blood groups in all the regions of Morocco. This study, done for the first time, aimed to provide the frequency of the Rhesus system and Kell (K) in more than 55000 blood donors from nine different regions around the country. In addition, the frequency of the Cellano, Duffy, Kidd, and MNS blood antigens was searched for 500 blood donors from the Rabat's region. Frequency of blood donors with rare blood groups was characterized for the first time in the country and compared to results found from other populations.

1. Introduction

Blood group phenotypes have been used for several applications as for blood transfusion practices and population genetic studies [1–3].

In Morocco, no study has identified yet the distribution and frequency of different blood groups. In this perspective we tried to identify the Rhesus phenotypes in nine different regions spanning the whole country. We have also conducted a study to determine the frequencies of the k (cellano), Fya, Fyb, Jka, Jkb, S, and s antigens in blood donors (BD) from the Rabat region.

2. Materials and Methods

Fifty-five thousand six hundred and thirty (N = 55630) BD who gave blood in nine different regions were phenotyped for the following Rhesus blood antigen D, C, E, c, and e. In addition, from the CRTS Rabat, we phenotyped 513 BD in the S and s antigens from the MNS system, Fya and Fyb antigens from the Duffy system, Jka and Jkb antigens from the Kidd system, and k (cellano) antigen from the Kell system.

For the determination of Rhesus and Kell typing, we used the OLYMPUS PK7300 Automated System and/or microplates by standard hemagglutination test using commercial monoclonal antisera IgM anti-D, anti-C, anti-c, anti-E, anti-e, and anti-K monoclonal antibodies (Diagast). All samples that showed negative agglutination with monoclonal/polyclonal IgM/IgG anti-D and the Fy (a−, b−) phenotype were confirmed using Coombs' test. Fya, Fyb, Jka, Jkb, S, s, and k (cellano) antigens were typed by commercially prepared polyclonal antisera (Seraclone) with microplates methods for S antigen and by hemagglutination in gel cards (BIO-RAD,ORTHO/BLISS, INVITROGEN) for other antigens.

Positive and negative control cells and Coombs' control cells were used for quality controls.

The allele frequencies were calculated using the gene counting method, which was described by Mourant et al. in 1976 [4].

Statistical analysis was carried out using Microsoft Excel and the program PASTE [5].

3. Results and Discussion

We characterized the Rhesus antigens distribution in 55630 randomly chosen BD from 9 regions, representing different ethnic groups of Morocco.

TABLE 1: Rhesus phenotypes found in the different regions of Morocco.

Regions	Rabat N (%)	Meknès N (%)	Tétouan N (%)	Safi N (%)	BeniMellal N (%)	Al-Hoceima N (%)	Oujda N (%)	Laayoune N (%)	Ouarzazate N (%)	Total (Moroccan population) (%)
N	48610	2138	1002	298	1231	462	1285	118	486	55630
CcDee	18825 (38.727)	794 (37.138)	344 (34.331)	102 (34.23)	499 (40.536)	181 (39.177)	463 (36.031)	48 (40.678)	148 (37.860)	38.54
ccDee	9444 (19.428)	436 (20.393)	164 (16.367)	59 (19.8)	229 (18.603)	59 (12.771)	214 (16.654)	28 (23.729)	111 (22.840)	19.31
CCDee	7396 (15.215)	307 (14.359)	200 (19.960)	52 (17.45)	200 (16.247)	87 (18.831)	232 (18.054)	17 (14.407)	84 (17.284)	15.41
ccDEe	4590 (9.442)	209 (9.775)	103 (10.279)	23 (7.718)	81 (6.580)	40 (8.658)	118 (9.1829)	8 (6.7797)	26 (5.350)	9.34
ccddee	3781 (7.778)	184 (8.606)	82 (8.184)	34 (11.41)	106 (8.611)	49 (10.606)	106 (8.249)	13 (11.017)	37 (7.613)	7.90
CcDEe	3660 (7.529)	165 (7.717)	87 (8.683)	22 (7.383)	97 (7.880)	40 (8.658)	109 (8.4825)	1 (0.8475)	28 (5.761)	7.57
ccDEE	529 (1.088)	22 (1.029)	14 (1.397)	2 (0.671)	11 (0.894)	3 (0.649)	21 (1.6342)	1 (0.8475)	10 (2.058)	1.10
Ccddee	270 (0.555)	17 (0.795)	5 (0.499)	2 (0.671)	7 (0.569)	1 (0.216)	7 (0.545)	2 (1.695)	3 (0.617)	0.56
CCDEe	38 (0.078)	3 (0.140)	2 (0.200)	1 (0.336)	1 (0.081)	2 (0.433)	3 (0.234)	0	1 (0.206)	0.09
ccddEe	62 (0.128)	1 (0.047)	1 (0.100)	1 (0.336)	0	0	2 (0.156)	0	2 (0.412)	0.12
CCddee	6 (0.0123)	0.000	0.000	0.000	0.000	0.000	10 (0.7782)	0.000	0.000	0.03
CcDEE	4 (0.0082)	0.000	0.000	0.000	0.000	0.000	0.000	0.000	0.000	0.01
CcddEe	3 (0.0062)	0.000	0.000	0.000	0.000	0.000	0.000	0.000	0.000	0.005
ccddEE	2 (0.0041)	0.000	0.000	0.000	0.000	0.000	0.000	0.000	0.000	0.004

The Rhesus antigens frequencies found were as follows: e (89.45%), D (70.65%), c (60.58%), C (38.54%), and E (9.59%). The observed phenotypes distributions are summarized in Table 1. The CcDee phenotype was represented in all the studied regions. Its frequency ranged from 34.23% in Safi to 40.67% in the south of the country at Laayoune. By contrast, three phenotypes (CcDEE, CcddEe, and ccddEE) were characterized only in Rabat BD with the lowest frequency in the country (0.0082%, 0.0062%, and 0.0041%, resp.).

Little data are available regarding the frequencies of the blood group antigens other than ABO and RhD in the Moroccan population. In this study, we examined the composition of RBC antigens in Moroccan BD. It is the first study in Morocco that involved such large number of BD (N = 55630). The D antigen is present in 70% of the BD population, thus showing an intermediate prevalence between those found in the African and European continents [6–8]. The e antigen (89%) and c antigen (61%) are most frequent in Morocco; this is concordant with Tagny et al.'s, 2010 [9].

The most common Rhesus haplotypes in Morocco are DCe, followed by Dce and then by dce, respectively, found at 0.38, 0.34, and 0.28. This prevalence is similar to our neighbor Algerians [10] and Tunisians [11]. While in Mauritania and in Sub-Saharan Africa, it is the Dce that shows the highest prevalence [6, 7, 12].

In addition, Principal Component Analysis showed a clear evidence of a north-to-south gradient for some Rhesus phenotypes. In fact the DCcEe, CCDee, and ccDEe are linked to the north regions (Tétouan, Oujda, and Al-Hoceima) while the Dccee is associated with the south provinces (Laayoune and Ouarzazate). This gradient was also found in a previous study by our group for the D antigen [1].

Other system (Kell, MNS, Duffy, and Kidd) phenotype frequencies showed that out of 513 Rabat's blood donors, only one donor (0.19%) was homozygote for the K. Cellano represented 99.80%. A north-to-south gradient was observed for the Kell antigen.

The S and s antigens were positive in 43.1% and 91.2%, respectively. Fy (a– b+) was the most common phenotype seen in about 42% of the studied subjects. The Duffy null or Fy (a– b–) phenotype was observed in 11.11%. This latter phenotype is referred to in the African population as discussed by different authors [7, 13, 14].

For the Kidd system, about half (49.5%) of our BD have the Jk (a+ b+), as found in the European population [15]. The Jk (a– b–) was not found in the studied population. Jka and Jkb antigens were recorded in 84.21% and 65.3% of subjects, respectively (Table 2).

4. Conclusion

Since the current practice of providing compatible blood to patients in Morocco is still relaying on blind cross-matching of available red blood cell units, we initiated this study to map the distribution of the blood groups around Morocco, especially for better management of red cell unit delivery to highly alloimmunized patients.

The main result found here illustrated that the Moroccan population shares phenotypes with Sub-Saharan Africa and

TABLE 2: Kell, MNS, Duffy, and Kidd blood group frequencies (%) compared with other ethnic groups.

Phenotypes	Our donors (%) (N)	Caucasians [16]	Blacks [16]
K+k–	0.19 (**1**)	0.2	Rare
K+k+	9.16 (**47**)	8.8	2
K–k+	90.64 (**465**)	91	98
S+s–	8.77 (**45**)	11	3
S+s+	34.31 (**176**)	44	28
S–s+	56.92 (**292**)	45	69
Fy (a+ b–)	19.30 (**99**)	17	9
Fy (a+ b+)	27.88 (**143**)	49	1
Fy (a– b+)	41.72 (**214**)	34	22
Fy (a– b–)	11.11 (**57**)	Very rare	68
Jk (a+ b–)	34.70 (**178**)	28	57
Jk (a+ b+)	49.51 (**254**)	49	34
Jk (a– b+)	15.79 (**81**)	23	9
Jk (a– b–)	0	Very rare	Very rare

European populations, and a clear evidence of a north-to-south gradient for some Rhesus phenotypes.

Some particularities were also found as the higher frequency of "e" antigen blood group and the Fy (a– b–) which was represented at a significant frequency (11.1%).

Conflict of Interests

The authors declare that there is no conflict of interests regarding the publication of this paper.

Authors' Contribution

A. Benahadi, S. Boulahdid, B. Adouani, A. Laouina, K. Hajjout, M. Benajiba, and R. Alami were supported by the CNTS, Ministry of Health. A. Soulaymani and A. Mokhtari were supported by Ibn Tofaïl University, Kenitra. A. Benahadi collected thedata and performed the research. S. Boulahdid, B. Adouani and A. Laouina collected the data. A. Soulaymani and A. Mokhtari analyzed the data, K. Hajjout and M. Benajiba contributed reagents/materials/analysis tools, and R. Alami designed the research study, performed the research, and validated the paper.

Acknowledgments

The authors would like to thank all regional blood centers across the country for their precious contribution and all technical staff who participated in this study.

References

[1] A. Benahadi, R. Alami, S. Boulahdid et al., "Distribution of ABO and Rhesus D blood antigens in Morocco," *The Internet Journal of Biological Anthropology*, vol. 6, no. 1, article 1425, 2013.

[2] R. N. Makroo, A. Bhatia, R. Gupta, and J. Phillip, "Prevalence of Rh, Duffy, Kell, Kidd & MNSs blood group antigens in

the Indian blood donor population," *Indian Journal of Medical Research*, vol. 137, no. 3, pp. 521–526, 2013.

[3] C. Flickinger, T. Petrone, and A. Church, "Review: American rare donor program," *Immunohematology*, vol. 20, no. 4, pp. 239–243, 2004.

[4] A. E. Mourant, A.C. Kopec, and K. Domaniewska-Sobczak, *The Distribution of the Human Blood Groups and Other Polymorphisms*, Oxford University Press, London, UK, 1976.

[5] Ø. Hammer, D. A. T. Harper, and P. D. Ryan, "PAST: paleontological statistics software package for education and data analysis," *Palaeontologia Electronica*, vol. 4, no. 1, article 4, 9 pages, 2001, http://palaeo-electronica.org/2001_1/past/issue1_01.htm.

[6] Z. A. Jeremiah and C. Odumody, "Rh antigens and phenotype frequencies of the Ibibio, Efik, and Ibo ethnic nationalities in Calabar, Nigeria," *Immunohematology*, vol. 21, no. 1, pp. 21–24, 2005.

[7] B. M'Baya, T. Mfune, E. Mogombo, A. Mphalalo, D. Ndhlovu, and R. C. Knight, "The prevalence of red cell antigens and antibodies in Malawi," *Transfusion Medicine*, vol. 20, no. 3, pp. 196–199, 2010.

[8] F. F. Wagner, D. Kasulke, M. Kerowgan, and W. A. Flegel, "Frequencies of the blood groups ABO, Rhesus, D category VI, Kell, and of clinical relevant high-frequency antigens in South-Western Germany," *Infusionstherapie und Transfusionsmedizin*, vol. 22, no. 5, pp. 285–290, 1995.

[9] C. T. Tagny, S. Owusu-Ofori, D. Mbanya, and V. Deneys, "The blood donor in sub-Saharan Africa: a review," *Transfusion Medicine*, vol. 20, no. 1, pp. 1–10, 2010.

[10] H. Aireche, A. Gueguen, J. L. Golmard, and M. Benabadji, "Determination of gene frequencies in the Rhesus in Algeria system," *Revue Française de Transfusion et Immuno-Hématologie*, vol. 25, no. 4, pp. 383–387, 1982.

[11] S. Hmida, F. Karrat, N. Mojaat, R. Dahri, and K. Boukef, "Rh system polymorphism in Tunisian population," *Revue Francaise de Transfusion et d'Hémobiologie*, vol. 36, no. 2, pp. 191–196, 1993.

[12] C. T. Hamed, M. A. Bollahi, I. Abdelhamid et al., "Distribution of RH and Kell blood group frequencies in the Mauritanian population," *Blood Transfusion*, vol. 11, pp. 154–155, 2013.

[13] D. M. Langhi Jr. and J. O. Bordin, "Duffy blood group and malaria," *Hematology*, vol. 11, no. 5-6, pp. 389–398, 2006.

[14] J. J. Lefrère and P. Rouger, *Pratique Nouvelle de la Transfusion Sanguine*, Elsevier Masson, 2nd edition, 2006.

[15] R. R. Race and R. Sanger, *Blood Group in Man*, Blackwell Scientific Publications, Oxford, UK, 6th edition, 1975.

[16] M. Reid and C. Lomas-Francis, *The Blood Group Antigen Facts Book*, Elsevier Academic Press, New York, NY, USA, 2nd edition, 2004.

19

Blood Transfusion, Serum Ferritin, and Iron in Hemodialysis Patients in Africa

Leonard Kouegnigan Rerambiah,[1] Laurence Essola Rerambiah,[2] Armel Mbourou Etomba,[3] Rose Marlène Mouguiama,[1] Phanie Brunelle Issanga,[1] Axel Sydney Biyoghe,[1] Batchelili Batchilili,[4] Sylvestre Akone Assembe,[1] and Joel Fleury Djoba Siawaya[1,5]

[1]*Centre National de Transfusion Sanguine (CNTS), Libreville, Gabon*
[2]*Service d'Anesthésie-Réanimation du Centre Hospitalier Universitaire de Libreville, Libreville, Gabon*
[3]*Centre National d'Hémodialyse de Libreville, Libreville, Gabon*
[4]*Centre Hospitalier Universitaire d'Angondjè, Libreville, Gabon*
[5]*Unité de Recherche et de Diagnostic Spécialisé/Laboratoire National de Santé Publique (URDS/LNSP), Libreville, Gabon*

Correspondence should be addressed to Joel Fleury Djoba Siawaya; joelfleury@yahoo.com

Academic Editor: Rajendra Chaudhary

Background and Objectives. There is no data analyzing the outcome of blood transfusions and oral iron therapy in patients with kidneys failure in sub-Saharan Africa. The present study aimed to fill that gap and assess the value of ferritin in the diagnosis of iron overload and deficiency. *Design.* From January to February 2012, we prospectively studied 85 hemodialysis patients (78% of males and 22% of females aged 20 to 79 years) attending the Gabonese National Hemodialysis Centre. *Results.* Correlation studies showed (a) a strong positive linear relationship between the number of blood transfusions and high serum ferritin in hemodialysis patient (Spearman r : 0.74; P value: 0.0001); (b) a weak association between the number of blood transfusions and serum iron concentrations (Spearman r : 0.32; P value: 0.04); (c) a weak association between serum ferritin and serum iron (Spearman r : 0.32; P value: 0.003). Also, the strength of agreement beyond chance between the levels of ferritin and iron in the serum was poor ($\kappa = 0.14$). The prevalence of iron overload was 10.6%, whereas the prevalence of iron deficiency was 2.3%, comparing (1) patients with a maximum of one transfusion not on iron therapy; (2) patients with a maximum of one transfusion on iron therapy; (3) polytransfused patients not on iron therapy; and (4) polytransfused patients on oral iron therapy. The "Kruskal-Wallis test" showed that ferritin levels varied significantly between the groups (P value: 0.0001). *Conclusion.* Serum ferritin is not reliable as a marker of iron overload. For patients undergoing regular transfusion we recommend routine serum ferritin measurement and yearly measurement of LIC.

1. Introduction

Renal anemia due to iron-restricted erythropoiesis is common condition associated with chronic renal failure [1, 2]. Kidneys secrete erythropoietin, a protein involved in erythropoiesis. When kidneys are damaged, the secretion of erythropoietin decreases, resulting in renal anemia [3]. Because iron is also required for erythropoiesis, low iron may also cause anemia [3, 4]. Blood transfusion, erythropoietin (EPO), and iron therapy remain the principal means to treat renal anemia in most settings [3–6]. However, renal anemia correction in chronic renal failure patients not only carries a risk for iron overload [7, 8], but also increases the risk of adverse events such as hypertension, congestive heart failure, myocardial infarction, and vascular access thrombosis [3, 9].

Correction of renal anemia in the Gabonese setting continues for the big part to be done by iterative blood transfusions and oral iron therapy. Although transfusions are considerably safer nowadays [10], transfusion-related risks persist [11–13]. These risks include transmission of infectious

TABLE 1: Ferritin and iron ranges in the serum and interpretations.

	Iron deficiency	Normal	Indeterminate (moderately high)	Iron overload
Serum ferritin	<100 ng/mL		200–800 ng/mL	>800 ng/mL
Serum iron	<4 ng/mL	5–15 ng/mL		>15 ng/mL

TABLE 2: Patients' distribution according to their ferritin and iron levels in the serum.

	Serum ferritin			
	Iron deficiency (<100 ng/mL)	Indeterminate (200–800 ng/mL)	Iron overload (>800 ng/mL)	Total
Serum iron				
Iron deficiency (<4 ng/mL)	2	4	3	9
Normal (5–15 ng/mL)	12	22	24	58
Iron overload (>15 ng/mL)	1	8	9	18
Total	**15**	**34**	**36**	**85**

agents [11, 14, 15], the development of alloimmunization [16, 17], and iron overload [18]. Additionally, significant costs are associated with blood transfusions and EPO therapy to which few patients have access.

Currently there is no data in sub-Saharan Africa analyzing the outcome of blood transfusions and oral iron therapy in patients with kidneys failure. The present study aimed to evaluate iron status in patients with renal failure undergoing hemodialysis and assess the value of ferritin in the diagnosis of iron overload and iron deficiency in an African setting.

2. Material and Methods

From January to February 2012, in a prospective cross-sectional study, we studied 85 hemodialysis patients (78% males and 22% females aged 20 to 79 years) attending the Gabonese National Hemodialysis Centre. Patients were divided into four (4) groups. Group one (1) consists of patients with zero (0) or one (1) transfusion under no iron therapy; group two (2) consists of patients with zero (0) or one (1) on iron therapy; group three (3) consists of polytransfused patients under no iron therapy; group four (4) consists of polytransfused patients on oral iron therapy.

2.1. Sample Handling. Blood samples were taken before the hemodialysis session. 5 mL of venous blood was collected into plain tubes. The collected blood samples were then centrifuged (5000 rev/min for 10 minutes) and sera stored at −80°C pending analysis.

2.2. Enzyme-Linked Fluorescence Assay. Commercially available ELFA kits were used to measure iron and ferritin in the serum (Biomérieux, France). Samples were assayed according to the manufacturer's protocol. Samples were read using a mini-VIDAS reader set to 450 nm. The mini-VIDAS system software generated concentrations of the respective analytes.

2.3. Data Analysis. Table 1 shows ferritin and iron concentration ranges in the serum and the corresponding interpretations. The strength of agreement between serum concentrations of ferritin and iron was assessed based on the Kappa coefficient (κ) that was calculated using the formula $\kappa = (P_o - P_e)/1 - P_e$, where P_o is the relative observed agreement among raters and P_e is the hypothetical probability of chance agreement. All other statistical analyses were performed using Prism 6 software from GraphPad Software (San Diego, California, USA). The differences between the groups were analyzed using the Kruskal-Wallis multiple comparison test and Dunn's post test. A P value below 5% was considered significant.

2.4. Ethics. The National Laboratory of Public Health board and the National Blood Transfusion Centre board approved the study. All patients consented to participate in the study.

3. Results

3.1. Correlation between Transfusion, Ferritin, and Iron Levels. Data showed a positive and significant correlation between the number of transfusions and ferritin levels (Spearman r : 0.74; P value: 0.0001) (Figure 1(a)). Although weak, the correlation between the number of transfusions and serum iron levels was positive and significant (Spearman r : 0.32; P value: 0.04) (Figure 1(b)). Further correlation analysis showed a significant association between serum ferritin and serum iron concentrations (Spearman r : 0.32; P value: 0.003) (Figure 1(c)). However, the observed Spearman r coefficient suggested that although significant, the correlation between serum ferritin and serum iron concentrations is weak.

3.2. Strength of Agreement between Ferritin and Iron Levels in Establishing Iron Overload. Table 2 shows patients distribution according to their ferritin and iron levels in our setting. The prevalence of iron overload based on serum ferritin was 42.3%. When assessed based on serum iron level iron overload prevalence was 21.2%. The prevalence of iron overload based on both ferritin and iron concentration in the serum was 10.6%. The prevalence of iron deficiency based on serum ferritin was 17.4%, whereas the prevalence of iron deficiency based on serum iron concentration was 10.6%. 2.3% was the prevalence of iron deficiency when both ferritin and iron concentration were crossed.

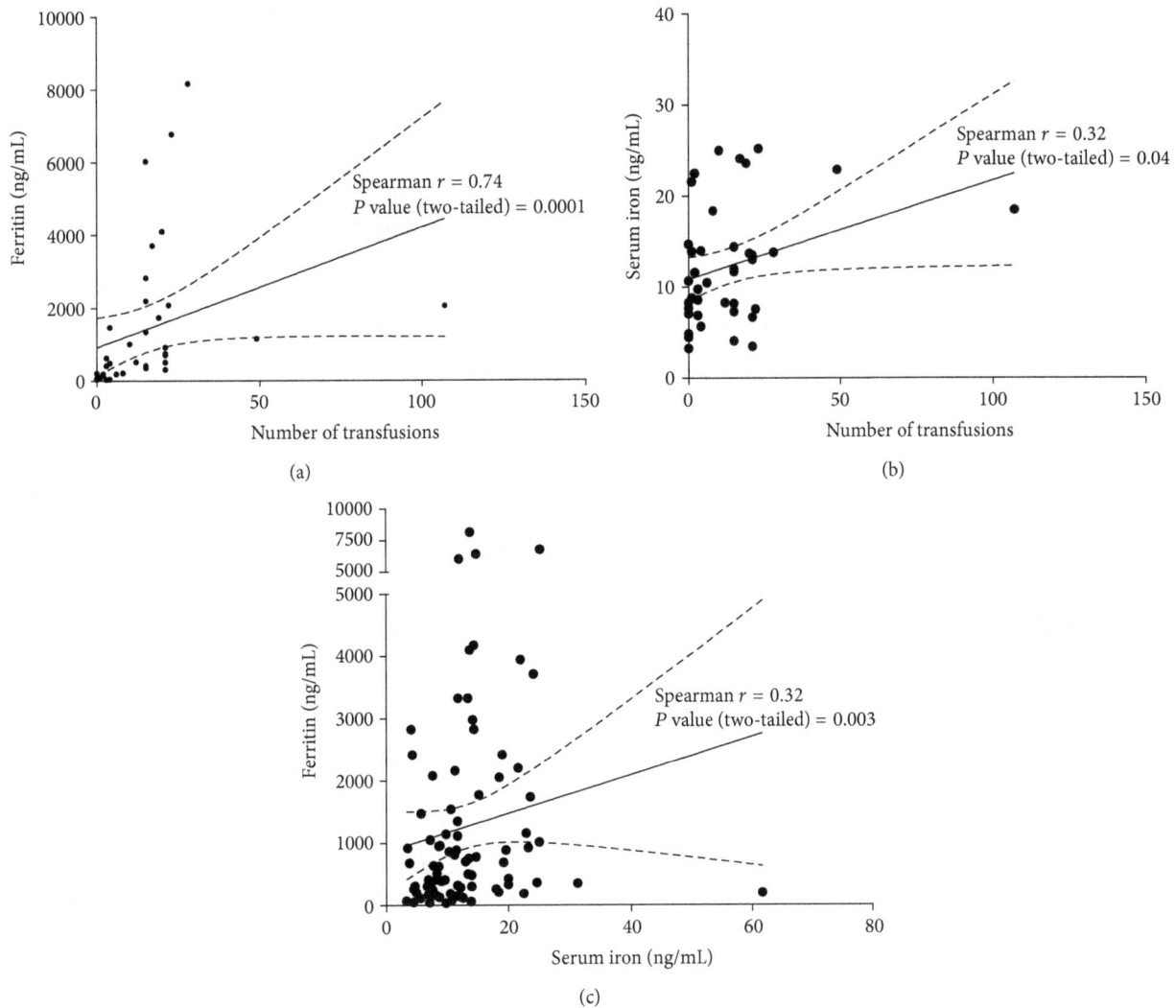

FIGURE 1: Correlation between (a) serum ferritin and the number of blood transfusions: the graph shows strong positive linear relationship between the number of blood transfusions and high serum ferritin in hemodialysis patient (Spearman r : 0.74; P value: 0.0001); (b) serum iron and the number of blood transfusions: the graph shows a weak association between the number of blood transfusions and serum iron concentrations (Spearman r : 0.32; P value: 0.04); (c) serum ferritin and serum iron: the graph shows a weak association between serum ferritin and serum iron (Spearman r : 0.32; P value: 0.003).

Applying Cohen's Kappa (κ) formula we got a κ coefficient of 0.14. Therefore strength of agreement beyond chance between the levels of ferritin and iron in the serum was weak or poor.

3.3. Transfusion and Serum Ferritin and Iron. Comparing patients with zero (0) or one (1) transfusion (on iron therapy and not on iron therapy) to polytransfused patients (on iron therapy and not on iron therapy), the "Kruskal-Wallis test" showed that ferritin levels varied significantly between the groups (P value: 0.0001). "Dunn's Multiple Comparison Test" showed that (1) in patients not on iron therapy ferritin level was significantly higher in polytransfused patients than patients with zero (0) or one (1) transfusion (P value: 0.0001), (2) in patients on iron therapy ferritin level was significantly higher in polytransfused patients than patients who had zero (0) or one (1) transfusion (P value < 0.05), (3) polytransfused patients on iron therapy had significantly higher levels of ferritin compared to patients who had zero (0) or one (1) transfusion who were not on iron therapy (P value: 0.001), and (4) polytransfused patients who were not on iron therapy had significantly higher levels of ferritin compared to patients who had zero (0) or one (1) transfusion and who were on iron therapy (P value < 0.05) (Figure 2). Comparing the same groups of patients for their serum iron concentrations, the "Kruskal-Wallis test" showed no significant differences between the groups.

4. Discussion

In the developing world the serum level of ferritin in patients is still used as the principal marker for diagnosis of iron overload or deficiency in hemodialysis patients. Monitoring iron status using serum ferritin may be subtle for hemodialysis

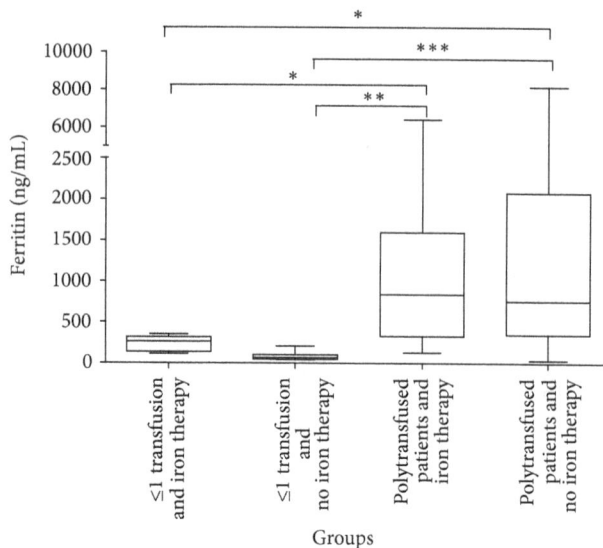

FIGURE 2: Serum ferritin levels in (1) patients with zero or one transfusion under no iron therapy; (2) patients with zero or one under iron therapy; (3) polytransfused patients under no iron therapy; (4) polytransfused patients under oral iron therapy. The star (*) marks significant differences between groups. *** P value of 0.0001; ** P value of 0.001; * P value < 0.05.

services workers, as there are confounding factors such as acute, chronic inflammation and malnutrition that could lead to differential when interpreting serum ferritin values [19]. Here we showed a strong positive linear relationship between the number of blood transfusions and high levels of serum ferritin. We also showed a weak association between the number of blood transfusions and the concentrations of iron in the serum. The strength of agreement between ferritin and iron levels in the serum was poor. Data suggests that multiple transfusions increase substantially serum ferritin and to a lesser extent serum iron.

We found that in hemodialysis patients serum ferritin greatly overestimates iron burden. Serum ferritin overestimates also iron deficiency, but to a lesser extent. Indeed, in our setting, the prevalence of iron overload based on serum ferritin was 42.3 whereas the prevalence of iron overload based on serum iron levels was 21.2%. The prevalence of iron deficiency based on serum ferritin and serum iron was, respectively, 17.4% and 10.6%. Data also showed that 65% of patient who had moderately high serum ferritin levels and 67% of patients who had very high serum ferritin levels had their serum iron level within the normal range. Therefore, our results denote and confirmed that high serum ferritin is not a reliable marker of iron overload [20, 21].

Because the use of serum ferritin as marker for iron overload or deficiency could lead to (1) withholding iron therapy in patients that need it and (2) giving iron treatment to patients who do not require it, accurate assessment of the body iron load is essential to prevent iron toxicity and to manage iron chelation therapy. Although we did not assess liver iron concentration (LIC) by magnetic resonance imaging (MRI), based on the published report [3, 22–25],

we could recommend it for the management of hemodialysis patients in developing countries. However, MRI-based methods are still relatively expensive in that part of the world. Therefore the accurate diagnosis and management of iron overload in developing countries remain challenging. In these countries, for patients undergoing regular transfusion therapy we would suggest to associate with the routine serum ferritin measurement, a yearly measurement of LIC as proposed by Hoffbrand and colleagues [22].

Conflict of Interests

The authors declare that there is no conflict of interests.

Authors' Contribution

Leonard Kouegnigan Rerambiah has conducted study design, samples collection, samples and data analysis supervision, and paper preparation; Laurence Essola Rerambiah, Armel Mbourou Etomba, Rose Marlène Mouguiama, Phanie Brunelle Issanga, Batchelili Batchilili, and Sylvestre Akone Assembe have conducted samples and data collection; Joel Fleury Djoba Siawaya has conducted study design, supervision, data analysis, and paper preparation.

Acknowledgments

The authors acknowledge the Gabonese National Hemodialysis Center for its participation in this study by giving them access to its patients. They also acknowledge the Gabonese National Blood Transfusion Center for logistics and financial supports.

References

[1] E. Urrechaga, L. Borque, and J. F. Escanero, "Erythrocyte and reticulocyte indices in the assessment of erythropoiesis activity and iron availability," *International Journal of Laboratory Hematology*, vol. 35, no. 2, pp. 144–149, 2013.

[2] L. T. Goodnough, E. Nemeth, and T. Ganz, "Detection, evaluation, and management of iron-restricted erythropoiesis," *Blood*, vol. 116, no. 23, pp. 4754–4761, 2010.

[3] C. E. Lankhorst and J. B. Wish, "Anemia in renal disease: diagnosis and management," *Blood Reviews*, vol. 24, no. 1, pp. 39–47, 2010.

[4] V. Ramanath, D. Gupta, J. Jain, K. Chaudhary, and R. Nistala, "Anemia and chronic kidney disease: making sense of the recent trials," *Reviews on Recent Clinical Trials*, vol. 7, no. 3, pp. 187–196, 2012.

[5] T. Kapoian, "Challenge of effectively using erythropoiesis-stimulating agents and intravenous iron," *The American Journal of Kidney Diseases*, vol. 52, pp. S21–S28, 2008.

[6] W. H. Hörl, Y. Vanrenterghem, B. Canaud et al., "Optimal treatment of renal anaemia (OPTA): improving the efficacy and efficiency of renal anaemia therapy in haemodialysis patients receiving intravenous epoetin," *Nephrology Dialysis Transplantation*, vol. 20, supplement 3, pp. iii25–iii32, 2005.

[7] P. Van Buren, R. L. Velez, N. D. Vaziri, and X. J. Zhou, "Iron overdose: a contributor to adverse outcomes in randomized

trials of anemia correction in CKD," *International Urology and Nephrology*, vol. 44, no. 2, pp. 499–507, 2012.

[8] H. Ghoti, E. A. Rachmilewitz, R. Simon-Lopez et al., "Evidence for tissue iron overload in long-term hemodialysis patients and the impact of withdrawing parenteral iron," *European Journal of Haematology*, vol. 89, no. 1, pp. 87–93, 2012.

[9] K. S. Gill, P. Muntner, R. A. Lafayette et al., "Red blood cell transfusion use in patients with chronic kidney disease," *Nephrology Dialysis Transplantation*, vol. 28, no. 6, pp. 1504–1515, 2013.

[10] W. H. Dzik, H. Corwin, L. T. Goodnough et al., "Patient safety and blood transfusion: new solutions," *Transfusion Medicine Reviews*, vol. 17, no. 3, pp. 169–180, 2003.

[11] L. T. Goodnough, "Risks of blood transfusion," *Critical Care Medicine*, vol. 31, no. 12, pp. S678–S686, 2003.

[12] L. T. Goodnough, A. Shander, and M. E. Brecher, "Transfusion medicine: looking to the future," *The Lancet*, vol. 361, no. 9352, pp. 161–169, 2003.

[13] Y. C. Tanhehco and J. S. Berns, "Red blood cell transfusion risks in patients with end-stage renal disease," *Seminars in Dialysis*, vol. 25, no. 5, pp. 539–544, 2012.

[14] L. K. Rerambiah, L. E. Rerambiah, C. Bengone, and J. F. Djoba Siawaya, "The risk of transfusion-transmitted viral infections at the Gabonese National Blood Transfusion Centre," *Blood Transfusion*, vol. 12, no. 3, pp. 330–333, 2014.

[15] C. T. Tagny, E. L. Murphy, and J.-J. Lefrère, "The Francophone Africa blood transfusion research network: a five-year report (2007–2012)," *Transfusion Medicine*, vol. 23, no. 6, pp. 442–444, 2013.

[16] M. Baby, S. Fongoro, M. Cissé et al., "Frequency of red blood cell alloimmunization in polytransfused patients at the university teaching hospital of Point G, Bamako, Mali," *Transfusion Clinique et Biologique*, vol. 17, no. 4, pp. 218–222, 2010.

[17] J. S. Shukla and R. K. Chaudhary, "Red cell alloimmunization in multi-transfused chronic renal failure patients undergoing hemodialysis," *Indian Journal of Pathology and Microbiology*, vol. 42, no. 3, pp. 299–302, 1999.

[18] R. M. Hakim, J. C. Stivelman, G. Schulman et al., "Iron overload and mobilization in long-term hemodialysis patients," *American Journal of Kidney Diseases*, vol. 10, no. 4, pp. 293–299, 1987.

[19] J. B. Wish, "Assessing iron status: beyond serum ferritin and transferrin saturation," *Clinical Journal of the American Society of Nephrology*, vol. 1, supplement 1, pp. S4–S8, 2006.

[20] K. Kalantar-Zadeh and G. H. Lee, "The fascinating but deceptive ferritin: to measure it or not to measure it in chronic kidney disease?" *Clinical Journal of the American Society of Nephrology*, vol. 1, supplement 1, pp. S9–S18, 2006.

[21] K. Kalantar-Zadeh, F. C. Luft, M. H. Humphreys, J. W. Eschbach, and J. W. Adamson, "Moderately high serum ferritin concentration is not a sign of iron overload in dialysis patients," *Kidney International*, vol. 56, no. 2, pp. 758–759, 1999.

[22] A. V. Hoffbrand, A. Taher, and M. D. Cappellini, "How I treat transfusional iron overload," *Blood*, vol. 120, no. 18, pp. 3657–3669, 2012.

[23] T. G. St. Pierre, P. R. Clark, and W. Chua-Anusorn, "Measurement and mapping of liver iron concentrations using magnetic resonance imaging," *Annals of the New York Academy of Sciences*, vol. 1054, pp. 379–385, 2005.

[24] T. G. St. Pierre, P. R. Clark, W. Chua-Anusorn et al., "Noninvasive measurement and imaging of liver iron concentrations using proton magnetic resonance," *Blood*, vol. 105, no. 2, pp. 855–861, 2005.

[25] T. G. St. Pierre, A. El-Beshlawy, M. Elalfy et al., "Multicenter validation of spin-density projection-assisted R2-MRI for the noninvasive measurement of liver iron concentration," *Magnetic Resonance in Medicine*, vol. 71, no. 6, pp. 2215–2223, 2014.

20

Assessment of Vascular Endothelial Growth Factor in Fresh versus Frozen Platelet Rich Plasma

Nada Hosny, Fikry Goubran, Basma BadrEldin Hasan, and Noha Kamel

Clinical Pathology Department, Faculty of Medicine, Suez Canal University, Ismailia 41522, Egypt

Correspondence should be addressed to Noha Kamel; nkamel30@yahoo.com

Academic Editor: Pär Johansson

Platelet rich plasma (PRP) is hemoconcentration with platelets concentration above baseline values and high concentration of many growth factors. The aim of this study was to assess freezing effect on vascular endothelial growth factor (VEGF) release from PRP using two different activation methods to simplify its use in different clinical applications. PRP was prepared using two-centrifugation steps method from 12 qualified blood donors. VEGF concentrations were measured in fresh PRP and after freezing/thawing for one and three weeks with two methods of activation using (i) calcium gluconate and (ii) calcium gluconate and thrombin. Platelets count was significantly increased compared to baseline whole blood values in all fresh and frozen PRP samples (p value was <0.05). No significant difference was found between VEGF concentrations after activating fresh and frozen-thawed PRP samples for one and three weeks by calcium alone or calcium with thrombin, and also no significant difference was found when freezing period was extended from one to three weeks. Our results showed that platelets count does not correlate with variable levels of VEGF. PRP could be prepared once and preserved frozen for at least three weeks for the next treatment sessions and activation with thrombin addition to calcium will not augment the growth factor release.

1. Introduction

Platelet rich plasma (PRP) is a generic term referring to any sample of autologous or allogeneic plasma with platelets concentrations above baseline blood values. PRP has been known as a powerful adhesive and hemostatic agent since the 1970s and as a rich source of autologous growth factors since the 1990s [1, 2].

The use of blood components for nontransfusional purposes started in 1998 [3]. Platelet concentrate component has gained a central role for nontransfusional use. As it is a source of growth factors, it can be used, in both liquid and gel forms, to promote the regeneration of damaged tissues [4].

Being an autologous product, it is an attractive therapy due to the theoretical reduced risks and side effects compared to those commonly approved traditional commercial drugs [5].

Platelets contain growth factors in their alpha granules, such as transforming growth factor-beta (TGF-β), fibroblast growth factor-2 (FGF-2), platelet-derived growth factors (PDGF-AB), insulin-like growth factor-1 (IGF-1), epidermal growth factor (EGF), hepatocyte growth factor (HGF), and vascular endothelial growth factor (VEGF). These factors are thought to produce beneficial effects on the healing process in soft and hard tissues and are the most applicable way to administer a biological stimulus to several damaged tissues that might benefit from this treatment option [6].

The ultimate goal of PRP treatment is to concentrate these growth factors and reintroduce them to the site of injury [6]. Numerous types of platelet products, such as platelet rich plasma, platelet-leukocyte gel, platelet rich fibrin, and platelet gel, derived from autologous or allogeneic peripheral blood, have been used for tissue repair [7].

The effect of platelet concentrates on stimulating the regeneration of bone and soft tissues led to these blood components being used in other clinical settings, in particular in maxillofacial surgery, in dentistry (dental implants, sinus augmentation, and cleft palate), in orthopaedics and traumatology (soft tissues lesions, nonunion, and loss of bone substance following trauma or excision of cysts), in ophthalmology (lesions to the corneal epithelium), in heart surgery (sternal wound dehiscence), and in other specialities following numerous reports which suggested that the product is effective, is easy to use, and does not cause adverse reactions [4]. There is no evidence of standardization of PRP preparation and its use [6]. The most argued aspects that led to a different effect on target tissues are platelets count, methods of preparation (single- or double-centrifugation, speed, timing, and temperature), activation methods (calcium chloride/gluconate; calcium chloride/gluconate and human thrombin; calcium chloride/gluconate and batroxobin; or calcium chloride/gluconate and centrifugation) [4], leukocytes/red blood cells content, and variable therapeutic protocols (amount applied, number of injections, and intervals between injections) [5].

PRP storage is also a hot topic as the freezing/thawing allows more applicable patient management, but it is thought to impair platelet function, alter the growth factor release pattern, favor the accumulation of pyrogenic cytokines, and increase the risk of bacterial proliferation [5].

For these reasons, fresh administration of PRP is preferred (thus necessitating blood collection for each injection, in case of multiple treatment sessions) [8]. Since fresh platelets are valid for only 5 days, they are difficult to be used in therapeutic uses for their regenerative ability by outpatient doctors in different indications, which need repeated sessions. Therefore, this study aimed to assess VEGF concentration in both fresh PRP and $-40°C$ stored PRP. In addition, we investigated a possible correlation between the platelet count and VEGF concentration.

2. Materials and Methods

The study is a comparative cross-sectional analytical study.

Twelve healthy subjects (10 males and 2 females, their age ranging from 21 to 37 years) who met allogeneic blood donor requirements (according to AABB guidelines, 2011) were enrolled in this study, after giving informed consents. The Institutional Research Review Board of Faculty of Medicine, Suez Canal University, approved the study protocol and the consent forms.

Donors who had infections and used nonsteroidal anti-inflammatory drug within 5 days prior to blood donation, with haemoglobin values ≤ 12 g/dL, or with platelet values $\leq 150 \times 10^3/\mu L$ were excluded.

2.1. PRP Preparation. Each subject donated approximately 450 mL of whole blood into triple blood bags used for platelets storage for 5 days containing 63 mL CPDA-1, purchased from JMS (Ang Mo Kio, Singapore), using routine whole blood donation procedures. These bags are used routinely at our blood bank centre.

Platelet concentrates were prepared from the donated whole blood within two hours of collection. The whole blood was centrifuged at 750 g for 7 minutes (start to finish), with 5 minutes of brake time to prepare PRP which was then transferred to a satellite bag. Then, PRP was centrifuged at 5,300 g for 10 minutes to prepare a platelet concentrate (centrifuge model: RC 12BP plus, Thermo scientific Inc., Waltham, USA). Leukoreduction of platelet concentrates was

not done. Most of the plasma was transferred to another satellite bag. An average of 50 ± 5 mL of plasma was left with the platelet concentrate.

2.2. Thrombin Preparation. Ten mL of venous blood was collected in plain Vacutainer tubes from each donor, was put aside to clot, and was centrifuged at 3,000 rpm for 10 minutes. Serum was separated.

2.3. Evaluation of Platelet Count and VEGF Released from PRP. Platelets counts were assessed in whole blood and PRP (fresh and frozen) using fully automated hematology analyzer (Horiba ABX Micros 60, France). Platelets count concentration factor (platelet yield) was calculated by dividing platelets count of PRP by platelets count of whole blood.

One hour after separation, 14 mL of PRP was collected from each PRP unit after gentle mixing by inversion and was aliquoted into three tubes. One tube was assayed immediately for baseline VEGF concentration, while the other two aliquots were kept frozen in $-40°C$. One of the aliquots was stored for one week, and the other for three weeks.

For each of the three aliquots, PRP was divided into two parts and activated shortly before VEGF assay by either calcium gluconate or "calcium gluconate and thrombin" as follows:

two mL of PRP + 300 μL of calcium gluconate (0.05 gm/mL);

two mL PRP + 500 μL of thrombin + 300 μL of calcium gluconate (0.05 gm/mL).

All activated PRP samples (fresh and frozen/thawed) were incubated for 30 minutes at room temperature, without another centrifugation to get releasate for VEGF assessment.

VEGF was measured by commercially available Quantikine ELISA kits (R&D Systems, Minneapolis, USA), according to manufacturer's instructions.

2.4. Statistical Analysis. Data were analysed using SPSS software (SPSS Inc. version 17, Chicago, USA). Data were presented as mean ± standard deviation (SD).

Student's t-test was used to compare between fresh and frozen PRP samples after activation by calcium and calcium and thrombin. Regression analysis (Spearman rank correlation coefficient) was done to correlate between PRP platelet count and VEGF concentrations. Significant difference was defined as $p < 0.05$.

3. Results

The mean initial platelet count in whole blood ($n = 12$) was $282 \pm 56 \times 10^3/\mu L$. It was significantly increased in fresh PRP after separation to reach $991.4 \pm 378 \times 10^3/\mu L$.

RBCs and WBCs were remarkably depleted in PRP compared with the initial concentrations in whole blood samples (Table 1).

Platelet concentrations significantly increased after double-spin PRP preparation where mean platelet yield in

TABLE 1: Red blood cell and white blood cell counts in whole blood and fresh PRP.

	RBCs ($\times10^6/\mu$L) (mean ± SD)	WBCs ($\times10^3/\mu$L) (mean ± SD)
Whole blood	4.1 ± 0.3	7.7 ± 2.3
Fresh PRP	0.02 ± 0.01	0.1 ± 0.02

RBCs: red blood cells; WBCs: white blood cells.

TABLE 2: Platelet yield of fresh and one-week and three-week frozen/thawed PRP.

	Platelet count $\times10^3/\mu$L (mean ± SD)	Platelet yield (mean ± SD)	p value
Whole blood	282 ± 56		
Fresh PRP	991.4 ± 378	3.5 ± 0.9	<0.001*
Frozen PRP (1 week)	453.2 ± 158	1.7 ± 0.6	<0.001*
Frozen PRP (3 weeks)	441.6 ± 154	1.6 ± 0.6	0.001*

*Statistically significant difference ($p < 0.05$).

fresh PRP was 3.5. The platelet yield decreased after freezing PRP samples; yet it was still significant when compared to the initial whole blood platelets concentration (p value < 0.05) (Table 2).

A baseline measurement of VEGF concentration was done in each fresh PRP sample; its mean ± SD was 160.8 ± 88 pg/mL.

VEGF levels significantly increased after activating fresh and frozen/thawed PRP samples for one and three weeks with either calcium or calcium/thrombin. VEGF concentrations in calcium activated PRP samples significantly increased from 160.8 ± 88 to 545.2 ± 349 pg/mL (fresh plasma), 339.5 ± 190 pg/mL (after one week of freezing/thawing), and 339.9 ± 189 pg/mL (after three weeks of freezing/thawing) (p value < 0.05 each). Regarding the addition of thrombin to calcium as an activator, VEGF concentrations significantly increased in all PRP samples (fresh, one-week frozen, and three-week frozen) (p value < 0.05); they were 608.7 ± 494, 365.2 ± 189, and 365.6 ± 188 pg/mL, respectively.

VEGF in calcium activated fresh PRP samples was nonsignificantly higher than that in frozen/thawed PRP samples. In addition, there was nonsignificant difference in VEGF results in frozen samples for one or three weeks. The same results were revealed in VEGF concentration in calcium and thrombin activated PRP samples.

The mean values of VEGF concentration in calcium activated PRP samples are nonsignificantly lower (p value > 0.05) than those activated by calcium and thrombin in all types of samples (fresh, one-week freezing/thawing, and three-week freezing/thawing) (Table 3).

Using the Spearman rank correlation coefficient, variation in VEGF levels did not significantly correlate with variations in PRP platelets count (they showed only fair degree of linear relationship where R_s ranged from 0.34 to 0.50) (Figure 1).

TABLE 3: VEGF concentration (pg/mL) in calcium versus calcium and thrombin activated fresh and frozen/thawed PRP samples.

	Ca activated PRP VEGF concentration	Ca and thrombin activated PRP VEGF concentration	p value
Fresh	545.2 ± 349	608.7 ± 494	0.695 (NS)
Frozen/thawed (1 week)	339.5 ± 190	365.2 ± 189	0.743 (NS)
Frozen/thawed (3 weeks)	339.9 ± 189	365.6 ± 188	0.741 (NS)

NS: not significant.

4. Discussion

During the past two decades, numerous researches have been published in an attempt to characterize and classify the several techniques for PRP preparation (centrifugation speed and the used anticoagulant), content (leucocytes and growth factors), and applications with no consensus [9]. There is increasing awareness on the need for PRP standardization starting from their preparation up to their clinical application. Among the various factors that need more investigations is the possibility to store PRP. As some researchers avoid freezing/thawing, fearing of potential deleterious effects on platelet function and growth factor release pattern [5].

In this regard, our aim was to test whether PRP can be used either as fresh or frozen/thawed, in different clinical applications that need repetitive sessions with preserved VEGF content. Thus, we measured the level of VEGF in fresh and frozen/thawed PRP and investigated the activation with calcium alone compared to calcium and thrombin.

We used a two-centrifugation-step method; the first step was to deplete the product of red and white blood cells with minimal loss of platelets, and the second step was to obtain the highest recovery and the best yield of platelets in the smallest final plasma volume [10].

Platelets purity was monitored in PRP by quantifying other cell types. RBCs and WBCs were remarkably depleted in PRP and remained at a very low concentration compared with the initial mean concentrations for both cell types. Similar results were reported by Amable et al. [10], who observed that initial RBCs and WBCs concentrations were remarkably depleted and remained at very low concentrations (<0.24% for RBCs and <0.28% for WBCs) after PRP preparation.

There is a paucity of data in assessing frozen/thawed PRP platelet counts and growth factors release; our results revealed that the count decreased almost to half the baseline PRP platelets count for the one-week storage samples at −40°C and did not change when the storage period was extended to three weeks. This decrease in count may be due to effect of either time or temperature or both.

Our results also showed that VEGF concentrations in fresh PRP showed nonsignificantly higher values than in frozen/thawed PRP for one or three weeks at −40°C when calcium alone was used as an activator, while results after freezing for one and three weeks did not significantly change.

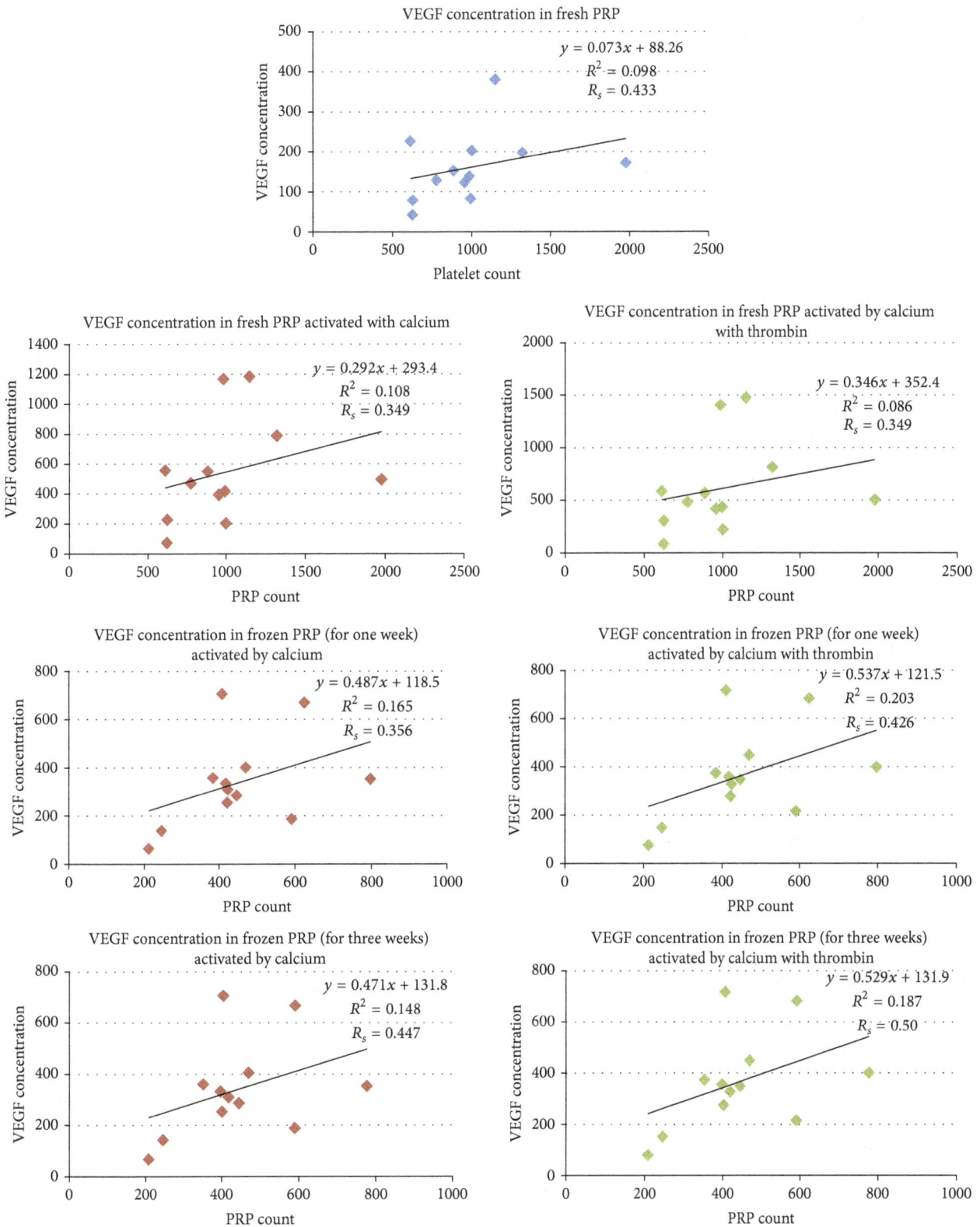

FIGURE 1: Correlations between VEGF concentrations and platelets count in different PRP activation and storage periods. R_s, Spearman rank correlation coefficient.

Furthermore, the same results were detected regarding values of calcium and thrombin activated PRP ($p > 0.05$).

Recently, Roffi and colleagues [11], who investigated whether PRP freezing/thawing affected the release of growth factors from platelets alpha-granules at two time points, obtained similar results, 1 hour (immediate release) and 7 days, as scheduled delivery time in the clinical application. No significant differences were detected for VEGF levels after freezing at one hour and at 7 days. They concluded that PRP cryopreservation is a safe procedure, which sufficiently preserves PRP quality and its biological activity.

Thus, freezing/thawing might still be a valid option to store PRP, although in this case frozen PRP might be less sensitive than fresh PRP to calcium, by not liberating the total amount of growth factors stored in the alpha-granules, and some platelets and bioactive molecules might be damaged [11].

We found that the mean VEGF concentrations in "calcium and thrombin" activated PRP showed no significant difference compared to the mean concentrations in calcium activated PRP, in either fresh or frozen/thawed PRP. To our knowledge, no other studies discussed the difference in growth factors release by PRP when activated by calcium alone and after activation by calcium and thrombin in either fresh or frozen PRP.

Our results showed that VEGF concentrations did not correlate with variations in PRP platelets count. In accordance, Bausset et al. [9] had reported that VEGF levels did not correlate with variation in platelets count. Similar observations were reported by Weibrich et al. [12], indicating that platelet count may not be an appropriate indicator to predict biological activity of platelets.

Therefore, there is no simple procedure available to obtain preoperative estimation of the content of individual growth factors in PRP. This information would be helpful to ensure a reliable and reproducible use of PRP for clinical treatment, since the regenerative potential of PRP undoubtedly depends on its growth factor levels [13]. Thus, the development of new strategies allowing preinjection testing of PRP biological activity is challenging, as there is a high interindividual variability in cellular production and storage of cytokines [9].

The actual challenge for PRP optimization is to determine the main bioactive components responsible for the clinical effects. Not the platelets count nor the platelet growth factors content but the synergy of both should be considered.

The limitation of this study is that freezing time was prolonged to only three weeks.

5. Conclusion

This study underlines two controversial issues. (1) PRP freezing/thawing does not significantly affect the release of VEGF. (2) The different release kinetics is not significantly influenced by the two investigated activating agents. However, until clinical studies explore and clarify the effects of PRP storage on patient symptoms and functional improvement, this study suggests that freezing/thawing does not significantly affect PRP and can be considered as a storage option and thus simplify the management of patients undergoing multiple injection sessions of PRP.

Conflict of Interests

The authors declare that they have no conflict of interests.

Authors' Contribution

All the authors have seen and approved the content and have contributed significantly to the work.

References

[1] S. Pauly, F. Klatte, C. Strobel et al., "Characterization of tendon cell cultures of the human rotator cuff," *European Cells and Materials*, vol. 20, pp. 84–97, 2010.

[2] M. González, M. Arteaga-Vizcaíno, A. Ruiz et al., "PDGF and VEGF levels in platelet-rich plasma," *Journal of Dentistry*, vol. 1, pp. 16–23, 2013.

[3] R. E. Marx, E. R. Carlson, R. M. Eichstaedt, S. R. Schimmele, J. E. Strauss, and K. R. Georgeff, "Platelet-rich plasma: growth factor enhancement for bone grafts," *Oral Surgery, Oral Medicine, Oral Pathology, Oral Radiology, and Endodontics*, vol. 85, no. 6, pp. 638–646, 1998.

[4] G. Aprili, G. Gandini, R. Guaschino, L. Mazzucco, L. Salvaneschi, and S. Vaglio, "SIMTI recommendations on blood components for non-transfusional use," *Blood Transfusion*, vol. 11, no. 4, pp. 611–622, 2013.

[5] E. Kon, G. Filardo, B. Di Matteo, and M. Marcacci, "PRP for the treatment of cartilage pathology," *The Open Orthopaedics Journal*, vol. 3, no. 7, pp. 120–128, 2013.

[6] A. D. Mazzocca, M. B. R. McCarthy, D. M. Chowaniec et al., "Platelet-rich plasma differs according to preparation method and human variability," *The Journal of Bone & Joint Surgery—American Volume*, vol. 94, no. 4, pp. 308–316, 2012.

[7] P. Rozman, D. Semenic, and D. M. Smrke, "The role of platelet gel in regenerative medicine," in *Advances in Regenerative Medicine*, S. Wislet-Gendebien, Ed., InTech, 2011.

[8] A. S. Wasterlain, H. J. Braun, and J. L. Dragoo, "Contents and formulations of platelet-rich plasma," *Operative Techniques in Orthopaedics*, vol. 22, no. 1, pp. 33–42, 2012.

[9] O. Bausset, L. Giraudo, J. Veran et al., "Formulation and storage of platelet-rich plasma homemade product," *BioResearch Open Access*, vol. 1, no. 3, pp. 115–123, 2012.

[10] P. R. Amable, R. B. V. Carias, M. V. T. Teixeira et al., "Platelet-rich plasma preparation for regenerative medicine: optimization and quantification of cytokines and growth factors," *Stem Cell Research & Therapy*, vol. 4, no. 3, article 67, 2013.

[11] A. Roffi, G. Filardo, E. Assirelli et al., "Does platelet-rich plasma freeze-thawing influence growth factor release and their effects on chondrocytes and synoviocytes?" *BioMed Research International*, vol. 2014, Article ID 692913, 10 pages, 2014.

[12] G. Weibrich, W. K. G. Kleis, and G. Hafner, "Growth factor levels in the platelet-rich plasma produced by 2 different methods: curasan-type PRP kit versus PCCS PRP system," *International Journal of Oral and Maxillofacial Implants*, vol. 17, no. 2, pp. 184–190, 2002.

[13] G. Weibrich, W. K. G. Kleis, G. Hafner, W. E. Hitzler, and W. Wagner, "Comparison of platelet, leukocyte, and growth factor levels in point-of-care platelet-enriched plasma, prepared using a modified Curasan kit, with preparations received from a local blood bank," *Clinical Oral Implants Research*, vol. 14, no. 3, pp. 357–362, 2003.

21

Questionnaire-Related Deferrals in Regular Blood Donors in Norway

Håkon Reikvam,[1] Kjersti Svendheim,[2] Anne S. Røsvik,[2,3] and Tor Hervig[2,3]

[1] Department of Haematology, Institute of Internal Medicine, University of Bergen, 5021 Bergen, Norway
[2] Department of Immunology and Transfusion Medicine, Haukeland University Hospital, 5021 Bergen, Norway
[3] Gades Institute, University of Bergen, 5021 Bergen, Norway

Correspondence should be addressed to Tor Hervig, Tor.Hervig@helse-bergen.no

Academic Editor: Silvano Wendel

Voluntary donation is a key issue in transfusion medicine. To ensure the safety of blood transfusions, careful donor selection is important. Although new approaches to blood safety have dramatically reduced the risks for infectious contamination of blood components, the quality and the availability of blood components depend on the willingness to donate and the reliability of the information given by the donors about their own health, including risk behavior. As donors who are deferred by the blood bank will be less motivated to return for donation, it is important to reduce the number of deferrals. The aims of the present study were to investigate the reasons for deferral of registered donors coming to the blood bank for donation, in order to identify areas of importance for donor education—as these deferrals potentially could be avoided by better donor comprehension. Deferral related to testing of donors is not included in this study as these deferrals are dependent on laboratory results and cannot be indentified by questionnaire or interview. Data were collected from all blood donors in a period for 18 months who came for blood donation at a large university hospital in Norway. 1 163 of the 29 787 regular donors, who showed up for donation, were deferred (3.9%). The main reasons were intercurrent illness ($n = 182$) (15.6%), skin ulcers ($n = 170$) (14.6%), and risk behaviour ($n = 127$) (10.9%). In a community, intercurrent illnesses, skin ulcers, and potential risk behavior are the most frequent reasons for deferral of regular donors. Strategized effort on donor education is needed, as "failure to donate" reduces donor motivation.

1. Introduction

The blood donor is the key to patient safety. The "ideal blood donor" is a voluntary, nonnumerated, repeat donor—as this donor will have the lowest risk of having an infection that may be transmitted through blood transfusion. Thus, a major task for the blood banks is to take care of the regular donors. An important part of this strategy is to avoid donor deferrals, as donor deferral imposes a risk of "no-return" of the donor. The more the donor knows about reasons for deferral, the better will the chance be that the donor will not appear in the donation room in a state related to temporary deferral. Thus, donor education is essential, as is also stated in the European Blood Directive [1]. Already in the early days of the HIV/AIDS epidemics, donor knowledge on risk factors was known to be important to avoid transmission of infection [2]. As the donor questionnaire has been more and more complicated, the donors need to have a broad knowledge on transfusion-related risks to avoid "dry visits" to the blood bank. This is also underlined by the extensive requirements for donor education as listed in the European Blood directive [1]. In Norway, the need to reduce donor deferral is especially important, as the country has a donor shortage even though the blood utilization is at average European level. During the last years, the yearly donation frequency has been between 2.4 and 2.2, far from the goal of 1.5–1.7 donations per year. Despite the need to minimize donor deferral, no national data enable us to reduce this negative factor for blood donation is available in Norway.

Thus, the purpose of this study was to provide useful information to improve the communication with the donors—both in contact with the registered donors and in "donor education sessions" for new donors [3].

2. Material and Methods

Data were collected from all donors who appeared at the Blood Bank, Haukeland University Hospital between June 15, 2008 and December 15, 2009. This is the largest Blood Bank in Western Norway, with approximately 23,000 donations, including platelet and red cell apheresis. As for all 41 Norwegian blood banks (total number of donations 220,000), all donors are repeat donors and only registration procedures are performed at the first visit to the blood bank.

At all 29,787 blood donations, a written questionnaire about on health condition and potential risk behaviour was filled in. The data presented in this study simply reflect the answers the donor filled in, with supplementary information obtained during the blood donor interview. The data collection was performed by going through all the questionnaires for the actual period. Persons who were deferred from donation because of low haemoglobin concentration, low ferritin concentration or blood pressure, and pulse outside the approved limits were not included in the study, as we consider these parameters to be beyond the topics that may be picked up by the questionnaire. Retrospectively all reasons for donor deferral were evaluated and classified. Descriptive statistics were performed by the use of SPSS (SPSS Inc., Chicago, IL, USA). Graphical presentations were made by using GraphPad Prism 4 (Graph Pad Software, Inc., San Diego, CA, USA).

3. Results

1163 donors (repeat donors) were deferred from donation. The total deferral rate was thus 3.9%. There were multiple reasons for donor rejection, as summarized in Figure 1. The main reason is *intercurrent illness* ($n = 182$) (15.6%), skin ulcers ($n = 170$) (14.6%), and risk behaviour ($n = 127$) (10.9%). Because intercurrent illnesses and risk behaviour are two of the largest groups among the refused donors, these two groups were further analyzed and subdivided. The underlying illnesses were classified according to aetiology or organ system affected (Figure 2). The most common reasons were respiratory tract infections ($n = 62$) (34.1%), gastrointestinal symptoms ($n = 24$) (13.2%), and exaggeration of season allergy ($n = 10$) (5.5%), in addition to a large group of unknown or unclassified reasons ($n = 58$) (31.9%). The group classified as "risk behaviour" was further analyzed (Figure 3). The dominant cause in this group was change of sexual partner ($n = 71$) (55.9%). Only 160 donors (0.6% of the total donations, 1.6% of the total donor base) were permanently excluded due to medical reasons during the registration period.

4. Discussion

The background for the blood donor criteria is to ensure that the donation does not pose any risk to the donor

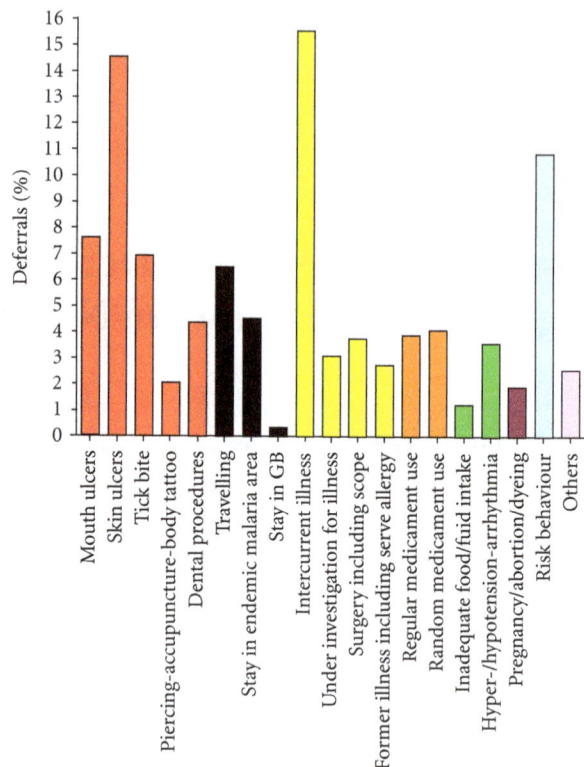

FIGURE 1: Reasons for refusing 1163 potential blood donors for donating. The figure demonstrates the classification of patients deferred from blood donation given as percentage of total deferrals. Red colour indicates deferrals reasons related to affection of skin barrier, blue indicates reasons related to abroad stay, yellow indicates disease-related deferrals, orange deferrals related to use of pharmacological agents, green physical reasons for deferral and pregnancy and related deferrals, and risk behaviour and others are indicated with own colours.

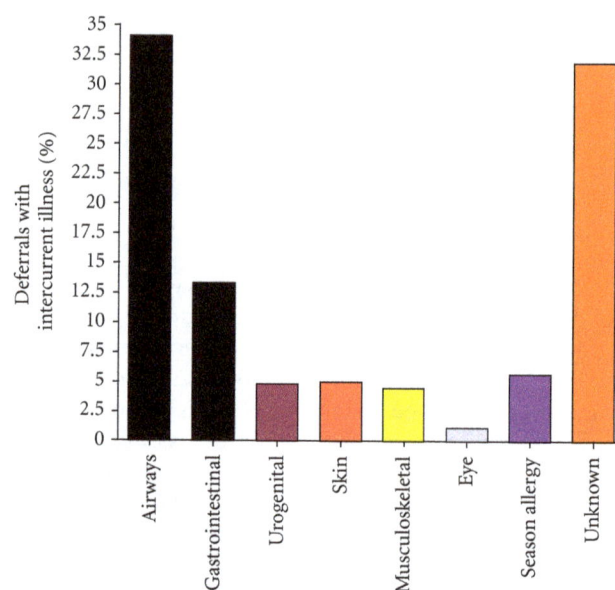

FIGURE 2: Subdividing of potential donors rejected because of intercurrent illness. The figure demonstrates the affected organ system or aetiology of the refused donors of intercurrent illness.

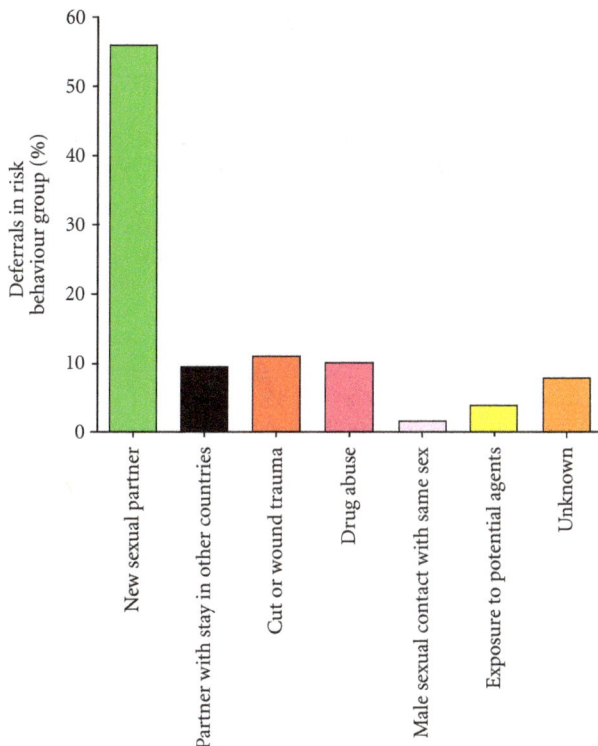

FIGURE 3: Subdividing of potential donors rejected because of risk behaviour. The figure demonstrates the reasons of the refusing donors with classified risk behaviour.

and to prevent the patient receiving blood components to be exposed to risk related to the donor [3]. Thus blood donor education is important as knowledge may prevent unsuitable individuals from becoming blood donors and the registered donors from coming to the blood bank when they may not be allowed to donate due to a temporary deferral reason [3]. Major reasons for temporary deferral are low haemoglobin concentration and/or depleted iron stores in the donor. As these factors are not directly related to donor education, these subjects are not discussed in this paper. We have implemented an "iron conservation program", which is referred to in other papers [4, 5]. The "donor education" principle is not new; on the contrary during all times of blood donation there have been a lot of pamphlets produced and verbal information has been given to the donors on many occasions [6]. The new aspect is the formal approach to blood donor education, as being highlighted in the European Blood directive [1]. Donor education is, however, no guarantee for better donor [7].

On the other hand, donor education must be precise to achieve reduced risks for the patients [8]. All in all, the total rejection rate of 3.9% as reported in this paper may seemingly be acceptable and in line with data from earlier reports [9]. The main reasons for rejections were intercurrent disease, mostly related to upper airway infection—and wound infection. The term "intercurrent disease" refers to several not severe diagnoses, as shown in Figure 2. Of these diagnoses, gastrointestinal disease may be the nearly

only of importance to the patient. It is well known that infection by Yersinia enterocolitica may cause only minor gastrointestinal symptoms in a person even if bacteraemia is present [10]. Accordingly, there are several reports of Yersina-infected donors leading to disease—and sometimes death—in the related blood recipient [11]. Therefore, several blood transfusion services introduced 2-3 weeks quarantine for donors with a history of diarrhoea. However, as this symptom is not well defined, and the frequency of "bad stomach" is high, this precaution has been abandoned by some blood services. "Skin problems" is another frequent cause of deferral of regular blood donors. There is established knowledge that wounds may be "subclinical infected"—and that this infection is followed by undiagnosed bacteraemia. The probability that a wound in a donor is related to bacteraemia is however minor [12].

Also, the importance of other causes of low-grade bacteraemia to blood transfusion is difficult to access. For Borrelia infections, which are common in Norway, no proof of blood transfusion-related transmission is available [13]. Even minor dental procedures may lead to temporary bacteraemia [14], but it would be impossible to implement quarantine periods for donors brushing their teeth.

Figure 3 shows the risk factors indentified—meaning the conditions where the donor has increased risk of carrying an infection that may be transferred through transfusion. The most frequent condition on this list is "change of sexual partner". In Norway, a blood donor who changes sexual partner is deferred for six months. If the new sexual partner does not belong to any risk group as listed in the donor questionnaire, the real impact on donor safety by this subject is disputable indeed. In Norway, it has earlier been reported that the blood donors have "low-risk behaviour" [15], thus contrasting a more recent report from Brazil [16]. It has also been indicated that the combination of a written questionnaire and an oral face-to-face interview does not ensure that the donors provide all relevant information [17]. In some countries, temporary deferral for change of sexual partner is for a very short period only or not implemented at all. Seemingly, there is need for more consensuses concerning new sexual partner as reason for donor deferral.

Other factors identified are related to "low risk". Again, in parallel with intercurrent skin disease, skin infection comes on the list. Sound identification of "wounds at risk" that is subclinical wound infections will probably be impossible. The best option may be to inform donors not to show up at the blood bank if the donor actually has a wound, although this may cause problems for donors working, for example, as carpenters. Thorough education of blood bank staff may also be of help, although it is difficult also for health professionals to identify "dangerous" wounds. Encouraging the donors to call back if infectious symptoms occur later may also be useful, also because this is a general principle not just only related to wound infections.

It is interesting that a few male donors report sex with other men. Even though disputed by some blood transfusion services, this is in general accepted as a real risk factor [18], and it is well communicated that males with male sexual contact should not donate blood. It is not known why this risk factor is sometimes overlooked by the donors—as the donors sometime forget recently holidays and appear in the blood bank shortly after being exposed to malarial infection—and do not inform the blood bank about it.

A limitation of the study is due to the practical approach we have used, and the study is therefore too small to provide data on factors as age, gender, and ethnicity in relation to donor deferral. For information concerning these matters we refer to a publication by Custer et al. [19].

In conclusion this survey of deferral reasons identifies that most rejections are not related to conditions which put the patient receiving blood components at high risk, but better donor knowledge on reasons for temporarily deferral could reduce the "dry visit" frequency, which again could improve donor motivation [20]. The reported results will be presented for our regular donors and a new survey after two years to see if there is reduction in donor deferral. Thus, we hope to avoid the negative effects of short-term deferral on future blood donations [21].

Conflicts of Interests

The authors report that they have no potential conflicts of interest.

Acknowledgments

The authors want to thank the staff at the Department of Immunology and Transfusion Medicine Haukeland University Hospital, Bergen, for helping collecting the data.

References

[1] Council of Europe, *Guide to Preparation, Use and Quality Assurance of Blood Components*, Council of Europe, 14th edition, 2008.

[2] "Joint statement on acquired immune deficiency syndrome (AIDS) related to transfusion," *Transfusion*, vol. 23, no. 2, pp. 87–88, 1983.

[3] A. K. Van Der Bij, R. A. Coutinho, and C. L. Van Der Poel, "Surveillance of risk profiles among new and repeat blood donors with transfusion-transmissible infections from 1995 through 2003 in the Netherlands," *Transfusion*, vol. 46, no. 10, pp. 1729–1736, 2006.

[4] A. S. Røsvik, T. Hervig, T. Wentzel-Larsen, and R. J. Ulvik, "Iron status in Norwegian blood donors: comparison of iron status in new blood donors registered in 1993—1997 and in 2005-2006," *Vox Sanguinis*, vol. 96, no. 1, pp. 49–55, 2009.

[5] A. S. Røsvik, R. J. Ulvik, T. Wentzel-Larsen, and T. Hervig, "The effect of blood donation frequency on iron status," *Transfusion and Apheresis Science*, vol. 41, no. 3, pp. 165–169, 2009.

[6] C. R. France, J. L. France, J. M. Kowalsky, and T. L. Cornett, "Education in donation coping strategies encourages individuals to give blood: further evaluation of a donor recruitment brochure," *Transfusion*, vol. 50, no. 1, pp. 85–91, 2010.

[7] T. T. Gonçalez, E. C. Sabino, N. A. Salles et al., "The impact of simple donor education on donor behavioral deferral and infectious disease rates in São Paulo, Brazil," *Transfusion*, vol. 50, no. 4, pp. 909–917, 2010.

[8] M. Goldman, Q. L. Yi, X. Ye, L. Tessier, and S. F. O'Brien, "Donor understanding and attitudes about current and potential deferral criteria for high-risk sexual behavior," *Transfusion*, vol. 51, no. 8, pp. 1829–1834, 2011.

[9] O. Arslan, "Whole blood donor deferral rate and characteristics of the Turkish population," *Transfusion Medicine*, vol. 17, no. 5, pp. 379–383, 2007.

[10] M. Arpi, K. T. Jensen, and W. Frederiksen, "Yersinia enterocolitica bacteremia: an analysis of thirty-six patients in Denmark and a review of the literature," *Contributions to Microbiology and Immunology*, vol. 12, pp. 260–264, 1991.

[11] A. Leclercq, L. Martin, M. L. Vergnes et al., "Fatal Yersinia enterocolitica biotype 4 serovar O:3 sepsis after red blood cell transfusion," *Transfusion*, vol. 45, no. 5, pp. 814–818, 2005.

[12] G. Jacobsson, S. Dashti, T. Wahlberg, and R. Andersson, "The epidemiology of and risk factors for invasive Staphylococcus aureus infections in western Sweden," *Scandinavian Journal of Infectious Diseases*, vol. 39, no. 1, pp. 6–13, 2007.

[13] U. Ljøstad, E. Skogvoll, R. Eikeland et al., "Oral doxycycline versus intravenous ceftriaxone for European Lyme neuroborreliosis: a multicentre, non-inferiority, double-blind, randomised trial," *The Lancet Neurology*, vol. 7, no. 8, pp. 690–695, 2008.

[14] I. Olsen, "Update on bacteraemia related to dental procedures," *Transfusion and Apheresis Science*, vol. 39, no. 2, pp. 173–178, 2008.

[15] H. Stigum, V. Bosnes, H. Ørjasæter, H. E. Heier, and P. Magnus, "Risk behavior in Norwegian blood donors," *Transfusion*, vol. 41, no. 12, pp. 1480–1485, 2001.

[16] G. M. Patavino, C. de Almeida-Neto, J. Liu et al., "Number of recent sexual partners among blood donors in Brazil: associations with donor demographics, donation characteristics, and infectious disease markers," *Transfusion*. In press.

[17] R. Fielding, T. H. Lam, and A. Hedley, "Risk-behavior reporting by blood donors with an automated telephone system," *Transfusion*, vol. 46, no. 2, pp. 289–297, 2006.

[18] A. M. Sanchez, G. B. Schreiber, C. C. Nass et al., "The impact of male-to-male sexual experience on risk profiles of blood donors," *Transfusion*, vol. 45, no. 3, pp. 404–413, 2005.

[19] B. Custer, J. A. Rios, K. Schlumpf, R. M. Kakaiya, J. L. Gottschall, and D. J. Wright, "Adverse reactions and other factors that impact subsequent blood donation visits," *Transfusion*. In press.

[20] B. Custer, K. S. Schlumpf, D. Wright, T. L. Simon, S. Wilkinson, and P. M. Ness, "Donor return after temporary deferral," *Transfusion*, vol. 51, no. 6, pp. 1188–1196, 2011.

[21] B. Newman, "Blood donor suitability and allogeneic whole blood donation," *Transfusion Medicine Reviews*, vol. 15, no. 3, pp. 234–244, 2001.

22

Knowledge, Attitude, and Practice of Voluntary Blood Donation among Healthcare Workers at the University of Benin Teaching Hospital, Benin City, Nigeria

Benedict Nwogoh,[1] **Usimenahon Aigberadion,**[1] **and Alexander Ikenna Nwannadi**[2]

[1] *Department of Haematology and Blood Transfusion, University of Benin Teaching Hospital, P.M.B 1111, Benin City 300283, Nigeria*
[2] *Department of Haematology, Benue State University, Makurdi 102119, Nigeria*

Correspondence should be addressed to Benedict Nwogoh; b.nwogoh@yahoo.com

Academic Editor: Silvano Wendel

Introduction. Adequate and safe blood supply has remained a challenge in developing countries like ours. There is a high dependency on family replacement and remunerated blood donors in our environment which carries an attendant increased risk of transfusion transmissible infection. *Objectives.* The objectives of this study were to assess the knowledge, attitude, and practice of voluntary blood donation among healthcare workers (nonphysicians) and to identify and recruit potential voluntary blood donors. *Methodology.* This was a cross-sectional descriptive study carried out at the University of Benin Teaching Hospital, Benin City. A total of 163 staffs were recruited. Pretest questionnaires were used to assess their knowledge, attitude, and practice of voluntary blood donation. *Statistical Analysis.* The responses were collated and analyzed with the Statistical Package for Social Sciences (SPSS) 16. The association between blood donation practice and gender of respondents, category of staff, and level of education was tested using Chi-square and Fisher's tests where appropriate. $P < 0.05$ were considered statistically significant. *Results.* The median age of the respondents was 32 years (18–56) with females accounting for 55.6% (90). A total of 74.8% (122) attained tertiary education, and 55.8% (91) of respondents were senior staffs. The majority has good knowledge and positive attitude towards donation; however, only 22.1% (36) have donated blood with 41.7% (15) of these being voluntary. Male workers were more likely to donate ($P < 0.05$). There is no significant association between blood donation and level of education. *Conclusion.* There is a strong disparity between the knowledge, attitude, and practice of voluntary donation amongst healthcare workers.

1. Introduction

In spite of extensive promising research, a true substitute for blood and blood components may not be available for many years [1]. Therefore, blood donation by humans will continue to be the major source for blood and blood components. There are no national data in Nigeria on blood donor demand and supply; however, available data suggest that over 7,000 units of blood are utilized annually at the University of Benin Teaching Hospital, most of which are provided by blood vendors [2, 3].

Donated blood can be lifesaving for individuals who have lost large volumes of blood from serious accidents, obstetric and gynecological hemorrhages, or surgery and stem cell transplant patients as well as for individuals who have symptomatic anemia from medical or hematologic conditions or cancers. Therefore, blood is an important concern to the society. The use of these life saving products may be complicated by infectious and immunological diseases some of which could be life threatening.

Blood banks are obligated to provide adequate and safe blood to the community. Generally, donors are classified into the following categories: voluntary, family replacement, remunerated or paid donors, and autologous donor. The safest donors are found among people who donate their blood voluntarily purely out of altruism and are self-aware of their unsuitability to serve as blood donors where there might be a slightest risk of causing health damage for blood recipients [4, 5]. The risk of transfusion transmissible diseases is highest with the use of blood procured from remunerated donors

[2, 3, 6–9]. A person in need for money is more likely to conceal his/her true state of health. Monetary remuneration, which is often offered as a donor motivating tool, might be highly appealing for people who live in desperate straits.

In developing countries like Nigeria, there is a dependency on family replacement and remunerated donors [3, 10–12]. Voluntary blood donation accounts for less than 5% of blood procured in most of our blood banks [13]. The World Health Organization advocates that member states should establish national blood transfusion services that will operate on the basis of voluntary, nonremunerable blood donation [14]. Despite the establishment of National Blood Transfusion Service (NBTS) in Nigeria, very little progress has been made in the direction of providing sufficient blood for our teaming populace.

The attitude, beliefs, and level of knowledge associated with blood donation may affect the disposition of potential donors to blood donation. Health workers are expected to have a good knowledge of blood usage, to be aware of the increasing demand and scarcity of the products, and are thus expected to donate as well as encourage voluntary blood donation among the public.

2. Study Objectives

The objectives of this study were to assess the knowledge, attitude and, practice of voluntary blood donation among healthcare workers (nonphysicians), to identify and recruit potential voluntary blood donors and to determine the association between blood donation, gender, category of staff, and level of education of the staffs.

3. Materials and Methods

This was a cross-sectional descriptive study carried out at the University of Benin Teaching Hospital, Benin City. The centre operates a hospital-based blood banking system which is highly dependent on blood procurement from vendors who operate paid-donor outlets. Their supplies are augmented by supply from the National Blood Transfusion Service (NBTS), family replacement, and very few voluntary donors. The hospital has over 3,000 health workers (nonphysicians) in various departments.

The staffs are categorized as junior or senior staffs based on their academic qualifications and their job descriptions. Senior staffs are employed into positions requiring higher qualifications such as scientists, nurses, engineers, and accountants, while junior staffs are employed into positions which often do not require a university degree qualification such as office assistants, record clerks, and technicians.

Pretested questionnaires were used to assess their knowledge, attitude, and practice of voluntary blood donation. The questionnaire was modeled after that used in our earlier research work on voluntary donations by physicians [15].

A total of 250 health workers were recruited from the various departments by quota sampling to participate in the study.

Statistical Analysis. The responses were collated and analyzed with the Statistical Package for Social Sciences (SPSS) 16.

The association between blood donation practice and gender of respondents, category of staff, and level of education was tested using Chi-square and Fisher's tests where appropriate. $P < 0.05$ were considered statistically significant.

4. Results

4.1. Demographic Parameters. A total of 163 health workers responded to the questionnaire giving a response rate of 65.2%. The age range of the respondents was 18–56 years (median age was 32 years). The male to female ratio is 1 : 1.3. Eighty-six (52.8%) were married, while 75 (46%) were singles. Most (74.8% of respondents) attained tertiary education; ninety-one (55.8%) were senior staffs, and 69 (42.3%) were junior staffs. Nursing staffs were 30 (18.4%), laboratory staffs 37 (22.7%), pharmacy staffs 19 (11.7%), and administrative workers 22 (13.5%) among others. Details of their demographic parameters are represented in Table 1.

4.2. Knowledge of Blood Transfusion. A total of 151 (92.6%) respondents expressed good knowledge of the common blood group types, and 153 (93.9%) knew their own blood groups. The blood groups of respondent were A Rhesus (Rh) positive (25) (15.3%), AB Rh positive (3) (1.8%), B Rh positive (16) (9.8%), O Rh negative (6) (3.7%), and O Rh positive (74) (45.4%). Thirty-five persons (21.5%) did not respond, and 4 (2.5%) responses were invalid.

Most respondents (157) (95.7%) were aware of the risk of transmission of infection by transfusion. The risk of transmission of HIV, HBV, HCV, and Syphilis was affirmed by 91.4% (149), 69.9% (114), 42.9% (70), and 27.0% (44), respectively.

Forty-four (27%) stated that the minimum interval between donations is 6 months, 35 (21.5%) said 3 months, and 13 (8.0%) said a month, while 33 (20.2%) said they have no knowledge of this.

The majority of the respondents had a good knowledge on who should and who should not donate. However, 6 (3.7%) of the respondents said vulnerable group (sex workers, intravenous drug users) should donate. Twelve (7.4%) and 10 (6.1%) respondents said people should not donate for religious and cultural reasons, respectively.

Only 66 (40.5%) knew the correct volume of blood collected in the process. Similarly, 59 (36.2%) knew that the donation process lasts less than 20 minutes. Details of the respondents knowledge of blood donation are shown in Table 2.

4.3. Attitude towards Blood Donation. A hundred and thirty-three (81.6%) respondents said blood donation was good. Voluntary donation was accepted as the best source of blood donors by 116 (71.2%), replacement donors by 11 (6.7%), remunerated by 3 (1.8%), and self donation by 3 (1.8%).

One hundred and twenty-five (71.2%) said blood donation may have adverse consequences. Twenty (12.3%) said a donor can contract infection, 99 (60.7%) said the donor may experience temporary weakness, and 9 (5.5%) said the donor may fall sick.

One hundred and forty-six (89.6%) feels that patient relatives should be asked to donate, and 149 respondents have

TABLE 1: Sociodemographic parameters of respondents.

(1) Age range (median age)	18–56 (32) yrs	
	N = 163	Percentage (%)
(2) Gender		
Males	69	42.3
Females	90	55.2
No response	4	2.5
(3) Marital status		
Single	75	46.0
Married	86	52.8
Widow	1	0.6
No response	1	0.6
(4) Educational status		
None	1	0.6
Primary	6	3.7
Secondary	29	17.8
Tertiary	122	74.8
No response	5	3.1
(5) Category of staff		
Junior	69	42.3
Senior	91	55.8
No response	3	1.8
(6) Department		
Nursing service	30	18.4
Administration	22	13.5
Pharmacy	19	11.7
Laboratory (pathology)	37	22.7
Records	10	6.1
Accounts	9	5.5
Dentistry	6	3.7
Engineering	6	3.7
Physiotherapy	9	5.5
Radiology	9	5.5
Others	6	3.7

asked relatives in the past to donate. Details of respondents' attitude to blood donation are shown in Table 3.

4.4. Practice of Blood Donation. Thirty-six (22.1%) have donated in the past. Only 5 (13.9%) were regular donors. Only 15 (41.7%) are voluntary, and 19 (52.8%) donated to a friend or relative in need of blood.

The reasons for nondonation by those who have not donated include nobody approached them for donation (32) (25.2%), unfit to donate (21) (16.5%), need to donate for a friend or relative in future (25) (19.7%), fear of needle (8) (6.3%), fear of knowing their viral status (4) (3.1%), the donated blood may be sold (5) (3.9%), nonremuneration (1) (0.8%), and their religion prohibits blood donation (1) (0.8%).

Sixty-seven (41.1%) respondents accepted to be invited to donate blood, but only 32 (19.6%) gave their contacts so that they can be reached.

There was a significant association between male gender and blood donation ($P = 0.003$) as shown in Table 4. The

TABLE 2: Knowledge on blood donation.

Do you know the common blood groups?	
Yes	151 (92.6%)
No	9 (5.5%)
No response	3 (1.8%)
Do you know your blood group?	
Yes	153 (93.9%)
No	7 (4.3%)
No response	3 (1.8%)
Blood group of respondent?	
A Positive	25 (15.3%)
AB Positive	3 (1.8%)
B Positive	16 (9.8%)
O Negative	6 (3.7%)
O Positive	74 (45.4%)
Invalid	4 (2.5%)
No response	35 (21.5%)
Can a person be infected by receiving blood transfusion?	
Yes (correct)	159 (97.5%)
No (incorrect)	2 (1.2%)
No response	2 (1.2%)
What diseases are transmissible by blood transfusion?	
HIV	149 (91.4%)
HBV	114 (69.9%)
HCV	70 (42.9%)
Syphilis	44 (27.0%)
Malaria	7 (4.3%)
No response	5 (3.1%)
How often can an individual donate?	
Weekly	3 (1.8%)
Monthly	13 (8.0%)
3 Monthly	35 (21.5%)
6 Monthly	44 (27%)
Annually	23 (14.1%)
Don't know	33 (20.2%)
Invalid	1 (0.6%)
No response	11 (6.7%)
Who should donate blood?	
Men (correct)	132 (81.0%)
Women (correct)	112 (81.0%)
Young (<18 yrs) (incorrect)	12 (7.4%)
Old (>60 yrs) (incorrect)	4 (2.5%)
Vulnerable group (incorrect)	6 (3.7%)
Healthy (correct)	111 (68.1%)
Diseased (incorrect)	1 (0.6%)

TABLE 2: Continued.

Who should not donate blood?	
Men (incorrect)	7 (4.3%)
Woman (incorrect)	13 (8.0%)
Young (<18 yrs) (correct)	58 (35.6%)
Old (>60 yrs) (correct)	82 (50.3%)
Vulnerable group (correct)	103 (63.2%)
Healthy (incorrect)	4 (2.5%)
Diseased (correct)	107 (65.6%)
Culture belief (incorrect)	10 (6.1%)
Religious belief	12 (7.4%)
No response	7 (4.3%)
What volume of blood is collected during each donation?	
≤500 mls (correct)	66 (40.5%)
500–1000 mls (incorrect)	37 (22.7%)
Don't know	52 (31.9%)
No response	8 (4.9%)
What is the duration of a donation process?	
<20 minutes (correct)	59 (36.2%)
20–60 minutes	43 (26.4%)
Don't know	52 (31.9%)
No response	9 (5.5%)

TABLE 3: Attitude and practice of blood donation.

	N (%)
Section C: Attitude towards blood donation	
What do you think about blood donation?	
Good	133 (81.6)
Bad	8 (4.9)
Neutral	20 (12.3)
No response	2 (1.2)
What do you think is the best source of blood donors?	
Voluntary donor	116 (71.2)
Replacement donor	11 (6.7)
Remunerated donor	3 (1.8)
Self donor	3 (1.8)
I don't know	8 (4.9)
No response	22 (13.5)
Can something harmful happen to a blood donor during or after donation?	
Yes	125 (76.7)
No	30 (18.4)
I don't know	8 (4.9)
What can happen to a blood donor during or after donation?	
Contract Infection	20 (12.3)
Temporary Weakness	99 (60.7)
Fall Sick	9 (5.5)
Should patient relatives be asked to donate?	
Yes	146 (89.6)
No	5 (3.1)
I don't know	5 (3.1)
No response	7 (4.3)
Section D: Practice of blood donation	
Have you donated before?	
Yes	36 (22.1)
No	127 (77.9)
How often do you donate?	
<1 time a year	26 (72.2)
1–3 times a year	5 (13.9)
>3 times a year	0 (0.0)
No response	5 (13.9)
Why did you donate?	
A friend or relative needed blood	19 (52.8)
Voluntary	15 (41.7)
Remuneration	1 (2.7)
To know my screening status	1 (2.7)
Will you donate if called upon or reminded to do so?	
Yes	67 (41.1)
No	51 (31.3)
No response	45 (27.6)
Number of those who stated their contact	32 (19.6)

level of education and category of staff have no significant association with the practice of blood donation ($P = 0.895$ and 0.334, resp.) as shown in Tables 5 and 6.

5. Discussion

The overdependence on family replacement and remunerated donors to meet the increasing demand for blood and blood products poses serious danger to potential recipient. Settings like ours which is still dependent on serological screening test for detection of transfusion transmissible infections in potential donors; who do not use pathogen nucleic acid detection technique; who do not practice pathogen inactivation; who do not leucodeplete nor irradiate blood products are more at risk. Hence, there is need to improve the recruitment and retention of voluntary-donor population to ensure a reasonably safe blood transfusion practice.

There are lots of publications assessing the knowledge, attitude, and practice of voluntary blood donation; however, very few studies have been published which assess the same on the healthcare workers in our environment and globally. This study has shown as expected that healthcare workers have a good knowledge of blood groups, possible transfusion transmissible infection, and the appropriate donor population but on the contrary exhibited a poor knowledge of the blood donation process.

The study also revealed a positive attitude of the workers towards blood donation, but there was a serious contradiction in the practice of voluntary blood donation. Though all study

TABLE 3: Continued.

	N (%)
Reasons for non donation by nondonors	
Not approached to donate	32 (25.2)
Unfit to donate	21 (16.5)
Need to donate for friends or relatives in future	25 (19.7)
Fear of needles	8 (6.3)
Fear of knowing my status	4 (3.1)
Religion forbids it	1 (0.8)
Donated blood may be sold	5 (3.9)
No remuneration	1 (0.8)
No response	39 (30.7)
Do you encourage relatives to donate?	
Yes	149 (91.4)
No	7 (4.3)
No response	7 (4.3)

TABLE 4: The association between gender and blood donation.

Gender	Donors (%)	Nondonors	Total
Males	23 (14.5)	46 (28.9)	69 (43.4)
Females	12 (7.5)	78 (49.1)	90 (56.6)
Total	35 (22.0)	124 (78.0)	159 (100)

$\chi^2 = 9.1$, $P = 0.003$.

TABLE 5: The association between staff category and blood donation.

Category of staff	Donors (%)	Nondonors (%)	Total (%)
Junior	15 (9.4)	54 (33.7)	69 (43.1)
Senior	19 (11.9)	72 (45.0)	91 (56.9)
Total	34 (21.3)	126 (78.7)	160 (100.0)

$\chi^2 = 0.017$, $P = 0.895$.

TABLE 6: The association between staff level of education and blood donation.

Level of education	Donors (%)	Nondonors (%)	Total (%)
Tertiary	25 (15.8)	97 (61.4)	122 (77.2)
Secondary	7 (4.4)	22 (13.9)	29 (18.3)
Primary	3 (1.9)	3 (1.9)	6 (3.8)
None	0 (0.0)	1 (0.6)	1 (0.6)
Total	35 (22.1)	123 (77.9)	158 (100.0)

Fishers exact test, $P = 0.334$.

participants are within the age range of potential donors, only 22.1% of them have donated blood in the past, out of which 52.8% were as family replacement and 41.7% voluntary. This is a far cry based on the knowledge and attitude displayed in this study and their experience of the increased demand for blood in the hospital. A total of 67 (41.1%) of the participants accepted to be invited in the future for voluntary donation but only 32 (19.6%) gave their contacts. This reflects the absence of commitment to their acceptance. Thus, there is a serious disparity in their knowledge, attitude, and practice.

In a similar study conducted on physicians in the same healthcare facility, a similar trend was observed, but higher proportion of donors and regular donors was reported in the physicians [15]. We recorded that 41.4% blood donation was by physicians, with 39.6% being regular donors and 53.4% of these were voluntary [15].

Study by Mullah et al. assessing the knowledge and perception of healthcare support staffs of a tertiary healthcare facility in Gujarat revealed a poor knowledge of donor eligibility among the staffs, 91% of them perceive blood donation as unsafe, and about 39% of them have donated blood [16].

In a similar study in Iran, Reza et al. assessed the knowledge of 122 healthcare workers and found that 51.6% (just above average) have acceptable knowledge on proper methods of blood and components transfusion [17]. Variation in knowledge of blood donation and transfusion processes may be attributable to the degree of enlightenment program available and the degree of involvement of staffs in blood and blood products management.

The major reason given by those who had never donated was that no one approached them to donate. This highlights the need for serious sensitization and education to all and sundry through the mass media to encourage the populace to approach the blood bank for a blood donation exercise.

This study found a significant association between blood donation and sex. Males in our society are more likely to donate blood than females. This is quite understandable since women within the donor age range usually may have one factor or another interfering with their chances of being suitable to donate. Factors such as their frequent menstrual cycles, pregnancy, and lactation may prevent them from donation. This is in affirmation of the WHO report that there are more male donors in Nigeria [18].

In conclusion, healthcare workers are reasonably informed and have positive perception towards blood donation; however, only few of them have donated and are positively disposed to donate blood. There is a need for active education program to encourage all, and sundry if adequate and safe blood will be guaranteed.

References

[1] K. C. Lowe and E. Ferguson, "Benefit and risk perceptions in transfusion medicine: blood and blood substitutes," *Journal of Internal Medicine*, vol. 253, no. 5, pp. 498–507, 2003.

[2] M. E. Enosolease, C. O. Imarengiaye, and O. A. Awodu, "Donor blood procurement and utilisation at the University of Benin Teaching Hospital, Benin City," *African Journal of Reproductive Health*, vol. 8, no. 2, pp. 59–63, 2004.

[3] B. Nwogoh, D. Ikponwen, and M. E. Isoa, "Donor blood procurement and the risk of transfusion transmissible viral infections in a tertiary health facility in South-South Nigeria," *Nigerian Medical Journal*, vol. 52, no. 4, pp. 227–229, 2011.

[4] A. M. Buyx, "Blood donation, payment, and non-cash incentives: classical questions drawing renewed interest," *Transfusion Medicine and Hemotherapy*, vol. 36, no. 5, pp. 329–339, 2009.

[5]   "Voluntary blood donation," http://www.who.int.

[6]   T. Eastlund, "Monetary blood donation incentives and the risk of transfusion- transmitted infection," *Transfusion*, vol. 38, no. 9, pp. 874–882, 1998.

[7]   C. L. Van der Poel, E. Seifried, and W. P. Schaasberg, "Paying for blood donations: still a risk?" *Vox Sanguinis*, vol. 83, no. 4, pp. 285–293, 2002.

[8]   O. A. Ejele, O. Erhabor, and C. A. Nwauche, "The risk of transfusion-transmissible viral infections in the Niger-Delta area of Nigeria," *Sahel Medical Journal*, vol. 8, no. 1, pp. 16–19, 2005.

[9]   S. A. Glynn, J. W. Smith, G. B. Schreiber et al., "Repeat whole-blood and plateletpheresis donors: unreported deferrable risks, reactive screening tests, and response to incentive programs," *Transfusion*, vol. 41, no. 6, pp. 736–743, 2001.

[10] Z. A. Jeremiah and B. B. Koate, "Anaemia, iron deficiency and iron deficiency anaemia among blood donors in Port Harcourt, Nigeria," *Blood Transfusion*, vol. 8, no. 2, pp. 113–117, 2010.

[11] A. O. Emeribe, A. O. Ejele, E. E. Attai, and E. A. Usanga, "Blood donation and patterns of use in southeastern Nigeria," *Transfusion*, vol. 33, no. 4, pp. 330–332, 1993.

[12] S. G. Ahmed, U. A. Ibrahim, and A. W. Hassan, "Adequacy and pattern of blood donations in north-eastern Nigeria: the implications for blood safety," *Annals of Tropical Medicine and Parasitology*, vol. 101, no. 8, pp. 725–731, 2007.

[13] "World Blood Donor Day: from ritual to implementation," *Nigerian Compass Newspaper*, 2010.

[14] "The Melbourne declaration on 100% voluntary non-remunerated donation of blood and blood components," Composed at World Blood Donor Day. Melbourne, Australia, 2009.

[15] B. Nwogoh, U. S. Aigberadion, I. A. Nwannadi, and I. Aigbe, "Knowledge, attitude and practice of voluntary blood donation among physicians in a tertiary health facility of a developing country," *International Journal of Blood Transfusion and Immunohematology*, vol. 2, pp. 4–10, 2012.

[16] F. Mullah, D. Kumar, D. Antani, and M. Gupta, "Study of knowledge, perceptions and practices related to blood donation among the healthcare support staff of a tertiary care hospital in Gujarat, India," *The Online Journal of Health and Allied Sciences*, vol. 12, 2, no. 1, 2013.

[17] P. A. Reza, S. V. Aziz, M. A. Ali, M. H. Marjan, and T. M. Reza, "Evaluation of knowledge of healthcare workers in hospitals of Zabol city on proper methods of blood and components transfusion," *Asian Journal of Transfusion Science*, vol. 3, no. 2, pp. 78–81, 2009.

[18] "WHO report on Gender distribution of blood donors by country," Data Reported by WHO Global Database on Blood Safety, 2011.

23

Blood Requisition and Utilization Practice in Surgical Patients at University of Gondar Hospital, Northwest Ethiopia

Tadesse Belayneh,[1] Gashaw Messele,[2] Zewditu Abdissa,[1] and Birehanemeskel Tegene[3]

[1] Department of Medical Anesthesiology, College of Medicine and Health Sciences, University of Gondar, Kebele 16, P.O. Box 196, Gondar, Ethiopia
[2] Department of Surgery, College of Medicine and Health Sciences, University of Gondar, Kebele 16, P.O. Box 196, Gondar, Ethiopia
[3] Department of Medical Microbiology, College of Medicine and Health Sciences, University of Gondar, Kebele 16, P.O. Box 196, Gondar, Ethiopia

Correspondence should be addressed to Tadesse Belayneh; tadbel20@gmail.com

Academic Editor: Silvano Wendel

Background. Although blood ordering is a common practice in surgical field, the average requirement for a particular procedure is usually based on subjective anticipation of blood loss rather than on evidence based estimates. Overordering with minimal utilization squanders technical time, reagent and imposes extra expenses on patients. This study was conducted to assess blood utilization practices. *Methods.* Cross-sectional study was conducted in Gondar Hospital. Five-month data were collected from all discharged surgical patients and blood bank registries. Blood utilization was calculated using crossmatch to transfusion ratio (C/T), transfusion probability (%T), and transfusion index (TI) indices. *Results.* A total of 982 patients were requested to prepare 1,072 crossmatched units. Of these, 468 units were transfused for 286 patients. The overall ratios of C/T, %T, and TI index were 2.3, 47%, and 0.77, respectively. Blood transfusion from the units crossmatched was 43.6%. Moreover, the highest C/T ratio was observed in elective surgical patients. *Conclusions.* The overall blood utilization was encouraging, but excessive crossmatching with minimal transfusion practice was observed in elective surgical patients. Blood ordering pattern for elective procedures needs to be revised and overordering of blood should be minimized. Moreover, the hospital with blood transfusion committee should formulate maximum surgical blood ordering policies for elective surgical procedures and conduct regular auditing.

1. Introduction

Blood transfusions play a major role in the resuscitation and management of surgical patients [1] and ordering of blood is usually a common practice in elective and emergency surgical procedures [2].

The preoperative request of blood units, especially in elective surgery, is often based on the worst case assumptions, demanding large quantities of blood or overestimating the anticipated blood loss, of which little is ultimately used [1]. This may cause exhaustion of valuable supplies and resources both in technician time, effort, and biochemical reagents. It also adds to financial burden for each patient undergoing a surgical procedure [3]. Increasing demand for blood and

blood products together with rising cost and transfusion associated morbidity led to a number of studies that review blood ordering and transfusion practice [4, 5].

Since the introduction of blood transfusion into clinical practice, its appropriate use has been the subject for debate. It has been reported that only 30% of crossmatched blood is used in elective surgery [6].

In addition, a number of studies in many countries of the world have shown overordering of blood by surgeons with utilization ranging from 5 to 40% [4]. In South Africa, for example, 7–10% of blood is wasted annually because of overordering of blood [7]. Reports from India, Kuwait, and Nigeria also showed utilization rate of 28% [1], 13.6% [8], and 69.7% [3], respectively. Even in trauma patients, utilization is less than 50% [9]. This study has also shown excessive cross matching of blood for elective surgeries with only 30.0% of blood utilized.

Common variations in rates of transfusion may be due to many factors, including differing opinions on the threshold level of hemoglobin below which a patient needs blood transfusion, differences in surgical and anesthetic techniques, cancellation of cases, differences in case mix, preoperative anemia, and lack of availability of transfusion protocols. This may reflect uncertainty about the relative benefits and risks of transfusion and the different perceptions of the value of minimizing blood loss and subsequent transfusion [10].

A number of indices are used to determine the efficiency of blood ordering and utilization system. Boral Henry was the first that suggested the use of crossmatch to transfusion ratio (C/T ratio) in 1975 [4]. Consequently, a number of authors used C/T ratio for evaluating blood transfusion practice. Ideally, this ratio should be 1.0, but a ratio of 2.5 and below was suggested to be indicative of efficient blood usage [3]. The probability of a transfusion for a given procedure is denoted by %T and was suggested by Mead et al. in 1980 [11]. A value of 30% and above has been suggested as appropriate [3]. The average number of units used per patient crossmatch is indicated by the transfusion index (TI) and signifies the appropriateness of number of units crossmatched. A value of 0.5 or more is indicative of efficient blood usage [3, 4].

Unnecessary ordering of blood for surgical patients can be reduced without having any detrimental effect on the quality of patient. Use of blood conservation policies such as the MSBOS has succeeded in limiting unnecessary transfusion practices [12]. Maximal Surgical Blood Order Schedule (MSBOS = 1.5 × TI) estimates the amount of blood that will be needed for the individual procedure. This is a criterion developed from institutional usage statistics providing a figure for the number of units to be crossmatched for any given surgical procedure [13]. In the surgeries which have insignificant blood loss, only blood grouping of the patient should be done and crossmatching can be avoided which can not only be rational and cost effective but also hasten the time lost in waiting for surgery. However, one must confirm the availability of blood for emergency situation before starting the surgery [4]. Many studies [1, 14] have shown that blood is generally over ordered and the implementation of MSBOS and the introduction of "T and S" procedure have led to a safe, effective, and economic solution to ordering of blood.

Evaluating blood ordering and transfusion practices and subsequent developing of a blood ordering schedule, which serves as a guide to anticipated normal blood usage for elective and emergency surgical procedures, can decrease overordering of blood. University of Gondar Hospital has no blood bank for its own, and it gets the necessary blood for its patients from Regional blood bank Branch of Ethiopian Red Cross Society. The Blood Bank has regular voluntary blood collection campaign schedule. But it does not fulfill the requirement of the need of patients in the hospital. Due to these, the patients are forced to collect their blood either from their relatives (family, friends) or paid donors. In this regard, studies assessing blood requisition and transfusion practices

are scarce in Ethiopia particularly in Gondar Hospital. Therefore, the aim of this study was to assess the efficiency of blood requisition and transfusion practices for patients undergoing both elective and emergency surgical procedures.

2. Materials and Methods

A hospital based cross-sectional study was conducted in those patients who underwent elective and emergency surgeries in University of Gondar Hospital over a period of five-months from November 2012 to March 2013. It is a 5000-bed tertiary teaching hospital performing 11,238 surgical procedures per year.

Blood requisition and transfusion of surgical, obstetrics, and gynecological cases were compiled and reviewed. Patient's age and sex, number of units prepared, crossmatched, and transfused, number of patients crossmatched and transfused, source of blood donation or collection, and type of anesthesia were collected from discharged patient medical records and blood bank registries.

Data were coded, entered, and analyzed using SPSS Version 16. Blood utilization indices were computed with the following equation.

 (i) Crossmatch to transfusion ratio (C/T ratio) = number of units crossmatched/number of units transfused. A ratio of 2.5 and below is considered indicative of significant blood usage.

 (ii) Transfusion probability (%T) = number of patients transfused/number of patients crossmatched × 100. A value of 30% and above was considered indicative of significant blood usage.

 (iii) Transfusion index (TI) = number of units transfused/number of patients crossmatched. A value of 0.5 or more was considered indicative of significant blood utilization.

 (iv) Maximal Surgical Blood Order Schedule (MSBOS) = 1.5 × TI.

 (v) In current study blood was wasted when a patient failed to use his/her already prepared blood in any case.

Ethical clearance was taken from Ethical Board of University of Gondar. Participants were communicated individually about the purpose of the study and verbal informed consent was taken before the interview. Confidentiality of the information was assured by using code numbers than personal identification names and keeping questionnaires locked.

3. Results

During the study period a total of 1,412 patients underwent major elective and emergency surgical procedures. Among these, 982 patients were requested to prepare 1,072 units of blood.

Majority of the patients were female (51.9%), underwent surgery in elective schedule, surgical cases in surgical department, underwent surgery under general anesthesia and prepared their blood from replacement donation, as shown in Table 1. Patients prepared blood ranging from 1 unit to 3 units; averagely it was 1.09. From 468 units transfused, 291 (62.2%) units were transfused postoperatively.

4. Blood Requisition and Utilization in Respective Departments

During the five months of study period, blood requisition was made to 644 patients undergoing surgery in surgical department and 428 from gynecologic and obstetrics department (Gyn/obs). From a total of 1,072 units of blood crossmatched, only 468 units were transfused. These showed that 43.6% of total blood crossmatched was utilized, leaving 56.4% of the units crossmatched not transfused to the patient who prepared, that is, wasted.

Gynecology and obstetrics department was the department with the highest number of both patients crossmatched (63.2%) and transfused (64.4%). On the other hand, surgery was the department with the highest number of both blood units crossmatched (60.1%) and transfused (59.8%). Of the 354 patients who underwent emergency operation, 418 units of blood were crossmatched and 209 patients received 230 units of blood transfusion. In case of patients who underwent elective operation, 654 units of blood were crossmatched, out of which only 77 patients received 238 units of blood for their procedures. Generally the highest crossmatched units but the least transfusion units were made for elective patients as compared to emergency cases, as shown in Table 2.

5. Blood Utilization Indices of Operated Patients in the Respective Departments

As shown in Table 3, generally the overall blood transfusion of the requested blood which was explained by indices of C/T ratio, %T, and TI were 2.3, 47%, and 0.77, respectively. These blood utilization indices showed a different value between each department.

In department of surgery, for instance, overall C/T ratio was 2.3 with high ratio in elective than emergency (2.6 versus 1.7). In addition, the overall %T was 46.2% with 35.0% in emergency and 79.3% in elective patients.

On the other hand, in department of gynecology and obstetrics, the overall C/T ratio was 2.3 with elective surgical patients having the highest C/T ratio (2.9) than emergency patients (1.8). Moreover, the overall %T and TI were 48.2% and 0.49, respectively.

6. Discussion

Blood and its component play a major role in the resuscitation and management of both elective and emergency surgical patients. Despite this advantage, currently there is a limited supply with increasing demand and underutilization of the requested blood worldwide [3].

Preoperative overordering of blood has been documented since 1976, when Friedman et al. published their findings. Subsequently, a number of studies have also showed over

TABLE 1: Sociodemographic and other characteristics surgical patients at University of Gondar Hospital, Ethiopia, 2013 ($N = 1,212$).

S.N	Characteristics	Total (no.)	Percent (%)
1	Sex		
	Male	472	48.1%
	Female	510	51.9%
2	Source of donation		
	Voluntary	176	17.9%
	Replacement	896	82.1%
3	Type of operation		
	Elective	628	63.9%
	Emergency	354	36.1%
4	Type of anesthesia		
	General	668	68.0%
	Spinal	314	32.0%
5	Department/cases		
	Surgery	599	60.9%
	Gynecology and obstetrics	383	39.1%
6	Total units of blood prepared	1,072	100%
7	Total units of blood crossmatched	1,072	100%
8	Total units of blood transfused	468	43.6%
9	Preoperative blood units replaced	34	7.2%
10	Intraoperative blood units replaced	143	30.6%
11	Postoperative blood units replaced	291	62.2%
12	Total units of blood wasted	604	56.4%

ordering of blood in different parts of the countries [1, 4]. Data from developing countries have shown gross over ordering of blood in 40% to 70% of patients transfused [8].

Since the introduction of blood transfusion into clinical practice, its appropriate use has been the subject of debate. It has been reported that only 30% of crossmatched blood is used in elective surgery [6, 15]. Generally the percentage of crossmatched patients receiving transfusion for general surgical procedures ranged from 5 to 40% [3]. Therefore, it is essential that the usage of blood and blood products should be rationalized and saved for crisis situations.

The current study revealed that 56.4% of the crossmatched blood was unutilized. This finding was almost comparable to that reported in northern India study where 59.0% of blood crossmatched was unutilized [16]. But it was relatively low compared to a study conducted in India (76.8%), Nigeria (69.7%), Nepal (86.4%), and Egypt (74.8%) [1, 3, 8, 17]. This might indicate that this malpractice is common in developing countries including our Ethiopia.

Boral Henry was the first, and a number of authors then after, used crossmatch to transfusion ratio [4] for evaluating blood transfusion practices. Ideally, this ratio should be 1.0, but a ratio of 2.5 and below was suggested to be indicative of efficient blood usage. According to this recommendation, the overall C/T ratio of 2.3 that was reported in current study was considered to be indicative of efficient blood usage. This ratio was comparable with that reported by a study conducted

TABLE 2: Comparison between number of units crossmatched and transfused in operated patients in University of Gondar Hospital, Ethiopia, 2013.

Department	Number of units		Number of patients	
	Crossmatched (N = 1072)	Transfused (N = 468)	Crossmatched (N = 602)	Transfused (N = 286)
Surgery (N = 599)				
Elective (N = 392)	412 (63.9)	154 (55.0)	54 (24.3)	43 (42.1)
Emergency (N = 207)	232 (36.1)	126 (45.0)	168 (75.7)	59 (57.9)
Subtotal	644 (60.1)	280 (59.8)	222 (36.8)	102 (35.6)
Gynecology and obstetrics (N = 383)				
Elective (N = 236)	242 (56.5)	84 (44.6)	146 (38.4)	34 (18.4)
Emergency (N = 147)	186 (43.5)	104 (55.4)	234 (61.6)	150 (81.6)
Subtotal	428 (39.9)	188 (40.2)	380 (63.2)	184 (64.4)

N: total number.

TABLE 3: Blood utilization indices of surgical patients at University of Gondar Hospital, Ethiopia, 2013 (N = 1, 212).

Department	Blood utilization indices								
	C/T ratio			%T			TI		
	N	D	I	N	D	I	N	D	I
Surgery									
Elective (N = 392)	412	154	2.6	43	54	0.79	154	54	2.85
Emergency (N = 207)	232	136	1.7	59	168	0.35	136	168	0.81
Subtotal	644	280	2.3	102	222	0.46	280	222	1.26
Gynecology and obstetrics									
Elective (N = 236)	242	84	2.9	34	146	0.23	84	146	0.57
Emergency (N = 147)	186	104	1.8	150	234	0.64	104	234	0.44
Subtotal	428	188	2.3	184	380	0.48	188	380	0.49
Total	1072	468	2.3	286	602	0.47	468	602	0.77

Abbreviations: N stands for numerator; D stands for dominator; I stand for index. C/T: crossmatch transfusion ratio, %T: the probability of transfusion, and TI: transfusion index.

in Nigeria (2.2) [3] and Indian (2.5) [18] but lower than that reported by a study conducted in Egypt (3.9) [17] and Malaysia (5.0) [19].

The present study also demonstrated that C/T ratio was similar across the emergency patients of surgical (1.7) and gynecology and obstetrics (1.8) departments. This was somewhat similar to that reported in Egyptian [17] and Nigerian studies [3]. In contrast, C/T ratio was widely varied and high across elective patients of surgery (2.6) and gynecology and obstetrics (2.9) departments. This was similar with study conducted in northern India [18]. Disparities in rates of transfusion in the current study are due to the fact that there is a great tendency to request more units of blood for elective procedures than what is actually required in each department. This over ordering of blood might due to subjective over blood loss estimation of a procedure by surgeons which usually explain for the provision of safety measure in the event of excessive unexpected blood loss during surgery.

Mead et al. [11] suggested the probability of transfusion for a given procedure (%T), which indicates efficient use of blood. Accordingly, a value of 30% and above has been suggested to be appropriate and signifies the appropriateness of number of units crossmatched [11]. Based on what is recommended in the above literature, the results of the present

study revealed an overall %T of 47.0%, which was indicative of appropriate utilization compared to unit crossmatched. This finding was higher than that which has been found in study conducted in Indian tertiary care hospital where %T ranged from 11.1% to 25% [1] and in Egypt where it was 36.9% [17]. Similarly, the probability of transfusion (%T) reported in different departments under the current study was considered appropriate except for elective patients in gynecology and obstetrics department (23.3%) which showed inefficient utilization.

Regarding transfusion index (TI), a value of 0.5 or more is indicative of efficient blood usage and signifies the appropriateness of number of units transfused [4]. The TI reported in the current study was 0.77. Transfusion index (TI) of elective and emergency patients under the study was considered appropriate in both departments except for emergency patients (0.44) in the department of gynecology and obstetrics. This finding was higher than that which has been found in a study conducted in Indian tertiary care hospital 0.36 [1] and Egypt in 0.69 [17]. Blood ordering pattern needs to be revised and overordering of blood should be minimized. This can be possible by the estimation of MSBOS for each procedure and requisition as calculated. Many studies [1, 14] have shown that blood is generally over ordered and the implementation of MSBOS and the introduction of "T and S" procedure have led to a safe, effective, and economic solution to ordering of blood.

In conclusion the overall ratio of C/T, %T, and TI index were considered to be optimal as compared with the standard figures, even though majority of the crossmatched blood was not utilized by the patient. In vast majority of elective surgical procedures routine crossmatch and preparation are not necessary. Moreover C/T ratios of elective patients in each department showed inefficient utilization of ordered blood. Developing a blood ordering policy, which is a guide to expect normal blood usage for surgical procedures, can decrease over ordering of blood thereby reducing unnecessary compatibility testing, returning of unused blood, and wastage due to outdating. It also allows for a more efficient management of blood inventory. In this respect, the hospital blood transfusion committee should formulate maximum surgical blood order schedules for selected cold surgical procedures, conduct regular auditing about effectiveness of the blood requesting policy using the crossmatch to transfusion ratio, and offer periodic feedbacks to improve blood ordering, handling, distribution, and utilization practices of this scarce resource.

Conflict of Interests

The authors declare that they have no conflict of interests.

Authors' Contribution

Tadesse Belayneh participated in the conception, design, acquisition of the data and statistical analysis interpretation of the data, drafting of the paper, and critical revision of the manuscript. Gashaw Messele, Zewditu Abddisa, and Birhanmeskel Tegene participated in the design and critical revision of the manuscript. All authors read and approved the final manuscript.

Acknowledgments

The authors would like to thank University of Gondar (financial support), data collectors, and study participants.

References

[1] M. Vibhute, S. K. Kamath, and A. Shetty, "Blood utilisation in elective general surgery cases: requirements, ordering and transfusion practices," *Journal of Postgraduate Medicine*, vol. 46, no. 1, pp. 13–17, 2000.

[2] R. L. Rund, A. R. Bird, and M. F. M. James, "Blood usage in elective surgery: a 3-month audit at groote schuur hospital, Cape Town," *South African Medical Journal*, vol. 81, no. 8, pp. 415–418, 1992.

[3] O. Ho and B. Bo, "Blood utilization in elective surgical procedures in Ilorin," *Tropical Journal of Health Sciences*, vol. 13, pp. 15–17, 2006.

[4] B. A. Friedman, H. A. Oberman, A. R. Chadwick, and K. I. Kingdon, "The maximum surgical blood order schedule and surgical blood use in the United States," *Transfusion*, vol. 16, no. 4, pp. 380–387, 1976.

[5] L. E. Silberstein, M. S. Kruskall, L. C. Stehling et al., "Strategies for the review of transfusion practices," *Journal of the American Medical Association*, vol. 262, no. 14, pp. 1993–1997, 1989.

[6] S. A. Sowayan, "Use of blood in elective surgery: an area of wasted hospital resource," *Annals of Saudi Medicine*, vol. 14, no. 4, pp. 326–328, 1994.

[7] K. Efraim, "Blood conservation in South Africa. A vital need," *Bloodless Medicine and Surgery*, vol. 43, pp. 7–9, 2001.

[8] R. B. Basnet, D. Lamichhane, and V. K. Sharma, "A study of blood requisition and transfusion practice in surgery at Bir Hospital," *Postgraduate Medical Journal of NAMS*, vol. 9, no. 2, pp. 14–19, 2009.

[9] P. O. Olatunji and H. O. Olawumi, "Transfusion in trauma," *African Journal of Trauma*, vol. 2, pp. 16–19, 2004.

[10] T. Chawla, G. N. Kakepoto, and M. A. Khan, "An audit of blood cross-match ordering practices at the Aga Khan University Hospital: first step towards a maximum surgical blood ordering schedule," *Journal of the Pakistan Medical Association*, vol. 51, no. 7, pp. 251–254, 2001.

[11] J. H. Mead, C. D. Anthony, and M. Sattler, "Hemotherapy in elective surgery. An incidence report, review of the literature, and alternatives for guideline appraisal," *American Journal of Clinical Pathology*, vol. 74, no. 2, pp. 223–227, 1980.

[12] W. G. Murphy, P. Phillips, A. Gray et al., "Blood use for surgical patients: a study of Scottish hospital transfusion practices," *Journal of the Royal College of Surgeons of Edinburgh*, vol. 40, no. 1, pp. 10–13, 1995.

[13] H. Dodsworth and H. A. F. Dudley, "Increased efficiency of transfusion practice in routine surgery using pre-operative antibody screening and selective ordering with an abbreviated cross-match," *British Journal of Surgery*, vol. 72, no. 2, pp. 102–104, 1985.

[14] S. A. Mujeeb, "An audit of blood crossmatch ordering practices at the Aga Khan University Hospital: first step towards a maximum surgical blood ordering schedule (MSBOS)," *Journal of the Pakistan Medical Association*, vol. 51, no. 10, pp. 379–380, 2001.

[15] M. Abdelhadi, A. M. Layla, and S. A. Bashawari, "Blood conservation in elective surgery," *Kuwait Medical Journal*, vol. 33, no. 3, pp. 232–234, 2001.

[16] A. Subramanian, K. Rangarajan, S. Kumar, K. Farooque, V. Sharma, and M. C. Misra, "Reviewing the blood ordering schedule for elective orthopedic surgeries at a level one trauma care center," *Journal of Emergencies, Trauma and Shock*, vol. 3, no. 3, pp. 225–230, 2010.

[17] S. Z. Ibrahim, H. M. Mamdouh, and A. M. Ramadan, "Blood utilization for elective surgeries at main University Hospital in Alexandria, Egypt," *Journal of American Science*, vol. 7, no. 6, pp. 683–689, 2011.

[18] A. Subramanian, S. Sagar, S. Kumar, D. Agrawal, V. Albert, and M. C. Misra, "Maximum surgical blood ordering schedule in a tertiary trauma center in northern India," *Journal of Emergencies, Trauma and Shock*, vol. 5, no. 4, pp. 321–327, 2012.

[19] S. Jayaranee, "An analysis of blood utilization for elective surgery in a tertiary medical centre in Malaysia," *The Malaysian Journal of Pathology*, vol. 24, no. 1, pp. 59–66, 2002.

24

How to Motivate Whole Blood Donors to Become Plasma Donors

Gaston Godin[1] and Marc Germain[2]

[1] *Research Group on Behavior and Health, Laval University, FSI-Vandry, Room 3493, Quebec City, QC, Canada G1V 0A6*
[2] *Medical Affairs, Héma-Québec, 1070, avenue des Sciences-de-la-Vie, Québec City, QC, Canada G1V 5C3*

Correspondence should be addressed to Gaston Godin; gaston.godin@fsi.ulaval.ca

Academic Editor: Erwin Strasser

This study tested the efficacy of interventions to recruit new plasma donors among whole blood donors. A sample of 924 donors was randomized to one of three conditions: *control; information only by nurse;* and *information plus self-positive image message by nurse* (SPI). Participants in the *control* condition only received a leaflet describing the plasma donation procedure. In the two experimental conditions the leaflet was explained face-to-face by a nurse. The dependent variables were the proportion of new plasma donors and the number of donations at six months. Overall, 141 (15.3%) new plasma donors were recruited at six months. There were higher proportions of new plasma donors in the two experimental conditions compared to the control condition ($P < .001$); the two experimental conditions did not differ. Also, compared to the *control* condition, those in the experimental conditions (all $Ps < .001$) gave plasma more often (*information only by nurse*: $d = .26$; SPI: $d = .32$); the SPI intervention significantly outperformed ($P < .05$) the *information only by nurse* condition. The results suggest that references to feelings of SPI such as feeling good and being proud and that giving plasma is a rewarding personal experience favor a higher frequency of plasma donation.

1. Introduction

In the USA, plasma intended for fractionation is obtained mainly from remunerated donors [1]. Therefore, the main challenge for commercial plasma collectors in the US is to apply procedures that will safeguard the quality and safety of the product. In many other countries, however, nonremunerated plasma donation is the usual practice. This means that specific interventions not based on monetary incentives are required to recruit plasma donors.

To our knowledge, in the scientific literature only a few studies have reported the impact of interventions on plasma donor recruitment [2–5]. Each of these interventions mainly provided information about the plasma donation procedure and was successful in recruiting a significant number of new plasma donors. Nonetheless, it was recently shown that one-on-one conversation was the best approach to motivate whole blood donors to become plasma donors especially if the conversation was donor-oriented, that is, focusing on "donor's needs and welfare" [5]. This latter observation is in agreement with the results reported by Ferguson et al. [6], showing that

committed blood donors are more willing to donate blood when exposed to a benevolence message. Moreover, their results were consistent with those of Weyant [7] who showed that when helping costs are high (e.g., giving plasma), beliefs in personal benefits are more important for promoting action.

Given the increasing importance for blood agencies to recruit new plasma donors without remuneration, the present research focused on (a) whether two interventions outperformed a *control* condition regarding the recruitment of new plasma donors, (b) whether any of the two interventions engendered a greater number of donations compared to a *control* condition, and (c) the moderating effects of gender, age, and donor status on the findings.

2. Methods

2.1. Participants and Procedure. The population targeted by this study was whole blood donors aged 18 to 70 years, who donated at one of the mobile blood drives organized by Héma-Québec, the blood establishment in Quebec. To be included in the study, donors had to be living near the fixed donation center in Quebec City, where apheresis plasma collections are performed. Thus, donors were included if they resided in the metropolitan area or if they gave blood at a mobile clinic within a driving distance of 45 minutes from the apheresis center. A total of 3,514 donors registered at one of the 33 different mobile blood drives held within the specified geographical area between February 14 and June 7, 2012. Donors were excluded if they self-reported plasma donation before ($n = 41$); were first time female donor ($n = 333$); or had blood types other than O+, B+, AB+, and AB− ($n = 1,753$) (see Figure 1). Thus 1,387 donors were eligible for the study.

Given the variability in size of the blood drives, at each site the number of donors to be recruited was predetermined and varied between 12 and 60. Recruitment of the donors was done at the time of registration, at a pace adapted to the flow of donors, and this is in order to avoid overloading the research nurses. For this latter reason, 396 were not included in the study. The other 991 eligible donors were asked at registration if they agreed to participate in a project aimed at better understanding the motivation of blood donors towards plasma donation. If yes, they were given one of three folders that were placed in a prerandomized order. This was the randomization method applied to allocate blood donors to one of the two interventions or the *control* condition.

Thus, 991 were randomized in one of the three groups. Subsequently, 37 donors were temporarily deferred from giving blood at the time of reviewing their screening questionnaire with the nurse, 25 donors had a history of apheresis according to the donor information system (*Progesa, Mak System*), and five registered twice during the study; thus, these 67 individuals were excluded from the study. In sum, data from 924 blood donors were included in the analyses. The number of blood donors in each condition was 303 (*information only by nurse*); 310 (*information plus self-positive image by nurse*); and 311 (*control*). This study, realized under the legal mandate of Héma-Québec, was conducted to evaluate possible changes in operational recruitment techniques that would have been applied to the donors in any case, except for randomization. Notwithstanding this observation, all standard American Psychological Association (APA) ethical procedures were applied.

2.2. Intervention. Participants in the *control* condition were given a folder containing the following: a leaflet explaining the plasma donation procedure (a paragraph of 95 words and a photograph showing someone giving plasma) and a registration form for a first plasma donation. They were only invited to read by themselves these documents. Participants in the *information only by nurse* condition received the same documents as those in the *control* condition but were told that the research nurse would provide further explanations at a later time during the donation process. Thus, upon completion of the donor eligibility questionnaire for blood donation, the trained research nurse briefly reviewed (in less than two minutes) the content of the leaflet describing the plasma donation and the procedure itself, including when, where,

and how donors could give plasma. They also answered any questions donors might have in this regard. Participants in the *information plus self-positive image by nurse* condition also reviewed the documents at the time they met the nurse, but the leaflet contained an additional paragraph (101 words) about feelings of self-positive image expressed by plasma donors. For both experimental conditions, five nurses were previously trained to deliver the messages on sites of mobile blood drives and to respond to any questions blood donors might have regarding plasma donation. At random, they met blood donors of both experimental conditions on each site. The review of the leaflet by nurses was done within the usual screening procedure for eligibility to give blood and did not require more than two minutes. Finally, before leaving the site of the blood drive, all donors of the three conditions could insert in an envelope their signed registration form providing consent to be phoned by the staff of the plasma donation center to set up an appointment for a first plasma donation, no earlier than 56 days after their whole blood donation.

2.3. Measurement of Donation Behavior. Objective measures of donation behavior were obtained for each participant. Thus, for each blood donor, whether s/he gave a first lifetime plasma donation and the number of plasma donations during the six-month period following the index donation were determined. This information was extracted from the donor information system (*Progesa, Mak System*). An anonymous research code was used to link individuals with their behavioral data.

2.4. Overview of Analyses. Data analyses proceeded in five stages. First, demographic and behavioral characteristics of the final sample are described. Second, representativeness and randomization checks are presented. Third, the omnibus tests for the effect of condition (experimental versus *control*) on the proportion of new plasma donors and the mean number of plasma donations over the study period of 6 months. Fourth, planned analyses were undertaken that compared the effect of each intervention on donation behavior, compared with the *control* condition. Analyses were undertaken according to the intention-to-treat analysis. Finally, tests for modification of intervention effects by gender, age, and donor status were conducted via moderated regression analysis.

3. Results

3.1. Demographic and Behavioral Characteristics of the Sample. The final sample ($N = 924$) consisted of 378 women (40.9%) and 546 men (59.1%). Participants were predominantly repeat donors (87.8%) and had a mean age of 41.5 years (SD = 14.9). Overall, 141 (15.3%) donors gave plasma at least once during the 6-month follow-up period. In total, they made 403 plasma donations.

3.2. Representativeness and Randomization Checks. To check on the success of randomization of participants, the three conditions (*control, information only by nurse,* and *information plus self-positive image by nurse*) were compared

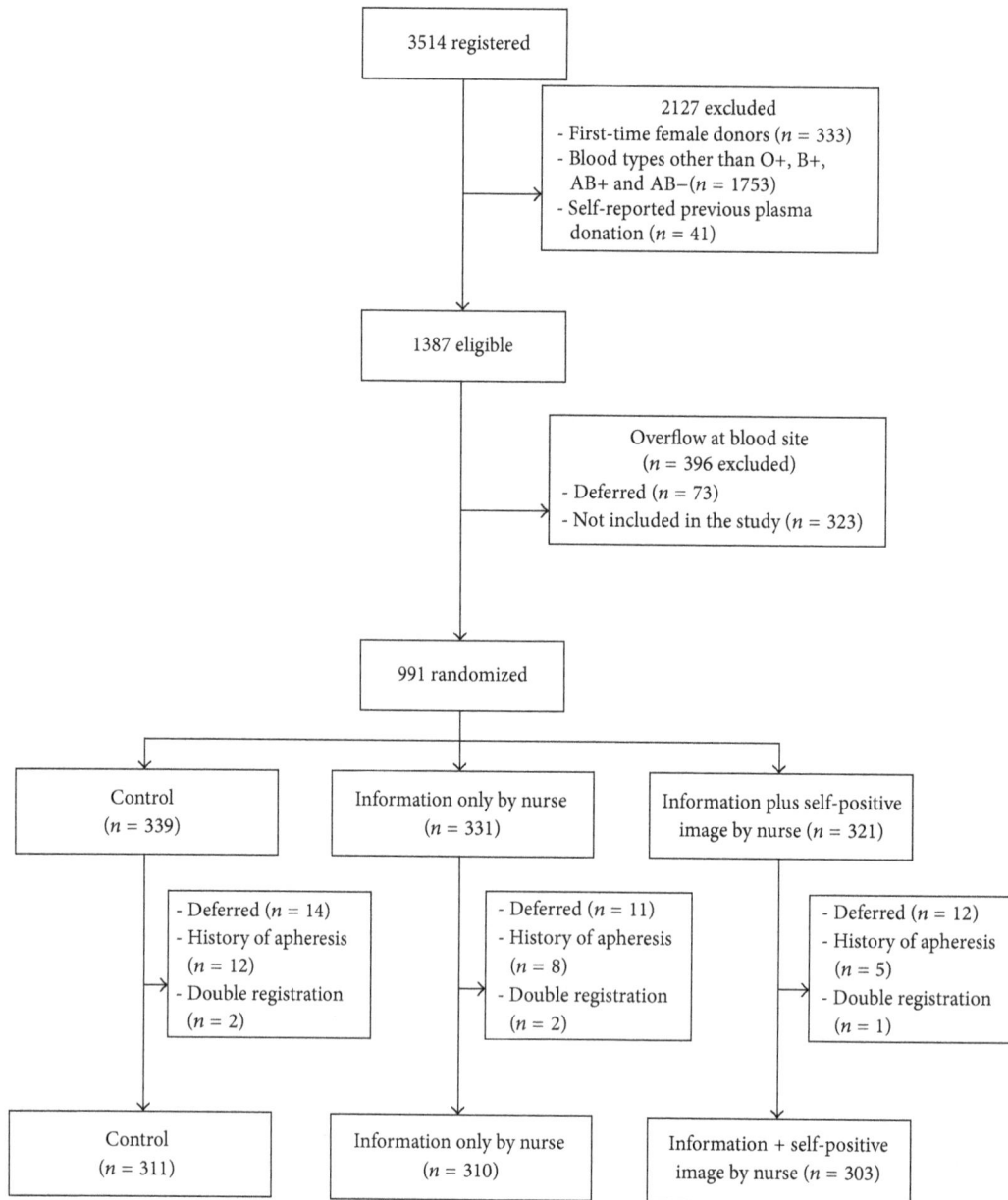

FIGURE 1

on sociodemographic variables (i.e., age, gender, and donor status) at the time of randomization. No difference was observed on any of the variables (gender, $\chi^2(2, N = 924) = 1.31$, $P = .518$; age, $\chi^2(4, N = 924) = 2.58$, $P = .63$; and donor status, $\chi^2(2, N = 924) = 2.83$, $P = .24$), suggesting randomization was successful. In addition, because correlations between these variables and donation (Spearman's coefficient: rho, ρ) were low (at 6 months: gender, $\rho = -.02$; age, $\rho = .06$; and donor status, $\rho = .10$), we did not control for these variables in subsequent analyses.

3.3. Omnibus Effect of Condition on Plasma Donation Behaviors. The use of a dichotomized measure refers to the number of individuals who gave plasma at least once. The

intention-to-treat analysis (GENMOD procedure, Binomial distribution: 1 = gave plasma; 0 = did not give plasma) showed a main effect on the proportion of blood donors in the experimental conditions who gave plasma at least once at 6 months compared to the *control* condition ($\chi^2(1, N = 924) = 31.97$, $P < .001$). For the frequency of plasma donation (GENMOD procedure, Poisson distribution), the analysis showed a main effect for the experimental versus *control* conditions at the 6-month follow-up, ($\chi^2(1, N = 924) = 5.04$, $P < .05$). These findings justify more focused contrasts to assess pairwise differences between conditions.

3.4. Pairwise Comparisons of the Impact of Conditions on Plasma Donation Behaviors. Contrast analyses indicated that

TABLE 1: Mean frequency of plasma donations at 6 months (N = 924).

Conditions	6 months	
	M	SD
Information only by nurse	0.327$_b$	0.819
Information plus self-positive image by nurse	0.439$_c$	1.191
Control	0.135$_a$	0.648

Note. Means within each column that do not share the same subscript differ significantly ($P < .05$, 2-tailed test).

information only by nurse ($\chi^2(1) = 25.15$, $P < .001$; 19.8%) and *information plus self-positive image by nurse* ($\chi^2(1) = 25.01$, $P < .001$; 19.7%) showed significant greater proportions of donors who gave plasma at least once compared to *control* (6.4%). The two experimental conditions did not differ ($\chi^2(1) = 0.00$, $P = .969$).

Table 1 presents the mean frequency of plasma donations for each condition at 6-month follow-up. As expected, the *control* condition exhibited the lowest mean donation ($M = .135$). At the 6-month follow-up, the *information only by nurse* ($\chi^2(1, N = 924) = 25.22$, $P < .001$, $d = 0.26$) and *information plus self-positive image by nurse* conditions ($\chi^2(1, N = 924) = 52.56$, $P < .001$; $d = 0.32$) showed significantly greater frequency of plasma donations compared to the *control* condition. Moreover, the *information plus self-positive image by nurse* significantly outperformed the *information only by nurse* ($\chi^2(1, N = 924) = 5.04$, $P < .05$, $d = 0.13$).

3.5. Tests for the Modification of the Intervention Effect on Plasma Donation Behaviors. As recommended by Aiken and West [8], a series of three-step hierarchical regressions were used to test whether gender, age, and donor status moderated the effect of each intervention at the 6-month follow-up. Behavior was regressed on the respective condition at step 1, the three moderator variables were entered on the second step, and the three condition × moderator interaction terms entered the equation on the third step.

Concerning the proportion of whole blood donors who gave plasma at least once, only donor status ($P < .05$) emerged as a moderator for one of the interventions: *information plus self-positive image by nurse*. This latter intervention was significant only among repeat whole blood donors ($B = 1.36$, SE = .28, $P < .001$).

Concerning the mean number of plasma donations, few moderation effects were observed. First, gender, age, and donor status (all $Ps < .01$) moderated the effect of the *information plus self-positive image by nurse* intervention. More precisely, this latter intervention was more efficient among men ($B = 0.81$, SE = .21, $P < .001$), although it remained significant among women ($B = 1.82$, SE = .33, $P < 001$), donors aged 35 year and more (35–49 years: $B = 1.23$, SE = .26, $P < .001$; 50 years and more: $B = 1.81$, SE = .38, $P < .001$), and repeat donors ($B = 1.24$, SE = .18, $P < .001$). Finally, it was observed that age ($P < .01$) moderated the effect of the *information only by nurse* intervention. This

intervention was more efficient among donors aged 50 years and more ($B = 1.78$, SE = .38, $P < .001$); it was not significant among the younger groups.

4. Discussion

The present study was quite successful and both interventions performed evenly in recruiting new plasma donors although the *information plus self-positive image by nurse* intervention outperformed the *information only by nurse* on the frequency of plasma donations. Three additional observations were noted regarding the moderation effects. First, the effect of both interventions on the frequency of plasma donation was moderated by age, being significant only among older aged groups. Second, the effect of the *information plus self-positive image by nurse* intervention on both outcomes (proportion of new plasma donors and frequency of donation) was moderated by donor status, the effect being significant only among repeat donors. Finally, the *information plus self-positive image by nurse* intervention was more effective to increase the frequency of plasma donation among men, although it was also significant among women.

It is quite interesting to note that only providing basic face-to-face information concerning the plasma donation procedure was sufficient to initiate this new behavior among a substantial proportion of blood donors. This observation runs contrary to the current trend observed in many public health policies to promote the adoption environmental change approaches instead of individuals change strategies. In the present study, our results suggest that providing information is a behavioral change technique that has the potential to change behavior of a significant proportion of blood donors. A number of reasons can explain this positive outcome. First, most blood donors were informed for the first time, face-to-face by a nurse, about the nature of this new behavior and given its similarity with blood donation, they likely evaluated having the capacity to adopt it. Second, the adoption of this new behavior was likely well aligned with the prevailing underlying motivations, for instance to help others. Third, there was a real opportunity to act, with the apheresis center being located within a driving distance of 45 minutes. In summary, in the present case, these above explanations would fit perfectly the COM-B System, a framework for understanding behavior [9]. According to this framework, when individuals have the capacity, are motivated, and have the opportunity to act, there is a high probability that they will take action. Notwithstanding all of these possible explanations, the present study showed that providing face-to-face information changed the behavior of blood donors.

The message referring to self-positive image did not have a significant effect above providing *information only by a nurse* on the recruitment of new plasma donors. However, our self-positive image message resulted in a higher number of donations in the group exposed to the *information plus self-positive image by nurse* intervention compared to *information only by nurse*. This suggests that reference to feelings of self-positive image such as feeling good and being proud and that giving plasma is a rewarding personal experience is a motivational approach to favor a higher frequency of plasma donation. This explanation would be supported by the results of Ferguson and colleagues [6] showing that donors exposed to a benevolent message (i.e., reading a leaflet) highlighting the personally rewarding nature of helping and of self-worth associated with donation significantly increased the willingness to give blood. Our findings are also aligned with the observation reported by Bagot et al. [5] suggesting that messages that emphasize the donor's needs and welfare are more effective to motivate whole blood donors to become plasma donors. Few explanations can be offered to explain this specific finding. First, donors in the SPI condition were described the plasma donation by a nurse as a rewarding experience and told that those who give plasma are proud of doing this, feel good about themselves, and hold personal positive affect (SPI). According to the theory of self-fulfilling prophecy [10], a positive expectation about the adoption of a given behavior (e.g., giving plasma) may affect a person's behavior toward this action in a manner that causes those expectations to be fulfilled. Therefore, once these new plasma donors were convinced that giving plasma really was a rewarding experience, they took very real actions in consequence and made more frequent donations than those who only received information.

Another possible explanation is offered by self-determination theory [11]. This theory would predict that an intrinsic source of motivation better support the adoption and maintenance of a given behavior. Thus, the information provided by nurses can be viewed as a source of external motivation. However, donors in the self-positive image condition may have retained the idea that doing the behavior makes you feel good and, in turn, this makes you do it again. This would then be an internal or intrinsic source of motivation that favors giving plasma again.

The three moderators analyzed, that is, age, gender, and donor status, carried some effect on the effectiveness of our interventions to initiate plasma donation among blood plasma donors. Overall, these moderating effects indicate that interventions to promote starting giving plasma among blood donors are more likely to be successful among a population of men aged 35 years and more and who have some experience with blood donation. There are a number of possible reasons for these moderating effects. For instance, men have a higher circulating blood volume, which enhances the total quantity of plasma that can be collected on the long term compared to women. Individuals aged 35 years and more might also be able to follow a rigorous collection schedule compared to younger individuals [12]. Finally, blood donors who have some experience with the procedure of blood donation likely have a better understanding of the ability required for giving plasma. In summary, this would provide support for policies targeting the recruitment of plasma donors only among those who have given whole blood at least once in their life, such as the case in Australia.

A few limitations of this study should be noted. First, our study was conducted on a sample of French speaking donors in Quebec, Canada, who might differ from other whole blood donors from different countries. Second, five nurses were trained for the present project. It is likely that the quality of the intervention varied from one nurse to another and it is not possible to know if the intervention was always delivered as planned.

5. Conclusion

Providing information on how, where, and when to give plasma is enough to convince a significant proportion of whole blood donors to start giving plasma. Moreover, a message highlighting self-positive image of giving plasma appears to enhance the frequency of donation. Blood agencies can therefore introduce this simple low cost promotional approach to recruit new plasma donors, especially among men, aged 35 years and more and who have some experience with giving blood.

Conflict of Interests

The authors declare that they have no conflict of interests relevant to the publication of this paper.

Acknowledgment

The authors would like to acknowledge the contribution of Sophie Dubuc for her assistance in data collection and data processing.

References

[1] R. C. James and C. A. Mustard, "Geographic location of commercial plasma donation clinics in the United States, 1980–1995," *American Journal of Public Health*, vol. 94, no. 7, pp. 1224–1229, 2004.

[2] D. M. Meyer, R. S. Hillman, and S. J. Slichter, "Plateletapheresis program. I. Donor recruitment and commitment," *Transfusion*, vol. 24, no. 4, pp. 287–291, 1984.

[3] D. G. Woodfield, A. Ramirez, A. Everard, and J. Kent, "Volunteer blood donors for a cell pheresis programme," *New Zealand Medical Journal*, vol. 98, no. 789, pp. 904–906, 1985.

[4] D. C. Bolgiano, S. Smith, and S. J. Slichter, "Strategies to recruit plateletpheresis donors from a registry of HLA- typed, unrelated, bone marrow donors," *Transfusion*, vol. 33, no. 8, pp. 675–678, 1993.

[5] K. L. Bagot, L. L. Bove, B. M. Masser, and K. M. White, "Asking for something different from our donors: factors influencing persuasion success," *Transfusion*, vol. 54, no. 3, pp. 848–855, 2014.

[6] E. Ferguson, K. Farrell, and C. Lawrence, "Blood donation is an act of benevolence rather than altruism," *Health Psychology*, vol. 27, no. 3, pp. 327–336, 2008.

[7] J. M. Weyant, "Effects of mood states, costs, and benefits on helping," *Journal of Personality and Social Psychology*, vol. 36, no. 10, pp. 1169–1176, 1978.

[8] L. S. Aiken and S. G. West, *Multiple Regression: Testing and Interpreting Interactions*, Sage, New Park, Calif, USA, 1991.

[9] S. Michie, M. M. van Stralen, and R. West, "The behaviour change wheel: a new method for characterising and designing behaviour change interventions," *Implementation Science*, vol. 6, no. 1, article 42, 2011.

[10] R. K. Merton, "The self-fulfilling prophecy," in *Social Theory and Social Structure*, pp. 475–490, Free Press, New York, NY, USA, 2nd edition, 1968.

[11] E. L. Deci and R. M. Ryan, *Intrinsic Motivation and Self-Determination in Human Behavior*, Plenum, New York, NY, USA, 1985.

[12] C. J. Julius and S. R. Sytsma, "Comparison of demographics and motivations of highly committed whole blood and platelet donors," *Journal of Clinical Apheresis*, vol. 8, no. 2, pp. 82–88, 1993.

25

Epidemiological Profiles of Foreign-Born and US-Born Hispanic Blood Donors in a Major Metropolitan Area in the United States

Adelbert B. James,[1] Cassandra D. Josephson,[1] Marta I. Castillejo,[1] George B. Schreiber,[2] and John D. Roback[1]

[1] Department of Pathology and Laboratory Medicine, Center for Transfusion and Cellular Therapies, Emory University School of Medicine, Atlanta, GA 30322, USA
[2] Independent Consultant, Bethesda, MD 20814, USA

Correspondence should be addressed to Adelbert B. James, abjames@emory.edu

Academic Editor: Silvano Wendel

Background. The explosive growth of Hispanics in the US makes this population a significant and untapped source for blood donation. *Methods.* A cross-sectional study was performed to evaluate blood donation behaviors and demographics of foreign-born and US-born Hispanic donors between 2006 and 2009 in metropolitan Atlanta, GA, USA. Bivariate analyses and multivariate logistic regression were used to assess factors associated with foreign-born donors. *Results.* 5,119 foreign-born and 11,841 US-born Hispanics donated blood. Foreign-born Hispanic donors were more likely than US-born donors to be blood group O (57.6% versus 52.0%; $P < .001$) and more frequent donors (2.2 versus 2.0; $P < .001$). Cuban-born donors had the highest rates of return donation (63.2%). In contrast, Mexicans, the most prevalent subpopulation among foreign-born Hispanic donors (31.8%), had the lowest rates of return donation (42.0%). *Conclusions.* The heterogeneity found among Hispanic donors in this study is valuable for the design of recruitment strategies to increase blood donations.

1. Introduction

In 2010, Hispanics accounted for more than half of the growth in the total US population between 2000 and 2010, making them the fastest growing ethnic group [1]. This expansion of Hispanics is largely due to the natural increase (births minus deaths) of the existing population. Since 2000, of the total Hispanic growth in the US, 40% of the increase was due to net international migration [2]. In numbers, Hispanics currently exceed African Americans and account for 15.1% of the total US population [2]. Particularly, the South has experienced a larger overall Hispanic growth than any other region in the US [2]. In Georgia, the Hispanic population increased 96.1% from 453,227 in 2000 to 853,689 in 2010; the overall total population increase between 2000 and 2010 was 18.3% [3].

This explosive growth of Hispanics in the US makes these residents a vital and underutilized source of potential blood donors. Currently, in Georgia, Hispanics donate at significantly lower rates than non-Hispanic whites and African Americans [4]. Approximately 1.4% of Hispanics donate blood each year when compared to 4.2% of non-Hispanic whites and 2.4% of African Americans [4]. The disparity between these groups' donation frequencies is especially vexing since a high percentage of Hispanics (57–70%) are blood group O [5] and their inclusion in the donor pool could significantly improve blood supply logistics.

In an effort to increase blood donation among Hispanics, an evaluation of their culture, education, language obstacles, and knowledge of blood donation is essential to understanding the observed donation differences. "Hispanics," however, are not a single monolithic culture. In the US, there are five primary Hispanic subgroups—Cuban, Central and South American, Mexican, and Puerto Rican [6, 7]. These subgroups are based upon geographic distributions of Hispanic populations within the US. For example, the majority of Cubans reside in Florida; Central Americans and South Americans reside mostly in the south, northeast, and the west; Mexicans reside primarily in the Southwest and the majority of Puerto Ricans live in the Northeast of the US [7]. Cultural differences exist between the primary Hispanic subgroups [8], and additional divergences exist with blending of Hispanics from distinct subgroups.

Acculturation is another important factor influencing Hispanics differently depending on whether one is born in, rather than immigrates to, the US. To this end, there is a need for more epidemiologic-based blood donor studies that focus on Hispanic subgroups.

Knowledge of the demographics of Hispanic donors could lead to a better understanding of Hispanic blood donation behaviors and is an important step for developing effective recruitment strategies that may help increase blood donations. Thus, the purpose of this study is to evaluate the demographics and patterns of blood donation of Hispanics, foreign-born, and US-born.

2. Materials and Methods

2.1. Study Population and Design. Data from the Retrovirus Epidemiology Donor Study-II (REDS-II) database at the American Red Cross Blood Services (ARC), Southern Region (Atlanta, GA), were included in this study. Donors were selected for this study based on their self-identification as being Hispanic from 19 Spanish-speaking countries and the US. The selection criteria also included ages between 16 and 82 years who gave between one and twenty-four whole blood donations from 2006 to 2009 at the ARC in metro Atlanta. Donors selected their country of birth from a list that included South American, Central American, and Caribbean countries. Since the US was included in the list to choose from, Hispanic donors could be categorized as either foreign-born or US-born. For purposes of this analysis, foreign-born donors were classified as Cuban, Central American, South American, Mexican, and Puerto Rican. (Donors from the Dominican Republic were classified as Central Americans.)

2.2. Statistical Analyses. Study variables consisted of date of donation, age, gender, highest level of education attained, history of deferral, history of blood transfusion, site of donations (fixed or mobile centers), and ever pregnant. This was a cross-sectional study using bivariate analyses for variables of interest. The mean donation frequency was calculated by dividing the total number of donations by the total number of blood donors. Donor rates were calculated as the total number of successful donations in counties where blood was collected over the total Hispanic subgroup population living in Georgia using data from the 2006–2008 US Census. Deferral rates were calculated by the number of deferrals divided by the total number of deferrals and successful presentations and expressed per 1,000 donor presentations. For this analysis, screening test positives rather than confirmatory testing results were used to calculate the proportion of deferrals. We used odds ratios (ORs), 95% confidence intervals (CI), and chi-square analyses to examine the relationships between foreign- versus US-born donors

and donation sites. In addition, multivariate logistic regression model was constructed to predict whether the donor was foreign-born versus US-born using gender, age, education, first-time donor status, history of transfusion and deferrals, and donation site as independent variables. Data were analyzed by SPSS statistics 19 (SPSS Inc., 2009, Chicago, IL).

3. Results

The study population consisted of 5,119 foreign-born (30.2%) and 11,839 US-born Hispanic blood donors (69.8%) between 2006 and 2009 (see Table 1). Foreign-born Hispanics represented 0.7% Cuban, 7% Central American 7.9% South, American, 9.6% Mexican, and 4.9% Puerto Rican of all Hispanic donors. More than half of all donors were females (56.2%), and donor ages ranged between 16 and 82 years with 73.7% of donors younger than 35 years. Overall, the mean age was 27.3 ± 12.4 years. The mean age among foreign-born donors was higher (30.8 ± 13.2 years) than US-born donors (25.8 ± 11.7 years) ($P < .001$).

Educational levels varied among subgroups. A greater percent of donors from Cuba (55.9%) and Puerto Rico (50.2%) represented the highest educated donors followed by South Americans (46.4%), US-born (35.0%), Central Americans (27.0%), and Mexican donors (14.3%). Mexican donors represented the highest percent of donors without a high school diploma (22.1%) followed by Central Americans (9.5%), US-born (3.8%), South Americans (3.2%), Cubans (2.9%), and Puerto Ricans (2.1%). The majority of donors with less than a 9th grade education were Mexicans (13.5%) and Central Americans (6.5%). There was no significant difference in earning a high school diploma or bachelor's degree between foreign-born and US-born donors.

The numbers of screening test positive donors for cytomegalovirus (CMV) (834), hepatitis B (104), syphilis (58), hepatitis C (HCV) (35), human immunodeficiency virus (HIV) (25), and Chagas disease (7) were relatively low. The majority of CMV (459) and HIV (23) infections were diagnosed among US-born Hispanics. Most HCV infections were diagnosed among US-born Hispanics (23), Puerto Ricans (5), and Mexicans (4). Overall, US-born Hispanics were more likely to be infected with HIV than foreign-born Hispanics (0.2% versus 0.0%, $P = .015$); less likely to be infected with hepatitis B (0.5% versus 1.0%, $P = .001$); less likely to be infected with syphilis (0.3% versus 0.6%, $P = .005$); less likely to be infected with CMV (49.9% versus 70.8%, $P < .001$); less likely to be infected with Chagas disease (0.0% versus 0.2%, $P = .002$). There was no statistically significant difference in HCV infection between US-born Hispanics and foreign-born Hispanics.

Figure 1 illustrates the rate of donor representation by subgroup in Georgia. Overall, the age-relevant donor rate including both foreign-born and US-born Hispanics was 34 per 1,000 population. Donor rates were sharply diminished among donors after the age of 24 years and were considerably varied across age groups. The rate among US-born donors (55 per 1,000 population) was higher when compared to foreign-born donors (18 per 1,000 population). The donor rate among younger Mexicans (16–24 yrs old) decreased

TABLE 1: Characteristics of US-born and foreign-born Hispanic donors.

	US-born		Foreign-born		
	Number	%	Number	%	P value
All donors	11,839	69.8	5,119	30.2	
Gender					<.001
Male	5,053	42.7	2,383	46.5	
Female	6,786	57.3	2,738	53.5	
Age groups (years)*					<.001
16–24	7,324	61.9	2,125	41.6	
25–34	1,925	16.3	1,117	21.9	
35–44	1,447	12.2	973	19.0	
45–54	789	6.7	606	11.9	
55–64	281	2.4	239	4.7	
65–82	64	0.5	52	1.0	
Mean age	25.8		30.8		<.001
Education*					<.001
9–12th grade, no diploma	4,566	42.2	1,516	34.3	
High-school graduate	1,526	14.1	686	15.5	
Some college or tech	2,768	25.6	1,136	25.7	
Bachelor's degree	1,950	18.0	1,079	24.4	
Mean donation frequency	2.0		2.2		<.001
First-time donor?*					<.001
Yes	5,389	48.8	2,148	45.7	
No	5,658	51.2	2,552	54.3	
History of blood transfusion?*					0.074
Yes	246	2.3	123	2.7	
No	10,516	97.7	4,466	97.3	
History of deferral?					.001
Yes	1,190	10.1	599	11.7	
No	10,649	89.9	4,520	88.3	
Donated at fixed sites?*					<.001
Yes	1,074	9.1	612	12.0	
No	10,763	90.9	4,506	88.0	
Infectious disease					
CMV	459	3.9	375	7.3	<.001
Hepatitis B	56	0.5	48	0.9	.001
Hepatitis C	23	0.2	12	0.2	.713
Syphilis	30	0.3	28	0.6	.005
HIV	23	.2	2	0.0	.015
Chagas disease	1	0.0	6	0.2	.002

* Missing data.

from 21 per 1,000 population compared to a rate of 2 per 1,000 population among older Mexicans (55–64 yrs old). The donor rates of Cuban, South American, and Puerto Rican donors were consistently higher than the rates of Central American and Mexican donors.

Overall, donor deferral rates ranged from 123 per 1,000 presentations among Puerto Ricans to 177 per 1,000 presentations among South Americans. The deferral rate among US-born Hispanics was 136 per 1,000 presentations.

The most common reasons for deferral were low hematocrit (Hct) or low hemoglobin (Hb), malaria travel, feeling unwell, and high blood pressure or pulse. South Americans (85 per 1,000 presentations), Cubans (74 per 1,000 presentations), and Central Americans (68 per 1,000 presentations) had the highest deferral rates due to low Hct or Hb; the deferral rate among US-born Hispanics was 60 per 1,000 presentations. Central Americans (17 per 1,000 presentations) and South Americans (10 per 1,000

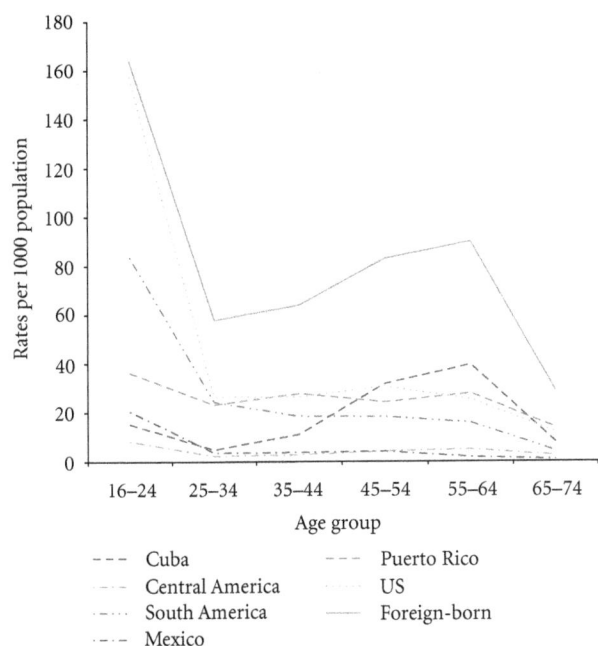

FIGURE 1: Blood donor rates among Hispanic subgroups in Georgia per 1,000 population.

presentations) had the highest deferral rates due to travel to a malaria endemic area; the deferral rate among US-born Hispanics was 6 per 1,000 presentations.

3.1. Hispanic Donors Born in the US. Women were the predominant US-born Hispanic donors (57.3%) of whom the majority were between 16 and 34 years old (62.0%). The prevalence of O type blood was 52.0%. At least 35.0% earned a bachelor's degree, and 17.4% received a high school diploma. Approximately 48.8% were first-time donors; 58.8% donated blood once; 10.1% had a history of deferrals; 9.1% donated at a fixed site. Overall, US-born donors were less likely to return than foreign-born donors (41.2% versus 46.5%, $P < .001$); 2 donations (20.6% versus 24.4%, $P < .001$); 3 donations (11.1% versus 14.8%, $P < .001$); 4 donations (6.7% versus 9.0%, $P < .001$); 5 donations, (4.7% versus 6.3%, $P < .001$); 6 donations (3.2% versus 4.4, $P < .001$); ≥7 donation.

3.2. Foreign-Born Donors. A preponderance of foreign-born Hispanic donors were female (53.4%), mostly between the ages of 16–34, (63.3%). Foreign-born donors were more likely to be male than US-born donors (OR = 1.13, 95% CI: 1.09–1.29) and less likely to be younger (16–34 years) than donors born in the US (OR = 0.48, 95% CI: 0.45–0.66). At least 34.1% earned a Bachelor's degree and 17.7% had received a high school diploma. As a group, foreign-born Hispanics were more likely to be blood type O and become repeat donors; 57.6% of foreign-born donors were blood type O, and these donors were 24% more likely to be repeat donors than US-born donors (OR = 1.24, 95% CI: 1.16–1.32). Foreign-born donors were more likely to have a

history of deferrals than US-born donors (OR = 1.18, 95% CI: 1.06–1.31).

The logistic regression model showed predictors for foreign-born donors. After adjustment of variables in the model, foreign-born donors were 20% more likely to use fixed donation centers than US-born donors (OR = 1.20; 95% CI: 1.06, 1.35). Foreign-born donors were 17% more likely to be males than US-born donors (OR = 1.17, 95% CI: 1.09, 1.27); foreign-born donors were more likely to be first-time donors than US-born donors (OR = 1.30, 95% CI: 1.18, 1.42) (see Table 2).

Table 3 shows that foreign-born donor characteristics were not homogenous but rather varied with the country of birth. The highest percentage of group O donors were found among Mexicans (63%), followed by South American donors (57.2%), Central American donors (57%), Puerto Rican donors (50.3%), and Cuban donors (45.4%). Cuban-born Hispanics also had the highest rates of return donation; the percent of repeat donors between donating between 2 and at least 7 donations was 63.2%, 43.2%, 30.4, 22.4%, 15.2%, and 9.6%, respectively. The frequencies of repeat donations per year among the other foreign-born Hispanics are South American (51.6%, 27.3%, 17.1%, 10.8%, 7.8%, and 5.7%), Puerto Rican (49.2%, 29.6%, 18.8%, 11.4%, 8.6%, and 6.4%), Central American (43.4%, 24.1%, 16.0%, 10.0%, 7.3%, and 4.6%), and Mexican (42.0%, 18.0%, 9.0%, 5.0%, 3.0%, and 1.8%). Mexican donors had the lowest percentage of historical deferrals (9.3%), followed by Puerto Ricans (10.3%), Central Americans (12.2%), South Americans (14.6%), and Cubans (16%).

3.3. Mean Donation Frequency. The mean donation frequency (2.0 donations per year) varied by demographic group and ranged from 1.8 among Mexicans to 3.1 among Cubans. The mean donation frequency of foreign-born Hispanic donors was higher (2.2) when compared to US-born donors (2.0. $P < .001$). Donors who visited fixed donor centers had a higher mean donation frequency (3.1) compared to donors who visited mobile sites (1.0, $P < .001$). Donors who were older (35–82 years) had a higher mean donation frequency (2.6) compared to younger donors (1.8) ($P < .001$). During this study period, 603 repeat donors contributed, at a minimum, 7 donations per year. The highest frequency of donations (24) was offered by one donor. Of the donors evaluated, 9701 (57.2%) donated one time, while 7257 (42.8%) donated two times (median return time 6.2 months). Of the remaining donors, 21.7% donated 3 times, 12.2% donated 4 times, 7.4% donated 5 times, 5.2% donated 6 times, and 3.6% donated blood at least 7 times.

4. Discussion

The findings in this study reveal variations in blood donation patterns among Hispanic groups in the US. The diversity in demographics between Hispanics who are foreign-born and Hispanics born in the US may account for these differences in donation practices. Foreign-born donors were more likely to be male and older compared to US-born donors ($P < .001$).

TABLE 2: Logistic regression model examining factors associated with foreign-born Hispanic blood donors.

	Unadjusted OR (95% CI)	P value	Adjusted OR (95% CI)	P value
Gender				
Male	1.17 (1.09, 1.25)	<.001	1.17 (1.09, 1.27)	<.001
Females	1.0		1.0	
Age groups (years)				
16–24	1.0		1.0	
25–34	2.00 (1.83, 2.18)	<.001	2.47 (2.19, 2.78)	<.001
35–44	2.32 (2.11, 2.54)	<.001	2.85 (2.50, 3.25)	<.001
45–54	2.65 (2.36, 2.97)	<.001	3.46 (2.97, 4.03)	<.001
55–64	2.93 (2.45, 3.51)	<.001	4.11 (3.30, 5.10)	<.001
65–82	2.80 (1.94, 4.05)	<.001	3.61 (2.35, 5.54)	<.001
Education				
9–12th grade, no diploma	1.0		1.0	
High school graduate	1.35 (1.22, 1.51)	<.001	0.94 (0.83, 1.07)	.359
Some college or tech	1.24 (1.13, 1.35)	<.001	0.75 (0.67, 0.85)	<.001
Bachelor degree	1.67 (1.52, 1.83)	<.001	0.77 (0.67, 0.89)	<.001
First-time donor?				
Yes	0.88 (0.82, 0.95)	<.001	1.30 (1.18, 1.42)	<.001
No	1.0		1.0	
History of transfusion?				
Yes	1.18 (0.95, 1.47)	.134	0.88 (0.69, 1.11)	.276
No	1.0		1.0	
History of deferral?				
Yes	1.19 (1.07, 1.32)	.001	1.09 (0.96, 1.23)	.183
No	1.0		1.0	
Donation site				
Fixed site	1.36 (1.22, 1.51)	<.001	1.20 (1.06, 1.35)	.005
Mobile site	1.0		1.0	

Hispanics born abroad tend to be older and are therefore less likely to donate at school blood drives, the most common site for recruiting first-time donors. Hispanics born in the US tend to donate at a younger age and are more likely to participate as first time donors in school drives.

Further analysis suggests that foreign-born donors were more likely to donate and become repeat donors than those born in the US. Some have suggested that Hispanic immigrants are not a random sample of their home countries since they tend to have more resources, education, psychological strength, and motivation to emigrate [9–11], and may be more willing to donate blood. Other researchers have shown that age, gender, and education are strong predictors for blood donations [4]. The findings of this study show that the Hispanic donor population is more highly educated than the US Hispanic population [12]. This study echoes previous findings; the donor rates of non-Hispanic whites (68.9/1,000 population) and African Americans (34.9/1,000 population) are significantly higher than that of Hispanics (34.1/1,000 population) [4].

This study demonstrates that Mexicans were least likely to donate blood when compared to all Hispanic subgroups, including those born in the US. This is troubling since

Mexicans are the largest subgroup, representing 63% of the total Hispanic population living in the US in 2010 [1, 3, 13]. An estimated 32 million Mexicans account for three-fourths of the 15.2 million increase in the total Hispanic population between 2000 and 2010 [1], including more than half who represent undocumented immigrants [9]. The results of this current study, revealing the highest prevalence of Universal blood type O among Mexicans (63%) and the lowest rates of previous deferrals, emphasize the need for recruitment strategies targeted at this subgroup in an effort to expand the current blood supply.

Enrollment programs must necessarily address the immigration concerns in the wake of recently enacted immigration laws and the reluctance perhaps to show a photo ID needed to donate blood. The findings in this and other studies of the relatively low level of education among Mexicans [14] also support enlistment strategies that provide blood donor education to this subgroup, at least 22% of whom have not graduated from high school. Possible donor selection bias towards Hispanics should be evaluated that might be contributing to underrepresentation of Hispanics in the donor base, namely, of Mexicans. Factors such as lower education and economic status might be significant barriers

TABLE 3: Characteristics of foreign-born and US-born Hispanic donors by country/region of interest.

	Cuba		Central America		South America		Mexico		Puerto Rico		US-born	
	Number	%	Number	%	Number	%	Number	%	Number	%	Number	%
All donors	125	0.7	1,185	7.0	1,346	7.9	1,629	9.6	834	4.9	11,839	69.8
Gender												
Male	63	50.4	533	45.0	635	47.2	773	47.5	379	45.4	5,053	42.7
Female	62	49.6	652	55.0	711	52.8	856	52.5	455	54.6	6,786	57.3
Age groups (years)												
16–24	16	13.0	450	38.0	501	37.2	915	56.2	243	29.2	7,324	61.9
25–34	7	5.7	291	24.6	277	20.6	354	21.8	188	22.6	1,925	16.3
35–44	27	21.9	235	19.8	269	20.0	246	15.1	196	23.6	1,447	12.2
45–54	46	37.4	134	11.3	210	15.6	93	5.7	123	14.8	789	6.7
55–64	22	17.9	62	5.2	77	5.7	16	1.0	62	7.5	281	2.4
65–82	5	4.1	13	1.1	12	0.9	3	0.2	19	2.3	64	0.5
Mean age	45.0	—	31.4	—	32.3	—	26.1	—	35	—	25.8	—
M. donation freq.	3.1		2.1		2.4		1.8		2.4		2.0	
Hx. of Transfusion	6	4.8	29	0.0	33	2.4	31	1.9	24	2.9	246	2.1
Hx. of deferral	20	16.0	145	12.2	197	14.6	151	9.3	86	10.3	1,190	10.1
Donated at fixed	18	14.4	146	12.3	227	16.9	126	7.7	95	11.4	1,074	9.1
Ever pregnant	42	73.7	321	52.4	308	47.2	320	39.5	233	54.4	2,292	35.8
Infectious disease												
CMV	7	5.6	88	7.4	146	10.8	96	5.9	38	4.6	459	3.9
Hepatitis B	1	0.8	19	1.6	6	0.4	15	0.9	7	0.8	56	0.5
Hepatitis C	0	0	1	0.1	2	0.1	4	0.2	5	0.6	23	0.2
Syphilis	0	0	11	1.0	7	0.5	9	0.6	1	0.1	30	0.3
HIV	0	0	1	0.1	0	0	1	0.1	0	0	23	0.2
Chagas disease	0	0	0	0	1	0.1	5	0.3	0	0	1	0.0

M.: mean; Hx.: history.

to donation. To this end, mobile drive campaigns could target sites or areas that appear to represent potential recruiting grounds for prospective Hispanic donors. In addition, enlistment of all Hispanics should be offered in their native Spanish for both newly immigrants and older generations of potential donors to increase their degree of comfort and understanding of donating blood.

Among the Hispanic subgroups, Colombians, Cubans, and Puerto Ricans were more likely to, and consistently, donate ($P < .001$). For example, Cubans were among the highest to repeat with a second donation (63%) and donated most frequently (3.1). The high rates of Cuban blood donors may be due to the efficiency of Cuba's national blood system that may mandate blood donations. For instance, Cuba has the highest blood donation rate in Latin America and the Caribbean (439.6/10,000 inhabitants) [15]. The donation rates in Colombia and Mexico are 115.7/10,000 and 126.2/10,000 inhabitants, respectively [15].

The World Health Organization (WHO) and the International Federation of the Red Cross recognize that a country must collect the equivalent of 3%–5% of its population to ensure an adequate volunteer blood supply. In comparison, the US and Latin America collect blood from just slightly over 4.0% and 1.4% of their population, respectively [16]. Complicating recruitment planning, this analysis demonstrated that Cuban donors had the highest percentage of deferrals, with up to 50% of perspective donors having a low hemoglobin level—yet another fact to consider in donation planning strategies.

In another study finding, foreign-born donors were more likely to visit a fixed site than a mobile site, and return for repeat donations much earlier is probably due to the impact of recruitment efforts. Individuals who want to donate more frequently often make return visits to fixed sites [17, 18]. It can be speculated that higher donor rates occur at fixed sites because of the center's availability, whereas donors at a mobile must depend on the frequency and convenience of the mobile rather than the donor's. Sites such as workplaces might frequently underrepresent the Hispanics makeup of the areas. Thus, policy makers could consider areas of heavily populated Hispanics and perhaps survey potential donors in these areas to consider the most convenient times for the blood mobiles to visit these communities. Education on the importance and ease of blood donation could target the areas to stimulate reasons to donate.

The need to emphasize the need for and merit of altruistic blood donations is important in the Hispanic community. To approximate the rate of blood donation of non-Hispanic whites in the US, Hispanics would have to triple their blood donors each year [5]. It is known that there is a greater willingness among Hispanics to offer blood for family members [19] yet limit donations for the wider community as a consequence of a dearth of appropriate donor recruitment and a lack of knowledge and/or mistrust of the US blood system [20]. Since directed donation is deemphasized in the US, the need for family donations is limited. Fortunately, the last decade has seen a shift to promote voluntary donations in Latin America and the Caribbean, where blood safety can be assured. The proportion of voluntary blood donors in Latin America and the Caribbean increased from 15% in 2001 to 36% in 2003 [15, 21].

This study provides substantial insight into the complexities and diversities among Hispanic donors. While donors from this study are from a limited metropolitan area and might not represent Hispanic populations in other areas of the country, it demonstrates that donors from numerous countries have cultural, social, economic, and educational divergences that may have an impact on their blood donations in the US. While current epidemiologic data are not collected solely on cultural subgroups, studies could be proposed in predominantly Puerto Rican, Colombian, or Cuban communities that could help highlight and report their divergences from another subgroup with regards to their knowledge of blood donation. The limitations of this study consist in the small number of foreign-born donors to analyze per country, such as Cuba. The study was also unable to determine the number of years lived in the US by foreign-born donors that may have impacted their blood donation knowledge and practices. Additionally, distinct acculturation processes over time and among subgroups of Hispanics may have profoundly influenced donation practices.

A study of Hispanic donors, powered to reach a greater number of Hispanics and yield greater distinctions among the individual and subgroup demographics and cultural patterns, is needed. Blood donation recruiters are the yeomen of the blood supply chain who rely on information describing current Hispanic blood donation practices to guide them in the formulation of new recruitment strategies and programs. The growing size and importance of the Hispanic Community efforts, including education adapted to Hispanic subgroups, could render a larger and more diverse donor pool which offers the "priceless" gift of life.

Funding

1 P01 HL 086773: Mechanisms and interventions addressing serious hazards of transfusion and cellular therapies.

Conflict of Interests

The authors declare that there is no conflict of interests.

References

[1] US Bureau of the Census, "2010 Census shows nation's Hispanic population grew four times faster than total U.S. population," 2011, http://2010.census.gov/news/releases/operations/cb11-cn146.html.

[2] R. Fry, "Latino settlement in the new century," 2008, http://pewhispanic.org/files/reports/96.pdf.

[3] US Bureau of the Census, "Race and Hispanic origin and the 2010 Census," 2011, http://blogs.census.gov/censusblog/2011/03/race-and-hispanic-origin-and-the-2010-census.html.

[4] B. H. Shaz, A. B. James, K. L. Hillyer, G. B. Schreiber, and C. D. Hillyer, "Demographic variations in blood donor deferrals in a major metropolitan area," *Transfusion*, vol. 50, no. 4, pp. 881–887, 2010.

[5] America's Blood Center and Vanguard Comm, "Blood donations among African Americans and Hispanics: background, hypotheses, research questions. Multicultural donor recruitment and marketing plans," Secondary Research report Phases 1.1, Chicago, Ill, USA, 2006.

[6] B. W. Ward and J. S. Schiller, "Prevalence of complex activity limitations among racial/ethnic groups and Hispanic subgroups of adults: United States, 2003–2009," 2011, http://www.cdc.gov/nchs/data/databriefs/db73.htm.

[7] A. L. Hajat, J. B. Lucas, and R. Kington, "Health outcomes among Hispanic subgroups: United States, 1992–95," in *National Center for Health Statistics. Advance Data from Vital and Health Statistics*, vol. 310, 2000.

[8] The Diversity Data Project, "Composition of the hispanic population by hispanic subgroup," 2000, http://diversitydataarchive.org/Data/Rankings/Show.aspx?ind=103.

[9] L. N. Rubalcava, G. M. Teruel, D. Thomas, and N. Goldman, "The healthy migrant effect: mew findings from the Mexican family life survey," *American Journal of Public Health*, vol. 98, no. 1, pp. 78–84, 2008.

[10] A. F. Abraído-Lanza, B. P. Dohrenwend, D. S. Ng-Mak, and J. B. Turner, "The Latino mortality paradox: a test of the 'salmon bias' and healthy migrant hypotheses," *American Journal of Public Health*, vol. 89, no. 10, pp. 1543–1548, 1999.

[11] K. S. Markides and J. Coreil, "The health of Hispanics in the southwestern United States: an epidemiologic paradox," *Public Health Reports*, vol. 101, no. 3, pp. 253–265, 1986.

[12] US Bureau of the Census, "Educational attainment in the United States:2007–2009," P20-560, http://www.census.gov/prod/2009pubs/p20-560.pdf.

[13] US Bureau of the Census, "2010 Census data," 2010, http://2010.census.gov/2010census/data/.

[14] US Bureau of the Census, "Current population reports P20-550 and earlier reports: "Educational Attainment"," 2011, http://www.census.gov/population/www/socdemo/educ-attn.html.

[15] Pan American Health Organization and World Health Organization, "Blood transfusion safety: progress report," CE142/20, 2008, www.paho.org/english/gov/ce/ce142-20-e.pdf.

[16] P. Carolan and M. Garcia, "Gift Blood is the safest blood," *Perspectives in Health*, vol. 10, no. 2, 2005, http://www.paho.org/english/dd/pin/Number22_last.htm.

[17] B. Custer, K. S. Schlumpf, D. Wright, T. L. Simon, S. Wilkinson, and P. M. Ness, "Donor return after temporary deferral," *Transfusion*, vol. 51, no. 6, pp. 1188–1196, 2011.

[18] G. B. Schreiber, K. S. Schlumpf, S. A. Glynn et al., "Convenience, the bane of our existence, and other barriers to donating," *Transfusion*, vol. 46, no. 4, pp. 545–553, 2006.

[19] G. A. Schmunis and J. R. Cruz, "Safety of the blood supply in Latin America," *Clinical Microbiology Reviews*, vol. 18, no. 1, pp. 12–29, 2005.

[20] F. Gillum, A. F. Eder, and T. L. McLaurin-Jones, "Hispanic ethnicity, race and blood donation in the United States," *Transfusion Medicine*, vol. 18, no. 6, pp. 366–370, 2008.

[21] Pan American Health Organization, "Eligibility for blood donation," 2009, http://publications.paho.org/english/introduction_OP+211.pdf.

26

Alloimmunization in Patients with Sickle Cell Disease in French Guiana

Narcisse Elenga[1] and Loic Niel[2]

[1]Pediatric Unit, Cayenne Hospital, rue des Flamboyants, BP 6006, 97306 Cayenne Cedex, French Guiana
[2]French Guianese Blood Agency, Cayenne Hospital, rue des Flamboyants, BP 6006, 97306 Cayenne Cedex, French Guiana

Correspondence should be addressed to Narcisse Elenga; elengafr@yahoo.fr

Academic Editor: Maria Rios

This study in French Guiana assessed the frequency of alloimmunization to red cell antigens in sickle cell disease patients over 1995–2011 and identified the most common antibodies. A retrospective analysis of the transfusion history and medical records of 302 patients showed that 29/178 transfused patients had developed alloantibodies (16%). The most frequent alloantibodies were anti-LE1, anti-MNS1, anti-LE2, and anti-FY1 and were developed after transfusion of standard red cell units. The frequency of the clinically significant antibodies in this population of SCD patients was 11% (19/178). The antibodies found on those patients who had delayed hemolytic transfusion reaction were anti-K1, anti-FY1, and anti-MNS3. The strategies used to decrease alloimmunization in French Guiana are discussed.

1. Introduction

Sickle cell disease (SCD) is a major public health problem in French Guiana [1, 2]. In this French region located in South America, with 230,000 inhabitants, the standards of health are close to those of mainland France. French Guiana is also a crossroad for poor Caribbean and South American populations that emigrate there in search of better conditions of life. Infectious diseases and chronic diseases are both public health problems. Transfusion remains a major treatment in SCD management. The purpose of red blood cell transfusion (RBC) is to increase oxygen distribution in the tissues and to replace the rigid sickle cell shaped RBCs with healthy deformable RBCs. Yet, in French Guiana, since 2006, donation of blood products has stopped because of Chagas disease. Chagas disease (American trypanosomiasis) is caused by the protozoan *Trypanosoma cruzi*, mainly transmitted to humans by blood-sucking triatomine bugs (Hemiptera, Triatominae) but also transmitted by blood transfusion from infected donors and occasionally by transplacental mother-to-child transmission. It is an endemic disease in the large part of Latin America extending from Mexico to Argentina. In the majority of the cases, after an acute infection sometimes unapparent, the disease becomes chronic, which can be problematic, in case of blood donation.

In French Guiana, the overall prevalence of *T. cruzi* specific IgG was 0.5% [3–5]. All blood products used for transfusion in SCD patients come from Lille, in the north of France or Guadeloupe. Because they will frequently receive transfusions in their life, patients with SCD become exposed to RBCs alloantigens of donor units and alloimmunization. Alloimmunization in SCD has a reported incidence of 20% to 50% [6, 7]. Red cell alloimmunization is frequent because of the antigen disparities between patients of African descent and donors of European ancestry [8–11]. This study, therefore, aimed to estimate the frequency of alloimmunization in a cohort of SCD patients followed in the French Blood Agency of French Guiana from 1995 to 2011, in the particular context of French Guiana, where the blood units come mostly from Caucasian donors, and to describe the measures organized to decrease alloimmunization.

2. Methods

2.1. Study Population. 302 SCD patients (151 males and 151 females) followed in the French Blood Agency of French

Guiana from 1995 to 2011 were included. Data prospectively collected from the medical records monitoring transfusion included demographic and haematological characteristics. All transfused patients ($n = 178$) had received cross-matched red cell units at least compatible in the ABO, RH, and Kell systems.

2.2. Study Design. We reviewed the medical charts in the computerized blood transfusion database.

2.3. Ethical Consideration. Patients included in the database of the French Blood Agency gave informed consent for the use of their data. This data collection was approved by the Commission Nationale Informatique et Libertés (CNIL), a national committee that oversees research data.

2.4. Statistical Analysis. Data were analysed with STATA 10.0 (Stata Corp LP, College Station, TX, USA). We performed a descriptive analysis.

3. Results

Among these patients, 68% were homozygous for HbS, 24% had sickle-hemoglobin C, and 8% had HbS/β-thalassemia. The major ethnic origins were Creole (46%) followed by Haitian (27%) and Bushinenge (22%). The proportions of blood groups were group A: 21.80%, group B: 21.80%, group O: 51.50%, and group AB: 4.90%. The red cell blood transfusion was available for 178 patients (Hb SS), for 2494 red blood cell units. Among the sickle cell anemia patients who had received at least 1 transfusion, 29 had developed alloantibodies (16%). The most frequent alloantibodies were anti-LE1, anti-MNS1, anti-LE2, and anti-FY1 and were developed after transfusion of standard red cell units (Table 1). One patient had 4 alloantibodies while 3 patients had 3 alloantibodies. 12 patients had 2 alloantibodies and 13 patients had 1 alloantibody. There were 74 transfusions and 19 exchange transfusions. Transfusion was performed for acute chest syndrome (ACS) in 26 cases, cholecystectomy in 15 cases, splenectomy in 12 cases, severe infections in 12 cases, and stroke in 10 cases. The frequency of the clinically significant antibodies in this population of SCD patients was 11% (19/178). There were six cases of delayed hemolytic transfusion reaction (DHTR), in two children, two pregnant women, and two other adult SCD patients. The antibodies found on those patients who had DHTR were anti-K1, anti-FY1, and anti-MNS3.

4. Discussion

4.1. Prevalence of Alloimmunization. The prevalence of alloimmunization is high in French Guiana. Nevertheless in Martinique and in Guadeloupe, two other French overseas territories, this prevalence seems similar [12]. It is necessary to note that even if in these two territories the blood collection and distribution are realized on the spot, part of the blood units still come from metropolitan France, because the local production does not allow completely covering needs.

TABLE 1: Blood alloantibodies detected in 29 sickle cell disease patients who have developed alloantibodies.

Alloantibody	Number of patients
Anti-LE1	10
Anti-MNS1	6
Anti-LE2	5
Anti-FY1	5
Anti-RH2	4
Anti-RH3	3
Anti-JK1	3
Anti-MNS 3	2
Anti-K1	2
Anti-RH1	1
Anti-RH8	1
Anti-FY2	1
Anti-JK2	1
Anti-LE4	1
Anti-LU1	1
Anti-DB1	1

Closer to French Guiana, in Brazil, where the prevalence of the Chagas disease in the general population is raised, the alloimmunization rate is 12.9% [13].

There is a basic assumption that since blood cannot be collected locally, use of blood mostly from French Caucasian blood donors is causing alloimmunization in the Guianese population due to ethnic/genetic differences. This assumption, although intuitive, has recently been scientifically refuted by an article on the SCD transfusion policy in a USA SCD center where it was shown that "ethnically" compatible blood in fact brings a high risk of alloimmunization [14].

4.2. Consequence of the Alloimmunization. The major consequence of alloimmunization is the delayed hemolytic transfusion reaction (DHTR), a severe and potentially life-threatening complication that is characterized by a hemolytic anemia of transfused as well as patients' own red blood cells. The diagnosis of DHTR can be difficult because the clinical features could be easily misinterpreted as a severe vasoocclusive crisis. In French Guiana, we noted 6 cases of DHTR that represent a rate of 3.4% (6/178). This frequency seems very high when compared with Brazil [15]. In Brazil, in spite of high prevalence of Chagas disease, blood collection in the general population has not been interrupted. So, blood units come from donors whose origin is close to those of patients. However, the prevalence of antibodies to *T. cruzi* among blood donors has decreased to 0.2% (2012) and in a serosurvey done in 2007 with children of 0–5 years old no single seropositive subject was detected [16] showing that Chagas is a vanishing disease and a minor problem concerning blood transfusion. No case of transmission of Chagas by blood transfusion was reported since the introduction of mandatory testing in the nineties. So, prevention of transfusion-transmitted (TT) Chagas in Brazil is based on serological testing and specific questions included in the predonation interview like the following: "have you ever seen a reduviid bug?"

French Guiana could follow the Brazilian model, which has proven itself. While waiting for the implementation of the blood donation in French Guiana, we recommend for SCD patients who require repeated transfusions extended antigen-matched RBC from Afro-Caribbean donors living in Guadeloupe and taking into account the patient's immuno-hematologic characteristics.

5. Conclusion

In French Guiana, the alloimmunization for the clinically significant antibodies in the SCD patients had a frequency of 11%. The prevention of TT Chagas based on serological testing and specific questions included in the predonation interview like "have you ever seen a reduviid bug?" as done in Brazil could be followed. This strategy for prevention of TT Chagas disease needs a strong political engagement of the sanitary authorities. This study also underlines the interest of selecting blood from Caribbean donors for all programmed transfusion or exchange transfusion.

Conflict of Interests

The authors declare that they have no conflict of interests.

Acknowledgment

The authors would like to thank the members of the French Guianese Blood Agency for data collection.

References

[1] N. Elenga, E. Cuadro, É. Martin, N. Cohen-Addad, and T. Basset, "Associated factors of acute chest syndrome in children with sickle cell disease in French Guiana," *International Journal of Pediatrics*, vol. 2014, Article ID 213681, 4 pages, 2014.

[2] M. Etienne-Julan, G. Elana, G. Loko et al., "La drépanocytose dans les départements français d'outre-mer (Antilles, Guyane, la Réunion, Mayotte): données descriptives et organisation de la prise en charge," *Bulletin Épidémiologique Hebdomadaire*, no. 27-28, 2012.

[3] C. Aznar, G. La Ruche, S. Laventure, B. Carme, P. Liegeard, and M. Hontebeyrie, "Seroprevalence of *Trypanosoma cruzi* infection in French Guiana," *Memorias do Instituto Oswaldo Cruz*, vol. 99, no. 8, pp. 805–808, 2004.

[4] A. L. Ostermayer, A. D. C. Passos, A. C. Silveira, A. W. Ferreira, V. Macedo, and A. R. Prata, "The national Survey of seroprevalence for evaluation of the control of Chagas disease in Brazil (2001–2008)," *Revista da Sociedade Brasileira de Medicina Tropical*, vol. 44, no. 2, pp. 108–121, 2011.

[5] F. Nagajyothi, F. S. Machado, B. A. Burleigh et al., "Mechanisms of *Trypanosoma cruzi* persistence in Chagas disease," *Cellular Microbiology*, vol. 14, no. 5, pp. 634–643, 2012.

[6] J.-A. M. Talano, C. A. Hillery, J. L. Gottschall, D. M. Baylerian, and J. P. Scott, "Delayed hemolytic transfusion reaction/hyperhemolysis syndrome in children with sickle cell disease," *Pediatrics*, vol. 111, no. 6, part 1, pp. e661–e665, 2003.

[7] E. P. Vichinsky, "Current issues with blood transfusions in sickle cell disease," *Seminars in Hematology*, vol. 38, no. 1, pp. 14–22, 2001.

[8] N. Elenga, V. Mialou, K. Kebaïli, C. Galambrun, Y. Bertrand, and C. Pondarre, "Severe neurologic complication after delayed hemolytic transfusion reaction in 2 children with sickle cell anemia: significant diagnosis and therapeutic challenges," *Journal of Pediatric Hematology/Oncology*, vol. 30, no. 12, pp. 928–930, 2008.

[9] M. de Montalembert, M.-D. Dumont, C. Heilbronner et al., "Delayed hemolytic transfusion reaction in children with sickle cell disease," *Haematologica*, vol. 96, no. 6, pp. 801–807, 2011.

[10] F. Noizat-Pirenne and C. Tournamille, "Relevance of RH variants in transfusion of sickle cell patients," *Transfusion Clinique et Biologique*, vol. 18, no. 5-6, pp. 527–535, 2011.

[11] N. Elenga, "Delayed hemolytic transfusion reaction in sickle cell disease," *American Journal of Clinical Medicine Research*, vol. 1, no. 3, pp. 40–44, 2013.

[12] C. Le Turdu-Chicot, L. Foucan, and M. Etienne-Julan-Otto, "Viral seroprevalence, transfusion and alloimmunization in adult sickle cell patients in Guadeloupe," *Transfusion Clinique et Biologique*, vol. 9, no. 2, pp. 115–120, 2002.

[13] G. Moreira Jr., J. O. Bordin, A. Kuroda, and J. Kerbauy, "Red blood cell alloimmunization in sickle cell disease: the influence of racial and antigenic pattern differences between donors and recipients in Brazil," *American Journal of Hematology*, vol. 52, no. 3, pp. 197–200, 1996.

[14] S. T. Chou, T. Jackson, S. Vege, K. Smith-Whitley, D. F. Friedman, and C. M. Westhoff, "High prevalence of red blood cell alloimmunization in sickle cell disease despite transfusion from Rh-matched minority donors," *Blood*, vol. 122, no. 6, pp. 1062–1071, 2013.

[15] A. Fabron Jr., G. Moreira Jr., and J. O. Bordin, "Delayed hemolytic transfusion reaction presenting as a painful crisis in a patient with sickle cell anemia," *Sao Paulo Medical Journal*, vol. 117, no. 1, pp. 38–39, 1999.

[16] A. Moncayo and A. C. Silveira, "Current epidemiological trends for Chagas disease in Latin America and future challenges in epidemiology, surveillance and health policy," *Memorias do Instituto Oswaldo Cruz*, vol. 104, no. 1, pp. 17–30, 2009.

27

Factors Associated with Repeat Blood Donation at the Northern Zone Blood Transfusion Centre in Tanzania

Wilhellmuss I. Mauka,[1,2] **Michael J. Mahande,**[3] **Sia E. Msuya,**[1,3,4] **and Rune N. Philemon**[1,5]

[1]*Institute of Public Health, Department of Community Medicine, Kilimanjaro Christian Medical University College, P.O. Box 2240, Moshi, Tanzania*

[2]*Northern Zone Blood Transfusion Centre, P.O. Box 823, Moshi, Tanzania*

[3]*Institute of Public Health, Department of Epidemiology and Biostatistics, Kilimanjaro Christian Medical University College, Moshi, Tanzania*

[4]*Department of Community Medicine, Kilimanjaro Christian Medical Centre, Moshi, Tanzania*

[5]*Department of Pediatrics, Kilimanjaro Christian Centre, Moshi, Tanzania*

Correspondence should be addressed to Wilhellmuss I. Mauka; wilhemauka@yahoo.com

Academic Editor: Silvano Wendel

Background and Objective. The aim of this study was to determine factors associated with repeat blood donation. *Methods.* This was a cross-sectional study carried out among blood donors aged 18–65 years in northern Tanzania. The questionnaire was administered among 454 participants through the phone. *Results.* Of the 454 participants, the proportion of repeat donation was 63.9%. In the backward logistic regression analysis, the significant predictors were living in Arusha which had lower odds of repeat donation compared to those living in Kilimanjaro. Knowledge of time interval between donations increased odds of repeating donations. High intention increased odds of repeat donation compared to low intention. Altruistic score had minor effect on increasing odds of repeating donation. *Conclusion.* Repeat blood donation is affected by proximity of donating site, awareness of the blood donation interval, intention to donate, and experience on previous donation. We recommend continuous education concerning blood donors and donation among health workers and society as a whole; this will create awareness on motivational factors for repeat donations.

1. Introduction

Blood donation is an act of a healthy person giving blood which will be used by another person in transfusion therapy and since it is a nonpharmaceutical product it has to come directly from a human being through donation [1, 2]. Globally, nearly 108 million units of blood are collected every year and half of those collections are from developed countries which are only one-fifth of total world population. High-income countries have at least 9 times more donations than low-income countries [3]. According to WHO's standards, country's minimum total blood donation collections should be 1% of total population in order to meet blood transfusion requirements [4].

According to Tanzania National Blood Transfusion Services (NBTS), by 2013, the country needed almost 450,000 units of blood annually. Between September 2013 and September 2014, a total of 133,077 units of blood were collected which is almost 30% of national requirement. However, more than 80% of blood donors donated only once and did not return for more donations (unpublished reports by Tanzania NBTS, 2013-2014). For the assurance of safe, adequate, and constant supply of the blood worldwide there is a need to retain blood donors who will become voluntary repeat regular donors [4].

Despite establishment of NBTS in 2004, there is a challenge in recruiting and retaining of the potential blood donors for repeating blood donations. Lack of repeat donors who donate blood regularly impedes blood collection which is to be planned systematically to meet the requirements of blood, by blood groups and components. Consequently, it incapacitates the blood transfusion service in maintaining a constant and reliable supply of safe blood when required in every clinical setting practicing transfusion [5].

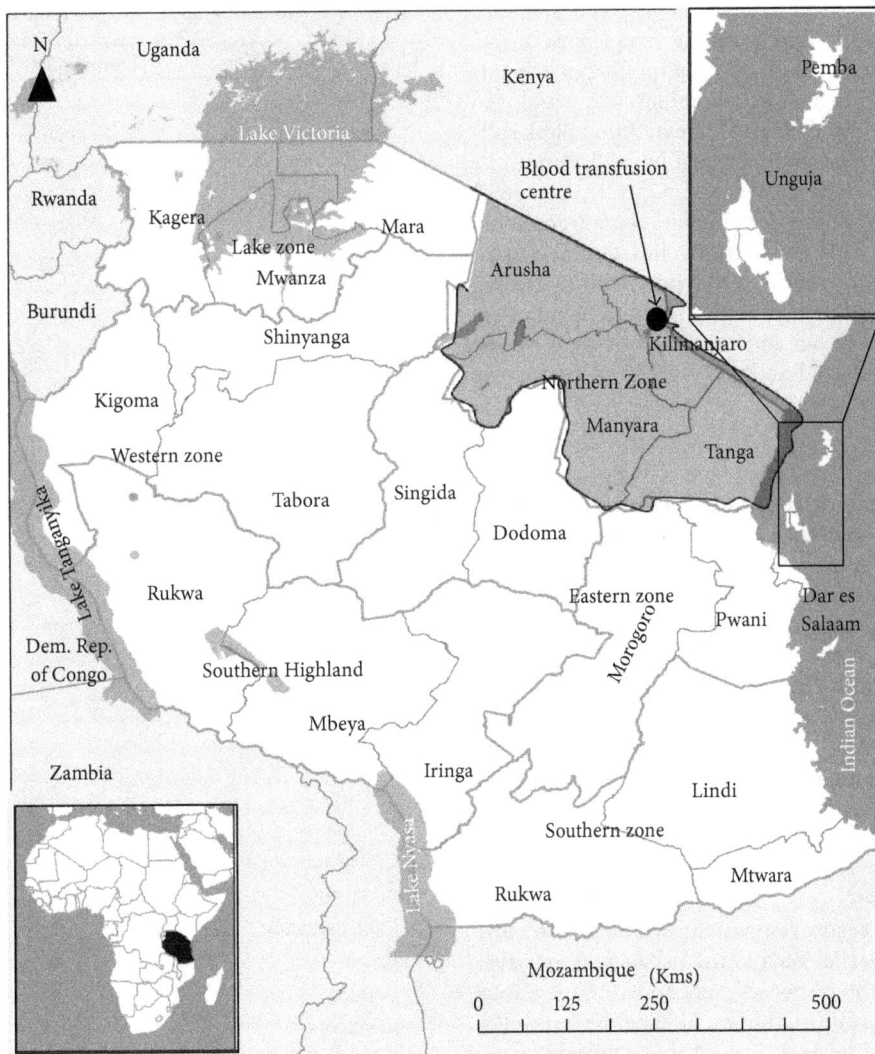

Tanzania Demographic Health Survey, 2010

FIGURE 1: Location of the study area in Tanzania.

There are several factors which have been associated with the return of blood donors for more donations. High intention and altruistic behavior have been pointed out to predict the repeat of blood donations [6, 7]. Knowledge concerning blood donation, convenient environment, and frequency of previous donation have been associated with repeat donations [8–10]. Sex and age have been associated with high turnover of repetition of donation whereby young males have higher chance of turning up for the repetition of blood donations than young females [9, 11].

To meet the demand for blood in the country, mobilization and sensitization activities have been commenced to recruit new and retain current blood donors. Because only a small proportion of eligible donors donate and an even smaller percentage return to give blood a second time or more; a better understanding of what motivates donors to give blood more than once is needed. This knowledge will help in planning, organizing, and implementation of donation activities in the country. Hence, the objective of this research was to determine different factors influencing repeat blood donation in our setting at Northern Zone Blood Transfusion Centre (NZBTC).

2. Methods

2.1. Study Design, Study Area, and Study Population. This was a cross-sectional study carried out between May 15 and June 15, 2015, at the Northern Zone Blood Transfusion Centre, Kilimanjaro, Tanzania. This centre is one of the six blood transfusion centers in Tanzania mainland, which serves four Northern regions in the country (Arusha, Kilimanjaro, Tanga, and Manyara) (Figure 1). The participants were blood donors registered between June 2012 and June 2014 in the donors' database, involving those who had donated once or more, aged 18 and above years, irrespective of gender and excluding those with no phone numbers.

2.2. Sample Size and Sampling. By using Kish Lisle formula for cross-sectional studies (Kish, 1967), the proportion of repeat donors was considered to be 50% in order to attain minimum sample size, with Z-score of 1.96 and standard error of 5%, plus 15% of nonresponse; a sample size of 442 participants was determined. But a total of 454 participants were recruited. Simple random sampling was employed whereby from donors' database (e-Delphyn Blood Bank software, version 5.7.0.0) registered between June 2012 and June 2014 and 34,115 donors were extracted. Only 12,969 (38%) who had telephone numbers documented were transferred into Microsoft Excel 2010, and RAND function was used to get random numbers which were reported in ascending order against the telephone numbers. Then participants were selected from top to bottom and contacted. A total of 460 participants were contacted and 454 agreed to participate making a response rate of 99%.

2.3. Data Collection. The participants were contacted through the phone and introduction of the study was done. For those who agreed to participate, date and time were set to conduct an interview at their convenience. The interview was conducted by four interviewers who were trained on questionnaire to have structured interview prior to the interview. By using questionnaire, the interview was done through the phone and the maximum time for interview was 20 minutes.

The participants were asked how many times they had donated blood in the past 5 years from the date of interview. The responses were ranging between 1 (once), 2 (twice), 3 (thrice), and 4 (more than 3 times). Those who reported more than 1 time were categorized as repeat donors [7]. The responses were not cross-checked with donors' database to confirm their responses.

Altruistic behavior score respondents were asked to score how often they had participated in the behavior from never (1) to very often (5); the responses were added to get a total score for each participant (minimum: 13; maximum: 65) [7]. Intention to donate in the next 12 months was reported from 1: "Very unlikely" to 5: "Very likely," and those who were in between 1 and 3 were graded as low intention; those graded 4 and 5 had higher intention [7]. The same applied to those who reported their experience during last donation who had to score from 1 to 5 (Very bad–Very good). In analysis, those who scored 1 to 2 were graded as "bad experience" and those scored 3 to 5 were graded as "good experience."

2.4. Data Analysis. Data was entered, cleaned, and analyzed with SPSS version 22 (IBM, NY, USA). Descriptive analysis was done whereby median for continuous data, frequency, and percentage were used to summarize the categorical data. Chi-square was used to test difference in categorical variables while Kruskal Wallis test was used for comparison of median scores of altruistic scores. The strength of association was determined by using crude and adjusted odds ratio (COR/AOR). Backward binary logistic regression model was employed to control the effect of confounding variables. P value less than 0.05 (2 tails) was considered statistically significant.

2.5. Ethical Consideration. Ethical clearance was sought and obtained from Kilimanjaro Christian Medical University College Research Ethical Committee. Permission was granted

TABLE 1: Sociodemographic characteristics of study participants.

Characteristics	Frequency ($n = 454$)	Percentage
Age (years)		
≤25	145	31.9
26–35	163	35.9
36–45	74	16.3
46–55	57	12.6
56 and above	15	3.3
Sex		
Male	327	72
Female	127	28
Area of residence (region)		
Kilimanjaro	248	54.6
Arusha	100	22
Tanga	44	9.7
Manyara	5	1.1
Outside Northern Zone	57	12.6
Marital status		
Single	231	50.9
Married	205	45.1
Others	18	4.0
Education Level		
No formal education	3	0.7
Primary	176	38.8
Secondary	155	34.1
College/university	120	26.4
Occupation		
Public servant	96	21.1
Private	81	17.8
Peasant	73	16.1
Business	79	17.4
Self-employed	44	9.7
Unemployed	11	2.4
Student	70	15.4

from National Blood Transfusion Service to access donors' database. Verbally informed consent was requested from each participant prior the interview. Participants identified details were not recorded on the questionnaire and collected information were used for this study purpose only.

3. Results

3.1. Sociodemographic Characteristics of Participants. A total of 454 blood donors participated in this study. The age of respondents was between 18 and 67 years. Median age was 29 (ranging between 24 and 39) years. Majority were males (72%). Most of respondents (54%) resided in Kilimanjaro region, followed by Arusha region (22%). At least half of respondents were single (50.9%). Primary education was mostly reported by respondents (38.8%) and the lowest proportion (0.7%) had no formal education. Profession-wise, the major group of respondents was public servants (21.1%) (Table 1).

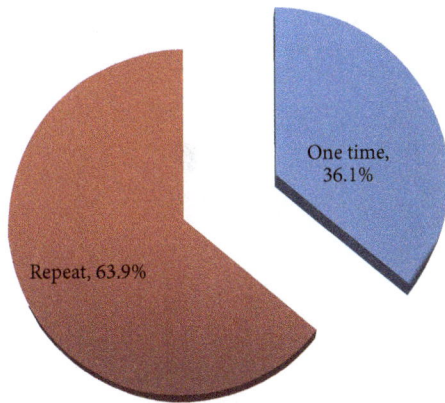

FIGURE 2: The proportion of donor's status.

TABLE 2: Sociodemographic and donor characteristics of the participants by donor status ($N = 454$).

Characteristics	Repeated blood donation		
	N	n (%)	
Age group (years)			0.004
18–25	145	81 (27.9)	
26–35	163	106 (36.6)	
36–45	74	50 (17.2)	
46–55	75	38 (13.1)	
56–67	15	15 (5.2)	
Area of residence			0.002^{Ω}
Kilimanjaro	248	161 (54.6)	
Arusha	100	50 (22)	
Tanga	44	29 (9.7)	
Manyara	5	5 (1.1)	
Outside NZ	57	45 (15.5)	
Sex			0.047
Male	327	218 (75.2)	
Female	127	72 (24.8)	
Level of education			0.035
No formal education	3	3 (1.0)	
Primary	176	99 (34.1)	
Secondary	155	107 (36.9)	
College/university	120	81 (27.9)	
Intention to donate			<0.001
Low	135	67 (23.2)	
High	318	222 (76.8)	
Knowledge on interval of blood donation			0.013
3–4 months	270	185 (63.8)	
Others	184	105 (36.2)	
Experience in last donation			<0.001
Bad	208	113 (39)	
Good	246	177 (61)	

$^{\Omega}$Fisher's Exact test otherwise χ^2 test.

Internal consistency of altruistic behavior scale (Cronbach's alpha, α) was 0.815. The minimum score was 18 and maximum was 65. The scores were unevenly distributed; hence, for more reliable measure of central tendency, median was employed, whereby the median was 47 (40–52).

Figure 2 shows the proportion of repeat donation which was 63.9%.

3.2. Factors Associated with Repeat Donation. Age and living place of the participants were significantly associated with donor status. Male had higher frequency (75.2%) of repeated donation compared to females ($P = 0.047$). Participants with secondary education (36.9%) had more repeated donations than others ($P = 0.035$). Majority (76.8%) had significant higher intention to donate compared to low intention ($P = 0.000$). Knowledge of donation interval (63.8 against 36.2%; $P = 0.013$) and good experience on last donation (61% against 39%; $P < 0.001$) had higher repeating donations prevalence compared to others (Table 2).

Majority of participants donated blood outside the blood centre, the reason being that the first donation was voluntary and for public use. Main concern or fear on their first donation was fainting while donating and majority were aged between 26 and 35 years. Most were public servants and single. Large proportion (96.9%) reported at least one usage of blood and had family member(s) who had donated blood.

There was a significant difference in median scores of altruistic behavior among donor status, whereby the repeat donors tend to score higher than one time donors ($P = 0.035$, Mann-Whitney U test) (Figure 3).

In multivariate analysis, factors remained significant predictors of repeat donations. Those who were living in Arusha had lower odds of repeat donation by 0.466 times (AOR (95% CI); 0.47 (0.29–0.08)); $P = 0.002$; those living outside the Northern Zone had higher odds by 2.1-fold of repeat donations compared to those living in Kilimanjaro (AOR (95% CI) (1–4.34)); $P = 0.049$. Knowledge of time interval between donations increased odds of repeating donations by 55.4% than those who reported wrongly (AOR (95% CI): 1.52 (1.02–2.36)); $P = 0.039$. High intention increased odds of repeat donation by 2.1-fold (AOR (95% CI): 2.1 (1.34–3.24));

$P = 0.001$, compared to low intention. Good experience in previous donations increased odds of repeat donations (AOR (95% CI): 2.15 (1.42–3.25)); $P < 0.001$. Altruistic score had minor effect on increasing odds of repeating donations by 2.5% (AOR (95% CI): 1.03 (1–1.05)); $P = 0.036$ (Table 3).

4. Discussion

Proximity has a major role when it comes to motivating donors to return for more donations. The closeness of the donation site creates a convenient environment for the donors who are really intending to donate blood. This finding concurs with WHO strategy 16, on 100 % towards voluntary blood donation, in encouraging blood donation and repeat blood donation, whereby the long distance to the donation site may precipitate negative perception of inconvenience

TABLE 3: Factors associated with repeat donation among blood donors ($N = 454$).

Variables	Repeated donation			
	COR (95% CI)	P value	AOR (95% CI)	P value
Living area				
Kilimanjaro	1			
Arusha	0.54 (0.34–0.87)	0.01	0.47 (0.29–0.08)	0.002
Tanga	1.05 (0.53–2.05)	0.899		
Manyara	—	0.999		
Outside NZ	2.03 (1.02–4.03)	0.04	2.09 (1–4.34)	0.049
Intention to donate				
Low	1		1	
High	2.35 (1.55–3.55)	0.000	2.09 (1.34–3.24)	0.001
Donation interval				
Others	1		1	
3-4 months	1.64 (1.11–2.42)	0.01	1.56 (1.02–2.36)	0.039
Experience in last donation				
Bad	1		1	
Good	2.16 (1.46–3.18)	0.000	2.15 (1.42–3.25)	0.000
Altruistic score	1.03 (1.01–1.05)	0.01	1.03 (1–1.05)	0.036

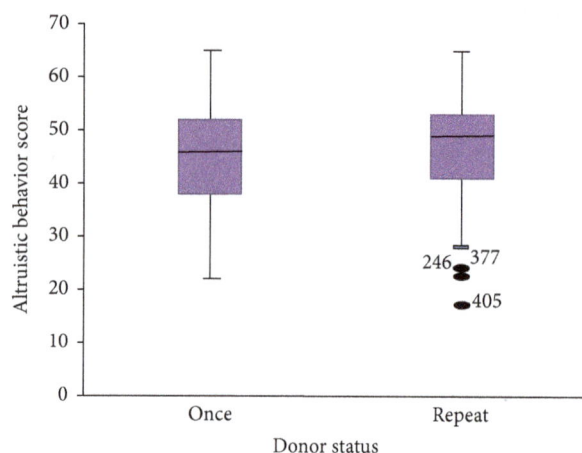

FIGURE 3: Altruistic behavior scores against donor status.

thus posing as barrier towards repeat donation [4]. Similar findings were reported by Schreiber et al., whereby majority of participants who could not routinely donate reported not having a convenient place to donate due to distance or transportation to the donation site [12].

In this study, majority of repeat blood donors reported high intention to donate in the next twelve months. Similarly, Godin and colleagues in their cohort study found that high intention was a strong predictor of returning for next donation [6]. Other literatures demonstrate that intention to donate is influenced by different factors such as sociodemographic characteristics [13, 14] and eligibility for donation [10]. In Zimbabwe, there has been an establishment of pledging system (Club 25) whereby the young people at the age of 16 are urged to pledge to donate blood almost 25 times in their life time [15]. This is one method of creating intention as in our social life pledging play a key role in making people commit to performing certain activity.

In the current study, awareness of time interval between donations was found to be significant information among repeat blood donors. Knowing the recommended time interval reminds the donors when to return for next donation. Similarly it has been reported by WHO that the donors who keep the pace or intervals of donation, as recommended by WHO [16], do develop habitual practice on the long run thus becoming potential voluntary repeat donors [6]. This leads to high frequency donation which has been demonstrated by other literatures, and that increases the likelihood of continuing to return for more donations [7, 8].

In our study, good experience in previous donation was significantly associated with repeat blood donation. It has been demonstrated by other studies that good handling of blood donors during the whole process of donation will increase the probability of returning of blood donors and building up the high intention to donate again [6, 8, 17]. Precounseling of blood donors on presumed adverse reactions may prepare the donors for unforeseen "bad experience."

In the current study there was a weak significant association of altruistic behavior score and repeat donation. The same observations have been noted in other literatures [7, 8, 11, 18]. Although in our setting altruistic behavior score items [19] are reflected in day to day life and thus may not reflect the blood donation activity, encouraging message on building up altruistic motivation is advisable to create voluntarism atmosphere of helping one another in the society when it comes to blood.

Strength and Weakness of the Study. This is the first study conducted in Tanzania among blood donors on factors associated with repeat blood donation. Thus it can be used as baseline information for further studies.

Since participants were contacted and interviewed through the phone, study included only blood donors who had their mobile phone numbers recorded who represented 1/3 of the blood donors registered. Two-thirds of blood donors were excluded from the study as we did not have their mobile phone numbers recorded. Since their characteristics are not known, they might have different characteristics compared to those we studied. So the exclusion of those blood donors and their effect on our result cannot be quantified.

5. Conclusion

Blood donation is affected by proximity of donation site; thus living away from the donation centre decreases the chances of repeating donation. Establishment of several donation sites will encourage returning of blood donors. Knowledge of the blood donation interval has positive impact on repeating of donation; thus dissemination of such knowledge is crucial in retaining the potential donors. Higher intention of donating blood is the strong predictor of going back for more donations. Good previous experience motivates donors to return for more donations. Altruistic behaviors may have influence on repeat blood donation. We recommend continuous education concerning blood donors and donation among health workers and society as a whole. This will create awareness and motivational factors for repeat donations.

Conflict of Interests

The authors declare that there is no conflict of interests regarding the publication of this work.

Acknowledgment

The authors would like to acknowledge the study participants for their readiness to provide data which makes this work possible.

References

[1] A. G. Salaudeen and E. Odeh, "Knowledge and behavior towards voluntary blood donation among students of a tertiary institution in Nigeria," *Nigerian Journal of Clinical Practice*, vol. 14, no. 3, pp. 303–307, 2011.

[2] WHO Expert Group, "Expert consensus statement on achieving self-sufficiency in safe blood and blood products, based on voluntary non-remunerated blood donation (VNRBD)," *Vox Sanguinis*, vol. 103, no. 4, pp. 337–342, 2012.

[3] WHO, *WHO 10 Facts on Blood Transfusion*, World Health Organization, 2014, http://www.who.int/features/factfiles/blood_transfusion/en/.

[4] WHO, "Towards 100% Voluntary Blood Donation A Global Framework for Action," 2010, http://www.who.int/bloodsafety/publications/9789241599696/en/.

[5] WHO, "More voluntary blood donations essential World Health Organization," 2012, http://www.who.int/mediacentre/news/releases/2012/blood_donation_20120614/en/.

[6] G. Godin, M. Conner, P. Sheeran, A. Bélanger-Gravel, and M. Germain, "Determinants of repeated blood donation among new and experienced blood donors," *Transfusion*, vol. 47, no. 9, pp. 1607–1615, 2007.

[7] W. R. Steele, G. B. Schreiber, A. Guiltinan et al., "The role of altruistic behavior, empathetic concern, and social responsibility motivation in blood donation behavior," *Transfusion*, vol. 48, no. 1, pp. 43–54, 2008.

[8] K. S. Schlumpf, S. A. Glynn, G. B. Schreiber et al., "Factors influencing donor return," *Transfusion*, vol. 48, no. 2, pp. 264–272, 2008.

[9] J.-P. Allain, F. Sarkodie, P. Boateng, K. Asenso, E. Kyeremateng, and S. Owusu-Ofori, "A pool of repeat blood donors can be generated with little expense to the blood center in sub-Saharan Africa," *Transfusion*, vol. 48, no. 4, pp. 735–741, 2008.

[10] P. I. Pule, B. Rachaba, M. G. M. D. Magafu, and D. Habte, "Factors associated with intention to donate blood: sociodemographic and past experience variables," *Journal of Blood Transfusion*, vol. 2014, Article ID 571678, 7 pages, 2014.

[11] A. H. Misje, V. Bosnes, O. G. Gåsdal, and H. E. Heier, "Motivation, recruitment and retention of voluntary non-remunerated blood donors: a survey-based questionnaire study," *Vox Sanguinis*, vol. 89, no. 4, pp. 236–244, 2005.

[12] G. B. Schreiber, K. S. Schlumpf, S. A. Glynn et al., "Convenience, the bane of our existence, and other barriers to donating," *Transfusion*, vol. 46, no. 4, pp. 545–553, 2006.

[13] N. Z. A. Hamid, R. Basiruddin, and N. Hassan, "The intention to donate blood: an analysis of socio-demographic determinants," *International Journal of Social Science and Humanity*, vol. 3, no. 6, pp. 503–507, 2013.

[14] G. Mirutse, G. Fisseha, L. Abebe, Z. Birhanu, and M. Alemayehu, "Intention to donate blood among the eligible population in mekelle city, northern Ethiopia: using the theory of planned behavior," *American Journal of Health Research*, vol. 2, no. 4, pp. 158–163, 2014.

[15] WHO, "Celebrating a gift of life, Club 25-where blood donors love lives 2005 World Blood Day," 2006, http://apps.who.int/iris/bitstream/10665/69363/1/WBD_2006_kit_eng.pdf.

[16] WHO, *Blood Donor Selection: Guideleines on Assessing Donor Suitability for Blood Donation*, World Health Organization, 2012.

[17] D. D. Nguyen, D. A. DeVita, N. V. Hirschler, and E. L. Murphy, "Blood donor satisfaction and intention of future donation," *Transfusion*, vol. 48, no. 4, pp. 742–748, 2008.

[18] E. Karacan, G. Cengiz Seval, Z. Aktan, M. Ayli, and R. Palabiyikoglu, "Blood donors and factors impacting the blood donation decision: motives for donating blood in Turkish sample," *Transfusion and Apheresis Science*, vol. 49, no. 3, pp. 468–473, 2013.

[19] J. P. Rushton, R. D. Chrisjohn, and G. D. Fekken, "The altruistic personality and the self-report altruism scale," *Personality and Individual Differences*, vol. 2, no. 4, pp. 293–302, 1981.

28

Infiltration of Autologous Growth Factors in Chronic Tendinopathies

Antonio Crescibene,[1] **Marcello Napolitano,**[2] **Raffaella Sbano,**[3]
Enrico Costabile,[4] **and Hesham Almolla**[5]

[1]*Orthopedics and Traumatology Unit, San Francesco di Paola Hospital, Via Promintesta, 87027 Paola, Italy*
[2]*Immunohaematology and Transfusion Medicine Unit, Cosenza Hospital, Via Migliori, 87100 Cosenza, Italy*
[3]*Radiology Unit, San Francesco di Paola Hospital, Via Promintesta, 87027 Paola, Italy*
[4]*Orthopedics and Traumatology Unit, Cosenza Hospital, Via Migliori, 87100 Cosenza, Italy*
[5]*Radiology Unit, Cosenza Hospital, Via Migliori, 87100 Cosenza, Italy*

Correspondence should be addressed to Antonio Crescibene; antonio.crescibene@libero.it

Academic Editor: Erwin Strasser

Achilles tendinopathy and patellar tendinopathy are among the most frequent diagnoses in sports medicine. Therapeutic treatment of the disease is difficult, particularly in chronic cases. In literature, several studies suggest the employment of Platelet-Rich Plasma as a therapeutic alternative in tendinopathies. The choice of employing this method is based on the activity of growth factors contained in platelets which activate, amplify, and optimize the healing process. We selected 14 patients affected by Achilles tendinopathy and 7 patients affected by patellar tendinopathy, with a two-year final follow-up. These patients underwent a cycle of three tendinous infiltrations, after clinical and instrumental evaluation carried out by means of specific questionnaires and repeated ultrasound scans. Ultrasound scans of 18 patients showed signs of reduction in insertional irregularities. The result is confirmed by complete functional recovery of the patients, with painful symptomatology disappearing. The patients showed a clear pain reduction, along with an enhanced VISA score after the 24-month follow-up, equal to 84.2 points on a scale of 0 to 100. In conclusion, the present study provides evidence to suggest that PRP infiltration is a valid option to patients with chronic tendinopathy who did not benefit from other treatments.

1. Introduction

In the last three decades, a considerable increase in the incidence of excess functional load pathologies has been reported. Not only did this occur because of the growing number of amateur sportspersons, but this also occurred because of lengthier and tougher trainings and sport events among professionals. Repeated traumas and microtraumas have been identified as the major cause of such pathologies, which affect those practising basketball, volleyball, tennis, skiing, and soccer [1, 2].

Achilles tendon inflammation was predominantly present in 11% to 24% of joggers, whereas patellar tendinopathy was found in 32% to 45% of basketball and volleyball players [3].

In nonresponsive conditions, before deciding on a surgical solution, it is worth considering an eco-guided PRP intratendinous infiltration.

Tendon tissue recovery is rather long, and this limited capacity of recovery is supposed to be caused by poor tendinous vascularisation [4].

In the region of the lesion, platelet degranulation occurs; this releases several growth factors such as TGF (Transforming Growth Factor), PDGF (Platelet Derived Growth Factor), EGF (Epidermal Growth Factor), VEGF (Vascular Endothelial Growth Factor), and IGF (Insulin-Like Growth Factor).

The first three, in particular, encourage cellular proliferation and migration through protein synthesis in the extracellular matrix.

TABLE 1: Laboratory values of Achilles tendinopathy.

Patient	RBC $10^6/\mu L$	HGB g/dL	HCT %	PLT $10^3/\mu L$	WBC $10^3/\mu L$
SL	5.15	13.8	43.6	236	9.49
MF	4.91	12.9	40.7	336	9.2
GG	3.85	12.5	36.3	321	6.21
SP	5.02	15.4	46.1	201	5.5
MML	5.90	11.7	37.5	301	8.0
MF	4.81	14.7	40.2	218	5.36
BR	5.23	15.0	44.2	204	4.0
NP	5.17	15.2	44.5	252	8.1
BM	4.21	13.6	38.2	264	7.55
CG	3.67	12.0	35.1	304	7.2
CD	5.52	16.0	44.2	215	6.14
IGA	4.88	14.5	43.3	261	7.58
PG	5.06	15.5	43.1	174	5.35
CR	4.73	13.1	38.7	284	8.6

RBC: red blood cells; HGB: hemoglobin; HCT: hematocrit; PLT: platelets; WBC: white blood cells.

TABLE 2: Laboratory values of patellar tendinopathy.

Patient	RBC $10^6/\mu L$	HGB g/dL	HCT %	PLT $10^3/\mu L$	WBC $10^3/\mu L$
CM	4.08	12.3	37.1	253	5.21
BG	4.32	13.6	39.0	197	5.07
SD	5.81	16.0	47.9	243	4.74
CG	5.27	15.1	44.5	278	6.54
ME	4.45	13.9	40.6	183	6.05
OR	5.12	14.8	44.2	227	6.0
DZ	4.75	13.9	41.0	265	6.0

Some other cytokines are released, such as HGF (Hepatocyte Growth Factor) and bFGF (Basic Fibroblast Growth Factor); they are chemotactic and mitogenic to endothelial cells and encourage angiogenesis and revascularization, two fundamental processes in tissue regeneration [5].

In literature, several studies suggest the employment of PRP as a successful therapeutic alternative in tendinopathies [6–8] because growth factors activate, amplify, and optimize the healing process [9–11].

2. Materials and Methods

We selected 21 patients affected by chronic tendinopathy, with persisting symptomatology for at least six months. Between September 2010 and March 2012, they underwent treatment of PRP infiltration.

The first stage involved visit, medical history reconstruction, and evaluation of the hemochromocytometric profile of the outpatients.

We considered as discriminating factors hemoglobin values <11 g/dL, a number of white blood cells >$10 \times 10^{\wedge 3}/\mu L$, and a number of platelets <$120 \times 10^{\wedge 3}/\mu L$.

All patient presented value in range of normality (Tables 1 and 2).

The inclusion criteria for the study were the presence of patellar or Achilles tendinopathy, pain at palpation and during physical activity for at least four months, insertional irregularity in ultrasound scanning [7].

All patients had previously undergone other treatments: intake of NSAIDs, rehabilitation programme, laser therapy, corticosteroids injections, with unsatisfactory outcome.

We also excluded patients with systemic pathologies such as diabetes mellitus, cancer, severe cardiovascular pathologies, immunodepression, anticoagulating, or antiaggregating therapy [7].

These conditions do not allow the application of the technique in the limits of safety for the patient that may develop infective complications and adverse effects.

The patients (14 men and 7 women) had an average age of 40, ranging from 16 to 70.

The average Body Mass Index (BMI) was 25, ranging from 23 to 26. In 13 cases, the left-hand side of the body was affected, with the remaining 8 patients affected in their right-hand side; the patients' blood tests were all normal, with no contraindications.

We treated 14 cases of Achilles tendinopathy and 7 cases of patellar tendinopathy.

All of the patients were sportspersons; there were 10 professionals among them. They underwent a cycle of three infiltrations, one per week.

During the initial pretreatment evaluation we administered some suitable questionnaires: the Numeric Rating Scale (NRS) [12] for measuring subjective pain, as well as

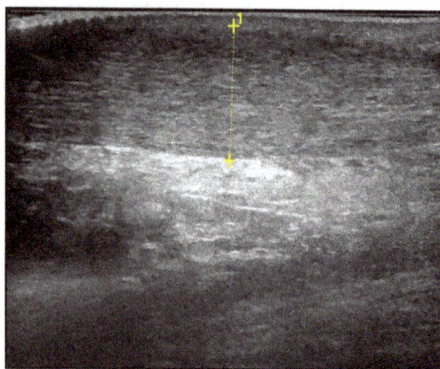

FIGURE 1: Pretreatment ultrasound image of the Achilles tendon.

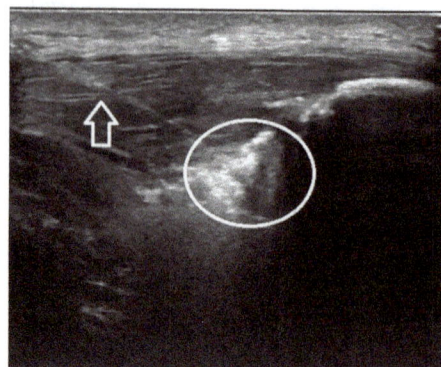

FIGURE 2: The arrow indicates the needle and the circle shows the PRP infiltration point in a case of patellar tendinopathy.

the Victorian Institute of Sport Assessment-Achilles (VISA-A) questionnaire [13] and the Victorian Institute of Sport Assessment-Patellar (VISA-P) questionnaire [14], designed for Achilles and patellar tendinopathies, respectively.

These evaluations were repeated at the end of the cycle and throughout the follow-up.

The VISA score measures the ability to practise sports activities by means of a 0–100 score, in which the highest score represents full activity.

All patients read and signed informed consent and the paper was performed in accordance with the Ethical standards of the 1964 Declaration of Helsinki as revised in 2000.

All procedures were performed in accordance with the ethical standards of the institutional and/or national research committee.

For statistical analyses we used the Mann-Whitney U or Wilcoxon Rank-Sum Test for Difference in Medians (t-test two samples).

In order to reduce intrinsic variables in ultrasound scanning, we decided on making use of the usual X-ray specialist and a *Logiq E9* scanner (Figure 1) with a 4 MHz multifrequency linear probe.

Any kind of sports activity was forbidden during this therapy. The patients followed a personalized therapeutic program consisting of an initial stage with cautious active mobilization of the region and hydrokinesitherapy, followed by eccentric exercises with constant check from the physiotherapist, for one month.

At the end of this program, patients could gradually resume their usual sports activities, by encouraging patients to perform stretching and eccentric exercises, in an average period of six weeks.

All the procedures were performed under control of the Chief Immunohematologist at the Hospital Department of Immunohematology and Transfusional Medicine, in accordance with Decree number 191/2005 [15], with prior acquisition of informed consent.

Each infiltration session encompassed a preparation stage. We collected a venous blood sample of about 8 cc into a RegenLab Fibrin Polymer 2 test tube and then centrifuged it at 3100 rpm for eight minutes.

By doing so, we obtained the separation through physical principles of erythrocytes from plasma, while platelets sedimented on the surface of separation [10].

We obtained in this way the PRP, to which we added 10% calcium gluconate [16], and then immediately apply the substance through infiltration; the gelification process occurred within 2–7 minutes due to body heat [17].

We use 1 cc of PRP in order to carry out quality controls and calculate the number of platelets in PRP.

We registered plasmatic platelet concentration of $276.8 \times 10^{\wedge 3} \mu L$, platelet recovery of 25.3%, and a concentration factor of 2.2.

After careful disinfection of the infiltration site with didecyldimethylammonium chloride, we anesthetized the cutaneous and subcutaneous tissue with 2 cc of 2% lidocaine and then inserted a needle 22 gauge into the tendon, with ultrasound scanning as guidance.

We now injected about half of the PRP into the tendon and the rest into the peritendinous area (Figure 2).

We removed the needle, disinfected the region, and applied a dressing. We left the limb to rest for fifteen minutes.

Throughout treatment we forbade patients to take non-steroidal anti-inflammatory drugs and suggested avoiding for at least two weeks intense sports activities which might involve use of the legs.

3. Results

18 patients completed the 24-month final follow-up, while 3 interrupted periodical visits after 12 months (one patient with Achilles tendinopathy and two affected by patellar tendinopathy).

The NRS scale for measuring subjective pain registered an average initial score of 6.6 ± 1.0 and a posttreatment average score of 1.2 ± 1.2 ($P < 0.01$).

We observed a VISA score enhancement, with an average pretreatment score of 46.4 ± 18.7 and an average posttreatment one of 82 ± 12.4.

The follow-up indicated an average score of 85.2 ± 3.0 after 12 months and an average one of 84.2 ± 2.9 after 24 months ($P < 0.01$).

TABLE 3: Clinical evaluation of Achilles tendinopathy (values are presented as mean).

Patient	NRS before	NRS after	VISA-A before	VISA-A after	VISA-A F.U. 12 months	VISA-A F.U. 24 months
SL	5	0	31	90	82	80
MF	7	1	33	84	89	81
GG	6	2	73	93	91	85
SP	5	0	69	87	87	86
MML	7	1	70	92	85	88
MF	8	2	35	85	81	89
BR	5	0	85	89	88	84
NP	6	1	46	86	87	80
BM	5	0	32	94	88	89
CG	6	0	64	92	89	88
CD	5	0	62	90	89	88
IGA	5	0	22	83	81	—
PG	7	2	43	89	85	85
CR	7	0	72	90	86	85

TABLE 4: Clinical evaluation of Patellar Tendinopathy (Values are presented as mean).

Patient	NRS before	NRS after	VISA-P before	VISA-P after	VISA-P F.U. 12 Months	VISA-P F.U. 24 Months
CM	7	2	23	56	81	—
BG	8	4	55	85	86	83
SD	7	0	17	90	88	86
CG	8	3	27	53	80	—
ME	6	2	52	82	85	83
OR	8	1	54	84	82	83
DZ	7	1	54	77	86	80

We noticed a significant improvement in patients with Achilles tendinopathy, whose VISA-A questionnaires showed, at each of the evaluation stages previously mentioned, the following results: 52.6 ± 20.1, 88.8 ± 3.4, 86.2 ± 3.1, and 85.2 ± 3.2 ($P < 0.01$).

The NRS scale for measuring subjective pain registered, in this group, a pretreatment average value of 6 ± 1 and a posttreatment average value of 0.6 ± 0.8 ($P < 0.01$) (Table 3).

We observed a less remarkable improvement in patients affected by patellar tendinopathy, whose VISA-P questionnaires suggested, at each of the evaluation stages, the following average scores: 40.2 ± 17.0, 75.2 ± 14.7, 84 ± 2.9, and 83 ± 2.4 ($P < 0.01$).

The NRS scale for assessment of pain intensity revealed, in this group, average results of 7.2 ± 0.8 and 1.8 ± 1.3 ($P < 0.01$) (Table 4).

Patients with Achilles tendinopathy showed the best scores of the study population and they accounted for 72% of the population studied.

We have noticed a score lowest in the population suffering from patellar tendinopathy; nevertheless, the patients have taken the sport with good final scores (Figure 3).

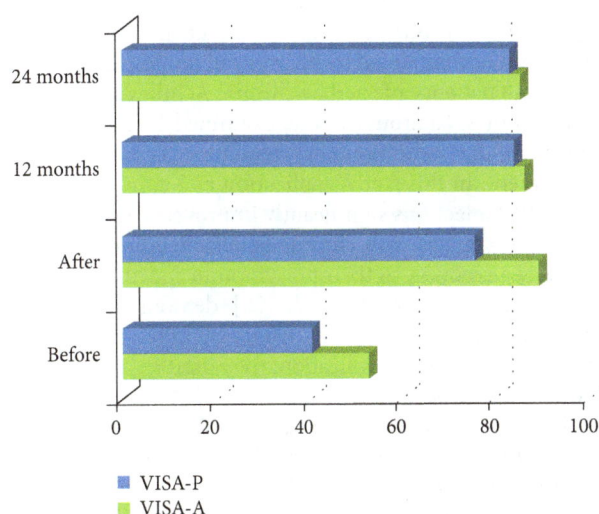

FIGURE 3: VISA evaluation of patellar and Achilles tendinopathy.

At the end of the follow-up, ultrasound scans of the 18 patients showed signs of reduction in insertional irregularities. This result is clinically confirmed by complete functional recovery of the patients, with painful symptomatology disappearing.

Moreover, a good tolerance to the use of PRP was observed, with the absence of any adverse effects related to such therapy.

4. Discussion

Achilles tendinopathy and patellar tendinopathy are among the most frequent diagnoses in sports medicine. Therapeutic treatment of the disease is difficult, particularly in chronic cases.

The most reliable and secure treatment is still the conservative recovery program, which encompasses eccentric specific and gradual muscular work, although the percentage of positive results in extreme chronic tendinopathies is about 50% [18, 19].

Since tendon tissue is avascularized, the healing process is bound to be disrupted and tendinopathies are bound to become chronic.

Tendon recovery with formation of scar tissue involves loss of the mechanical properties of elasticity and resistance which are typical of healthy tendon tissue.

The healing process takes place in three main phases: inflammatory phase, proliferative phase and remodeling.

In the first phase, platelets play the physiological role of starting and modulating the healing process.

Recent studies have proved that use of autologous growth factors might be helpful in a number of conditions.

The effect of individual growth factors in models of in vivo and in vitro tendon repair has already been described in literature [6–8, 20–22].

Deans et al. [6] obtained statistically remarkable results in terms of pain, various other symptoms, everyday activities, sports activities, and quality of life in a group of 26 patients with chronic Achilles tendinopathy. Ferrero et al. [7] reported a significant and long-term improvement in clinical symptomatology, accompanied by recovery of tendon matrix, in a group of 48 patients affected by chronic Achilles and patellar tendinopathies. Charousset et al. examined 28 athletes with chronic patellar tendinopathy refractory to nonoperative management. In this study, application of 3 consecutive US-guided PRP injections significantly improved symptoms and function in athletes with chronic patellar tendinopathy and allowed fast recovery to their presymptom sporting level [8].

Research by Sánchez et al. [23] demonstrated better results in a group of patients whose Achilles tendon was repaired through PRP application; they used a control group to compare results.

The present study on the use of PRP to treat chronic tendinopathies has been prompted by the safe autologous nature of this therapy, its mechanism of action based on basic biological principles, and promising works in scientific literature.

The group of patients we examined was regarded as a good model in evaluating the benefits of PRP application in chronic tendinopathies, but further randomized controlled studies performed on a larger sample size are warranted to confirm these preliminary results.

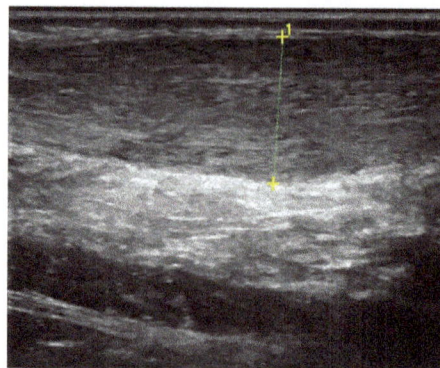

FIGURE 4: Ultrasound scan control of the Achilles tendon on 24-month follow-up.

The limitations of this study are the small number of patients and the lack of control group.

This process was integrated with a rehabilitation program and patients' progress was measured by means of the VISA score and evaluation of serialized ultrasound images.

5. Conclusions

The patients showed a clear pain reduction, along with a VISA score after the 24-month follow-up equal to 84.2 points on a scale of 0 to 100.

From ultrasound scans, we noticed a visible reduction in tissue irregularity in 86% of infiltrated tendons (Figure 4).

In conclusion, the present study provides evidence to suggest that PRP infiltration is a valid option to patients with chronic tendinopathy who did not benefit from other treatments.

Conflict of Interests

The authors declare that they have no conflict of interests.

Acknowledgment

The authors thank Sig. Massimo Rugna for his active collaboration.

References

[1] H. Alfredson, T. Pietilä, P. Jonsson, and R. Lorentzon, "Heavy-load eccentric calf muscle training for the treatment of chronic achilles tendinosis," *American Journal of Sports Medicine*, vol. 26, no. 3, pp. 360–366, 1998.

[2] J. S. Yu, J. E. Popp, C. C. Kaeding, and J. Lucas, "Correlation of MR imaging and pathologic findings in athletes undergoing surgery for chronic patellar tendinitis," *American Journal of Roentgenology*, vol. 165, no. 1, pp. 115–118, 1995.

[3] N. J. Wasielewski and K. M. Kotsko, "Does eccentric exercise reduce pain and improve strength in physically active adults with symptomatic lower extremity tendinosis? A systematic review," *Journal of Athletic Training*, vol. 42, no. 3, pp. 409–421, 2007.

[4] R. P. Nirschl and E. S. Ashman, "Elbow tendinopathy: tennis elbow," *Clinics in Sports Medicine*, vol. 22, no. 4, pp. 813–836, 2003.

[5] R. E. Marx, E. R. Carlson, R. M. Eichstaedt, S. R. Schimmele, J. E. Strauss, and K. R. Georgeff, "Platelet-rich plasma: growth factor enhancement for bone grafts," *Oral Surgery, Oral Medicine, Oral Pathology, Oral Radiology, and Endodontics*, vol. 85, no. 6, pp. 638–646, 1998.

[6] V. M. Deans, A. Miller, and J. Ramos, "A prospective series of patients with chronic Achilles tendinopathy treated with autologous-conditioned plasma injections combined with exercise and therapeutic ultrasonography," *Journal of Foot and Ankle Surgery*, vol. 51, no. 6, pp. 706–710, 2012.

[7] G. Ferrero, E. Fabbro, D. Orlandi et al., "Ultrasound-guided injection of platelet-rich plasma in chronic Achilles and patellar tendinopathy," *Journal of Ultrasound*, vol. 15, no. 4, pp. 260–266, 2012.

[8] C. Charousset, A. Zaoui, L. Bellaiche, and B. Bouyer, "Are multiple platelet-rich plasma injections useful for treatment of chronic patellar tendinopathy in athletes? a prospective study," *American Journal of Sports Medicine*, vol. 42, no. 4, pp. 906–911, 2014.

[9] R. T. Nguyen, J. Borg-Stein, and K. McInnis, "Applications of platelet-rich plasma in musculoskeletal and sports medicine: an evidence-based approach," *PM & R*, vol. 3, no. 3, pp. 226–250, 2011.

[10] D. M. Dohan Ehrenfest, I. Andia, M. A. Zumstein, C.-Q. Zhang, N. R. Pinto, and T. Bielecki, "Classification of platelet concentrates (Platelet-Rich Plasma-PRP, platelet-rich fibrin-PRF) for topical and infiltrative use in orthopedic and sports medicine: current consensus, clinical implications and perspectives," *Muscles, Ligaments and Tendons Journal*, vol. 4, no. 1, pp. 3–9, 2014.

[11] B. Dallaudière, L. Pesquer, P. Meyer et al., "Intratendinous injection of platelet-rich plasma under US guidance to treat tendinopathy: a long-term pilot study," *Journal of Vascular and Interventional Radiology*, vol. 25, no. 5, pp. 717–723, 2014.

[12] M. P. Jensen, P. Karoly, and S. Braver, "The measurement of clinical pain intensity: a comparison of six methods," *Pain*, vol. 27, no. 1, pp. 117–126, 1986.

[13] J. M. Robinson, J. L. Cook, C. Purdam et al., "The VISA-A questionnaire: a valid and reliable index of the clinical severity of Achilles tendinopathy," *British Journal of Sports Medicine*, vol. 35, no. 5, pp. 335–341, 2001.

[14] J. Zwerver, T. Kramer, and I. van den Akker-Scheek, "Validity and reliability of the Dutch translation of the VISA-P questionnaire for patellar tendinopathy," *BMC Musculoskeletal Disorders*, vol. 10, article 102, 2009.

[15] Decreto Legislativo 19 agosto 2005, no. 191, Attuazione della direttiva 2002/98/CE che stabilisce norme di qualità e di sicurezza per la raccolta, il controllo, la lavorazione, la conservazione e la distribuzione del sangue umano e dei suoi componenti, Gazzetta Ufficiale No. 221 del 22 Settembre 2005.

[16] M. Sánchez, J. Guadilla, N. Fiz, and I. Andia, "Ultrasound-guided platelet-rich plasma injections for the treatment of osteoarthritis of the hip," *Rheumatology*, vol. 51, no. 1, pp. 144–150, 2012.

[17] R. Zimmermann, R. Jakubietz, M. Jakubietz et al., "Different preparation methods to obtain platelet components as a source of growth factors for local application," *Transfusion*, vol. 41, no. 10, pp. 1217–1224, 2001.

[18] M. A. Childress and A. Beutler, "Management of chronic tendon injuries," *American Family Physician*, vol. 87, no. 7, pp. 486–490, 2013.

[19] B. L. Woodley, R. J. Newsham-West, and G. D. Baxter, "Chronic tendinopathy: effectiveness of eccentric exercise," *British Journal of Sports Medicine*, vol. 41, no. 4, pp. 188–198, 2007.

[20] E. Anitua, I. Andía, M. Sanchez et al., "Autologous preparations rich in growth factors promote proliferation and induce VEGF and HGF production by human tendon cells in culture," *Journal of Orthopaedic Research*, vol. 23, no. 2, pp. 281–286, 2005.

[21] M. B. Klein, N. Yalamanchi, H. Pham, M. T. Longaker, and J. Chang, "Flexor tendon healing in vitro: effects of TGF-β on tendon cell collagen production," *Journal of Hand Surgery*, vol. 27, no. 4, pp. 615–620, 2002.

[22] T. Natsu-ume, N. Nakamura, K. Shino, Y. Toritsuka, S. Horibe, and T. Ochi, "Temporal and spatial expression of transforming growth factor-β in the healing patellar ligament of the rat," *Journal of Orthopaedic Research*, vol. 15, no. 6, pp. 837–843, 1997.

[23] M. Sánchez, E. Anitua, J. Azofra, I. Andía, S. Padilla, and I. Mujika, "Comparison of surgically repaired Achilles tendon tears using platelet-rich fibrin matrices," *The American Journal of Sports Medicine*, vol. 35, no. 2, pp. 245–251, 2007.

29

The Value of Tranexamic Acid in Reducing Blood Loss following Hip Reconstruction in Children with Cerebral Palsy

I. Majid, S. Alshryda, B. Somanchi, E. Morakis, and A. Foster

Royal Manchester Children Hospital, Central Manchester University Hospitals, Oxford Road, Manchester M13 9WL, UK

Correspondence should be addressed to S. Alshryda; sattar26@doctors.org.uk

Academic Editor: Pär Johansson

This is a retrospective study of 51 consecutive hip reconstructions in children with cerebral palsy performed between 2011 and 2013. Tranexamic acid (TXA) was used in 14 hip reconstructions only. Transfusion rate was higher, postoperative Hb was lower, and patients stayed longer in the TXA group. This did not reach a statistical significance ($P = 0.75$, 0.5, and 0.71, resp.). More than half of the patients who had TXA underwent bilateral hip reconstructions in comparison with 27% only in the non-TXA group. Bilateral hip reconstructions mean more surgery, more blood loss, and more blood transfusion. The patients who had TXA were significantly more disabled as evident by the higher proportions of patient with worse GMFCS levels. Although we have not been able to demonstrate the value of TXA in reducing blood loss and transfusion rate in children with CP who underwent hip reconstruction, it is hoped that an interest in exploring the value of TXA in paediatric orthopaedic surgery is generated. Ideally this should be explored further in an adequately powered, randomised controlled trial where risk of bias is minimized.

1. Introduction

Cerebral palsy (CP) is caused by an injury to the immature brain usually occurring during or shortly after birth. Although all functions of the brain may be affected, the motor function is usually the most vulnerable [1]. The gross motor function classification system (GMFCS) categorises the functional capabilities of children with CP into 5 levels (Table 1) [2].

The initial treatment usually involves a combination of interventions such as medicines, braces, and adaptive and assistive equipment; however, surgery is sometimes warranted to control symptoms and maintain an optimum level of function and appearance. Hip joint dislocation is a common problem in children with CP that can cause significant pain and interference with personal care and hygiene. Surgical hip reconstruction reduces the hip joint through soft tissue releases and bony cuts of the femur and/or pelvis (Figure 1). Blood loss and subsequent blood transfusion are a normal consequence of hip reconstruction [3, 4].

Postoperative anaemia has been shown to impede functional ability and therefore delay discharge in this patient group. However allogeneic blood transfusion is associated with risks for the recipient (haemolysis, infection, immunosuppression, transfusion-related acute lung injury, and even death). The risk of postoperative wound infection correlates with the amount of transfused allogeneic blood and has significant cost implications. Thus surgeons aim to minimise blood loss at surgery.

There has been a recent surge in the use of tranexamic acid (TXA) in trauma and orthopaedic practice. TXA belong to a group of agents called "the antifibrinolytics" which has been used successfully to reduce blood loss. A Cochrane review scrutinised 252 trials that had used antifibrinolytics in elective surgery: 60 trials evaluated TXA. The reviewers concluded that antifibrinolytics are effective in reducing blood loss, the need for allogeneic red cell transfusion, and the need for reoperation due to continued postoperative bleeding after elective surgery [5]. Numerous other studies have confirmed the effectiveness of TXA in reducing blood loss and transfusion requirements in total joints replacements and spine

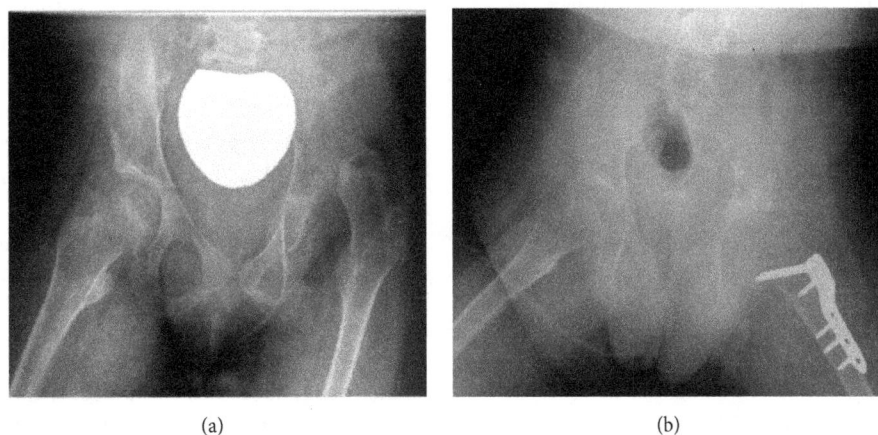

(a)   (b)

FIGURE 1: Preoperative and postoperative X-rays of a dislocated hip in a child with cerebral palsy. The left X-ray showed a dislocated left hip in a child with CP. The acetabulum has become shallow and is not covering the femoral head any more. There is a valgus deformity of the proximal femur. The postoperative pictures showed that the hip is reduced, the proximal femoral deformity is corrected (varus derotation corrective osteotomy), and the acetabulum is corrected by pelvic Dega osteotomy.

TABLE 1: The gross motor function classification system.

GMFCS	Descriptions
Level I	Children in this group can perform usual activities such as running and jumping almost as normal. There may be a decreased speed, balance, and coordination.
Level II	They have the ability to walk indoors and outdoors and climb stairs with a railing. They have difficulty with uneven surfaces, running, or jumping.
Level III	They need assistive mobility devices (such as canes, crutched, and walkers). They may be able to climb stairs using a railing.
Level IV	They use wheelchairs most of the time and may propel their own power wheelchair. They can participate in standing transfers.
Level V	There is severe limitation in all areas of motor function. They cannot sit or stand independently, even with adaptive equipment. They depend on others for mobility.

surgery [6–12]. However, there is very little published work on the use of TXA in paediatric orthopaedic practice.

In a multicenter, retrospective review of 84 patients with CP who underwent spinal deformity correction [13], the use of TXA was associated with less blood loss and length of stay. Very few surgeons use TXA in hip reconstruction surgery for children with CP and, to the best of our knowledge, there is no available report on its effectiveness and safety profile in this group of patients.

2. Methods

A retrospective observational study design, including 51 consecutive hip reconstructions performed between 2011 and 2013, was used to evaluate the use of tranexamic acid (TXA). The study was approved by the Institution's Audit Department (reference number 4942). Medical records were reviewed for age, date of birth, gender, medications, weight at surgery, blood loss in theatre, and the need for transfusion. The latter was cross-checked with the blood bank data base for confirmation. The preoperative laboratory results of complete blood count including hemoglobin (Hb), platelets, and haematocrit (Hct) were recorded. The estimated blood volume (EBV) was estimated from the following formula: (EBV = 80 mL $*$ body weight in kg). The estimation of red blood cell volume (RBCV) at preoperative Hct is as follows: $RBCV_{preop} = EBV \times Hct_{preop}$. The estimation of red blood cell volume (RBCV) at postoperative Hct is as follows: $RBCV_{Postop} = EBV \times Hct_{Postop}$. The total blood loss is calculated from the fall in red blood cell volume: Blood loss $= RBCV_{diff}/Hct_{Postop}$ [14, 15].

Data cleaning and analysis were performed using SPSS 20. The data were checked for normality using the Kolmogorov-Smirnov test (KST) and the Shapiro-Wilk test (SWT). When substantial nonnormality was indicated ($P < 0.05$), then nonparametric estimate was provided alongside the parametric findings. Moreover, a bootstrap estimate was provided to explore robustness of estimates [16]. Continuous outcomes were analysed (blood loss, volume transfused, length of stay, haemoglobin and Haematocrit, and overall cost), using independent samples t-test. Categorical outcomes were analysed by Fisher's exact test (blood transfusion required, GMFCS levels, and complications). The study main outcome was transfusion rate with other measures considered supportive.

3. Results

Fifty-one hip reconstructions were performed in children with CP in our institute: 14 received TXA, 37 did not. The two groups were similar in age, weight, gender distribution, and the ASA Physical Status (the American Society of Anesthesiologists) (see Table 2). Baseline mean operative Hb levels and Hct levels were similar, as were proportions of patients taking nonsteroidal anti-inflammatory drugs (NSAID) and

TABLE 2: Baseline characteristics of the study population.

Characteristics	No Tranexamic acid	Tranexamic acid	P value
Number	37	14	
Age (y)	10.2 (SD 3.3)	9.8 (SD 3.3)	0.74
Male (%)	21 (57%)	5 (36%)	0.22
Weight (kg)	30.2 (SD 11.8)	27.7 (SD 13.0)	0.54
GMFCS (low/high)	9/27	3/11	0.79
ASA (1/2/3/4/5)	3/18/8/0/0	1/6/5/0/0	0.32
Bilateral	10 (27%)	8 (57%)	0.06
Types of bony osteotomy (F, P, and B)	11/1/25	3/0/11	0.62
Prescribed NSAID (%)	19 (58%)	6 (50%)	0.74
Epilim (%)	5 (14%)	5 (36%)	0.12
Preoperative Hb (g/dL)	13.5 (SD 1.2)	13.3 (SD 1.4)	0.73
Preoperative Hct	0.397 (SD 0.032)	0.383 (SD 0.033)	0.19

GMFCS: gross motor function classification system, ASA: American Society of Anaesthetists, F: femoral osteotomy, P: pelvic osteotomy, B: both femoral and pelvic osteotomy, NSAID: nonsteroidal anti-inflammatory, Hb: hemoglobin, Hct: hematocrit, and SD: standard deviation.

Epilim: these are implicated with increased surgical blood loss [17, 18]. Patients in the tranexamic acid group had a higher GMFCS level (78% versus 75%: $P = 0.79$), more combined pelvic and femoral osteotomies (78% versus 67%: $P = 0.62$), and more bilateral surgery (57% versus 27%: $P = 0.06$). Although none of these differences reached a statistical significance, the latter had come quite close. Bilateral hip reconstruction was performed in 57% of children in the TXA group in comparison to 27% in the other group ($P = 0.06$); thus the TXA group may have more severe underlying disease. There is a borderline significant different in the pattern of gross motor function classification system (GMFCS) between groups, despite no systematic trend by level ($P = 0.79$).

3.1. Blood Transfusion. The proportion of children receiving blood transfusion was 42.9% in the TXA groups versus 36.1% in the non-TXA group, a statistically nonsignificant difference (RD: 6.7%, 95% CI: −21.3% to 36.1%, $P = 0.75$) (Table 3).

3.1.1. Blood Loss. The total blood loss was estimated using Gross's formula [14, 15]. The mean total blood loss was similar: TXA 969 mL versus no TXA 971 mL (RD: −2 mL, 95% CI: −536 mL to 531 mL, $P = 0.99$).

3.1.2. Postoperative Hemoglobin, Haematocrit, and Hb Drop. Hemoglobin (Hb) and hematocrit (Hct) were tested on postoperative day 2 unless there was a clinical need to do

these earlier. Levels were similar and differences between the two groups were not statistically significant.

3.1.3. Length of Stay. The duration of stay in hospital was similar between groups: TXA 8.17d versus no TXA 7.63 (difference: 0.54 d, 95% CI: −2.37 to 3.45), $P = 0.71$.

3.2. Adverse Events. There were 3 complications in the tranexamic acid group (2 fragility fractures and 1 paralytic ileus). The two fractures were treated nonoperatively in a resting cast. Two complications were recorded in the non-TXA group: one deep infection and a pressure sore. The former was treated with washout and antibiotic and the latter was treated with regular dressing. There were no reported thromboembolic events (see Table 4).

4. Discussion

This retrospective study was conducted to explore the transfusion rate in children with cerebral palsy who underwent hip reconstruction as a background work for a future trial. Blood transfusion rate is considered to be a reliable outcome measure and it is of great importance for patients, healthcare providers, and managers and hence it is chosen as the primary outcome for our study. A recent local audit showed that the our unit was 96% compliant with the national guidelines for blood transfusion [19, 20] supporting the findings and subsequent conclusions of this study. Out of 51 hip reconstructions, 13 patients (25.4%) received allogenic blood transfusion. Contrary to most studies [5, 11, 12] that used TXA, in children with CP and hip reconstruction, transfusion rate was higher, postoperative Hb was lower, and patients stayed longer in the TXA group. This did not reach a statistical significance ($P = 0.75, 0.5,$ and 0.71, resp.). This may be a true finding that TXA does not reduce blood loss in this group of patients or it may be a type II error where the study did not demonstrate the real positive effect of TXA on blood transfusion for various reasons.

The table of baseline characteristics of the study populations showed significant selection bias which disfavours TXA. It is apparent that TXA was used when larger blood loss was expected. More than half of the patients who had TXA underwent bilateral hip reconstructions in comparison with 27% only in the non-TXA group. Bilateral hip reconstructions mean more surgery, more blood loss, and more blood transfusion. The patients who had TXA were significantly more disabled as evident by the higher proportions of patient with worse GMFCS levels. It is expected that these factors would mean more transfusion rates in the TXA group and nevertheless this was not the case. Similar can be said on length of stay where patients who received TXA stayed longer in hospital.

Eipe and Ponniah [14] showed that surgical blood loss was underestimated by 64% using clinical methods assessing blood soaked mops and gauze pieces and measuring blood lost to suction bottles and the vacuum drain. They recommended using a biochemical method based on Hct. In our study, total blood loss was estimated using Gross's

TABLE 3: Primary and secondary outcomes.

	No tranexamic acid [1]	Tranexamic acid [2]	[2] – [1] (95% CI), P
Transfusion rate	13/36 (36.1%)	6/14 (42.9%)	6.7% (−21.3% to 36.1%), $P = 0.75$
Total blood loss, mL	971 (SD 766)	969 (SD 742)	−2 (−536 to 531), $P = 0.99$
Postop Hb, g/dL	9.4 (SD 1.76)	8.9 (SD 1.5)	−0.5 (−1.7 to 0.7), $P = 0.40$
Postop Hct	0.29 (SD 0.06)	0.27 (SD 0.04)	−0.02 (−0.06 to 0.02), $P = 0.36$
Hb drop, g/dL	4.1 (SD 1.9)	4.3 (SD 2.0)	0.2 (−1.1 to 1.6), $P = 0.72$
Length of stay, days	7.63 (SD 4.2)	8.17 (SD 3.9)	0.54 (−2.37 to 3.44), $P = 0.71$

Hb: hemoglobin, Hct: hematocrit, and SD: standard deviation.

TABLE 4: Adverse events.

Complications	No tranexamic acid	Tranexamic acid
Deep venous thrombosis	0	0
Pulmonary embolism	0	0
Deep infection	1	0
Paralytic ileus	0	1
Pressure sore	1	0
Fragility fracture	0	2
Total	2	3

formula [14, 15]. The difference was not clinically important and statistically was not significant.

There are several weaknesses to our study. It is a retrospective study where data were collected from medical records and hospital laboratory. Although this may undermine the accuracy of data, most primary outcomes (blood transfusion, HB level, and length of stay) are accurately and independently recorded in our center. The number of patients involved in our study is relatively small. It is estimated that 184 patients are required to have an 80% chance of detecting a 50% decrease in the transfusion rates of 36% in the non-TXA group at the 5% level. The rate of the type II error is closely related to the number of participants involved in a study (the study power).

In conclusion, although we have not been able to demonstrate the value of TXA in reducing blood loss and transfusion rate in children with CP who underwent hip reconstruction, it is hoped that an interest in exploring the value of TXA in paediatric orthopaedic surgery is generated. Ideally this should be explored further in an adequately powered, randomised controlled trial where risk of bias is minimized.

Conflict of Interests

The authors declare that there is no conflict of interests regarding the publication of this paper.

References

[1] J. Gage, *Gait Analysis in Cerebral Palsy*, Mac Keith Press, 1991.

[2] R. Palisano, P. Rosenbaum, S. Walter, D. Russell, E. Wood, and B. Galuppi, "Development and reliability of a system to classify gross motor function in children with cerebral palsy," *Developmental Medicine and Child Neurology*, vol. 39, no. 4, pp. 214–223, 1997.

[3] B. T. Carney and C. L. Minter, "Is operative blood loss associated with valproic acid? Analysis of bilateral femoral osteotomy in children with total involvement cerebral palsy," *Journal of Pediatric Orthopaedics*, vol. 25, no. 3, pp. 283–285, 2005.

[4] P. Nicolai, P. P. Leggetter, P. R. Glithero, and C. R. Bhimarasetty, "Autologous transfusion in acetabuloplasty in children," *The Journal of Bone and Joint Surgery—British Volume*, vol. 86, no. 1, pp. 110–112, 2004.

[5] D. A. Henry, P. A. Carless, A. J. Moxey et al., "Anti-fibrinolytic use for minimising perioperative allogeneic blood transfusion," *Cochrane Database of Systematic Reviews*, vol. 4, no. 1, Article ID CD001886, 2007.

[6] G. Benoni, H. Fredin, R. Knebel, and P. Nilsson, "Blood conservation with tranexamic acid in total hip arthroplasty: a randomized, double-blind study in 40 primary operations," *Acta Orthopaedica Scandinavica*, vol. 72, no. 5, pp. 442–448, 2001.

[7] E. Lemay, J. Guay, C. Côté, and A. Roy, "Tranexamic acid reduces the need for allogenic red blood cell transfusions in patients undergoing total hip replacement," *Canadian Journal of Anesthesia*, vol. 51, no. 1, pp. 31–37, 2004.

[8] H. Husted, L. Blønd, S. Sonne-Holm, G. Holm, T. W. Jacobsen, and P. Gebuhr, "Tranexamic acid reduces blood loss and blood transfusions in primary total hip arthroplasty: a prospective randomized double-blind study in 40 patients," *Acta Orthopaedica Scandinavica*, vol. 74, no. 6, pp. 665–669, 2003.

[9] S. Alshryda, J. Mason, P. Sarda et al., "Topical (intra-articular) tranexamic acid reduces blood loss and transfusion rates following total hip replacement: a randomized controlled trial (TRANX-H)," *The Journal of Bone and Joint Surgery—American Volume*, vol. 95, no. 21, pp. 1969–1974, 2013.

[10] S. Alshryda, J. Mason, M. Vaghela et al., "Topical (intra-articular) tranexamic acid reduces blood loss and transfusion rates following total knee replacement: a randomized controlled trial (TRANX-K)," *The Journal of Bone & Joint Surgery—American Volume*, vol. 95, no. 21, pp. 1961–1968, 2013.

[11] S. Alshryda, P. Sarda, M. Sukeik, A. Nargol, J. Blenkinsopp, and J. M. Mason, "Tranexamic acid in total knee replacement: a systematic review and meta-analysis," *The Journal of Bone & Joint Surgery—British Volume*, vol. 93, no. 12, pp. 1577–1585, 2011.

[12] M. Sukeik, S. Alshryda, F. S. Haddad, and J. M. Mason, "Systematic review and meta-analysis of the use of tranexamic acid in total hip replacement," *The Journal of Bone and Joint Surgery—British Volume*, vol. 93, no. 1, pp. 39–46, 2011.

[13] A. A. Dhawale, S. A. Shah, P. D. Sponseller et al., "Are antifibrinolytics helpful in decreasing blood loss and transfusions during spinal fusion surgery in children with cerebral palsy scoliosis?" *Spine*, vol. 37, no. 9, pp. E549–E555, 2012.

[14] N. P. Eipe and M. Ponniah, "Perioperative blood loss assessment-how accurate?" *Indian Journal of Anaestheisa*, vol. 50, no. 1, pp. 35–38, 2006.

[15] J. Duke, *Anaesthesia Secrets*, Mosby Elsevier, 3rd edition, 2006.

[16] S. G. Thompson and J. A. Barber, "How should cost data in pragmatic randomised trials be analysed?" *British Medical Journal*, vol. 320, no. 7243, pp. 1197–1200, 2000.

[17] S. L. Winter, R. L. Kriel, T. F. Novacheck, M. G. Luxenberg, V. J. Leutgeb, and P. A. Erickson, "Perioperative blood loss: the effect of valproate," *Pediatric Neurology*, vol. 15, no. 1, pp. 19–22, 1996.

[18] H. G. Chambers, C. H. Weinstein, S. J. Mubarak, D. R. Wenger, and P. D. Silva, "The effect of valproic acid on blood loss in patients with cerebral palsy," *Journal of Pediatric Orthopaedics*, vol. 19, no. 6, pp. 792–795, 1999.

[19] M. F. Murphy, T. B. Wallington, P. Kelsey et al., "Guidelines for the clinical use of red cell transfusions," *British Journal of Haematology*, vol. 113, no. 1, pp. 24–31, 2001.

[20] The British Committee for Standards in Haematology, *Guidelines on Clinical Use of Red Cell Transfusion*, The British Committee for Standards in Haematology, 2012, http://www.bcshguidelines.com/350_ARCHIVED_GUIDELINES.html?dtype=Transfusion&dpage=0&sspage=0&ipage=0#gl.

30

Postoperative Autologous Reinfusion in Total Knee Replacement

A. Crescibene,[1] F. Martire,[1] P. Gigliotti,[2] A. Rende,[3] and M. Candela[1]

[1]*Orthopedics and Traumatology Unit, San Francesco di Paola Hospital, Azienda Sanitaria Provinciale di Cosenza, Via Promintesta, 87027 Paola, Italy*

[2]*Kidney and Transplantation Research Center, Azienda Ospedaliera di Cosenza, Via Felice Migliori, 87100 Cosenza, Italy*

[3]*Transfusion Medicine Unit, San Francesco di Paola Hospital, Azienda Sanitaria Provinciale di Cosenza, Via Promintesta, 87027 Paola, Italy*

Correspondence should be addressed to A. Crescibene; antonio.crescibene@libero.it

Academic Editor: Erwin Strasser

Surgeries for total knee replacement (TKR) are increasing and in this context there is a need to develop new protocols for management and use of blood transfusion therapy. Autologous blood reduces the need for allogeneic blood transfusion and the aim of the present study was to verify the safety and the clinical efficacy. An observational retrospective study has been conducted on 124 patients, undergoing cemented total knee prosthesis replacement. Observed population was stratified into two groups: the first group received reinfusion of autologous blood collected in the postoperative surgery and the second group did not receive autologous blood reinfusion. Analysis of data shows that patients undergoing autologous blood reinfusion received less homologous blood bags (10.6% versus 30%; $p = 0.08$) and reduced days of hospitalization (7.88 ± 0.7 days versus 8.96 ± 2.47 days for the control group; $p = 0.03$). Microbiological tests were negative in all postoperatively salvaged and reinfused units. Our results emphasize the effectiveness of this procedure and have the characteristics of simplicity, low cost (€97.53 versus €103.79; $p < 0.01$), and easy reproducibility. Use of autologous drainage system postoperatively is a procedure that allows reducing transfusion of homologous blood bags in patients undergoing TKR.

1. Introduction

Total joint replacement usually represents the final route for treatment of degenerative disease of the knee. Joint replacements are more and more frequent and routine these days thanks to, for example, the consequent aging of the general population, increased functional requirements, and the development and use of new materials and more sophisticated surgical techniques.

In this context, there is a need to develop new protocols for management and use of transfusion therapies in the field of orthopedic surgery.

Transfusion of homologous blood are frequent and costly and expose patients to potential risks of infection [1, 2]; hence several methods have been proposed to avoid them [3, 4].

Preoperative blood donation and intra- and postoperative blood collection and administration of pharmaceutical agents to either reduce blood loss (e.g., tranexamic acid) or stimulate the production of erythrocytes (e.g., erythropoietin) have

been proposed as alternative techniques to transfusion of homologous blood in various studies [3, 4].

In the scientific literature, there are several reports of studies where reinfusion of blood collection in postoperative orthopedic surgery, especially in prosthesis surgery [5–14], is analyzed.

The aim of the present study was to verify the safety, the clinical efficacy, and the possible benefits of reinfusion of postoperatively collected autologous blood in total knee replacement procedures, with special emphasis on cost-benefit and reinfusion procedure, by comparing autologous blood transfusion with nonautologous blood transfusion.

2. Materials and Methods

2.1. Patients. Between 2011 and 2012, one hundred twenty-four patients with a mean age of 71.2 ± 6.8 years and a range between 50 and 84 years were included in the study.

All patients were diagnosed with primary osteoarthritis of the knee.

The first group consisted of a series of sixty-four consecutive patients (male to female ratio 1 : 5, range of age between 62 and 84 years), who underwent one stage unilateral total knee arthroplasty using a blood reinfusion device in 2012.

Fifty-eight of these patients received autologous transfusion and six patients were excluded, five due to systemic pathologies.

The control group consisted of sixty consecutive patients (male to female ratio 1 : 3, age ranging from 50 to 79 years). This population was operated on consecutively in 2011 but is not subjected to autologous blood reinfusion because we have been using this device since January 1, 2012.

Before any study-related measures were taken all patients read and signed informed consent for any possible transfusion of homologous red blood cell and a specific consent for reinfusion, after adequate information on possible risks and benefits of both methods.

The manuscript was performed in accordance with the ethical standards of the 1964 Declaration of Helsinki as revised in 2000; for this type of study formal consent is not required.

2.2. Surgical Procedure. Antibiotic prophylaxis was obtained by administration of ceftriaxone 1 g intramuscular injection once daily and teicoplanin 800 mg intravenous injection once daily, 30 minutes before inducing anaesthesia.

Antithrombotic prophylaxis was obtained by administration of enoxaparin sodium 4,000 I.U. once daily by subcutaneous injection for 35 days, 12 hours before surgery; two patients had an urticarial reaction and therefore it has been replaced with fondaparinux sodium 2.5 mg once daily by subcutaneous injection for 35 days.

Patients were subjected to surgical intervention for unilateral primary arthroplasty knee, by implanting a Zimmer's Nexgen cemented prosthesis or How Medical's Triathlon prosthesis.

All patients received subarachnoid anesthesia.

Surgery was carried out by the same surgeon on all patients; a standard surgical procedure was performed including a longitudinal medial skin incision and median parapatellar quadriceps splitting approach.

The hole drilled in the femoral canal was plugged.

Limb ischemia was achieved through temporary leg loop tire located at the root of the limb and the tourniquet was deflated after the step of cementing.

Postoperative pain was controlled with paracetamol 100 mL/10 mg endovenous with a 4-hour minimum interval between each administration.

2.3. Blood Salvage and Reinfusion. Bellovac ABT is a drainage system for postoperative collection, filtration, and reinfusion of shed autologous blood. It consists of all components required for collection and reinfusion of one unit of shed autologous blood.

The initial negative suction pressure is 90 mmHg (12 kPa), generating safe and efficient drainage.

Once the recovery of shed blood is completed (within <6 hours) the transfusion bag can be replaced with a collection bag for evacuation only, thus serving as a simple wound drainage (Card System Technical Bellovac ABT for drainage and the recovery of the blood postoperative manufacturer: Astra Tech AB, Via Cristoni, Casalecchio di Reno (BO)).

The minimal drained blood to be transfused is 100 cc.

2.4. Transfusion Trigger. For all patients, we decided that a homologous transfusion therapy was only indicated for haemoglobin values below 8 g/dL [15].

2.5. Clinical Data. The study group consisted of a series of sixty-four consecutive patients with mean age 73.3 ± 5.7 years (14 males and 50 females), while the control group consisted of sixty consecutive patients with mean age 69 ± 7.2 years (18 males and 42 females).

We excluded patients with systemic pathologies such as uncompensated diabetes mellitus, cancer, severe cardiovascular pathologies, immunodepression, anticoagulating or antiaggregating therapy, coagulation disorders including deep venous thrombosis, and ongoing infections.

We considered as discriminating factors hemoglobin values <12 g/dL for women and <14 g/dL for men.

Length of surgery was 2.24 ± 0.38 hours in the study group versus 2.06 ± 0.32 hours ($p = 0.17$).

2.6. Laboratory Data. Hemoglobin values (Hb; g/dL) were checked preoperatively, immediately after surgery, on the first day and the second day after the operation, and on discharge. They were later compared between groups.

In the study group, patients were subjected to a microbiological culture of a blood sample (20 mL) from the bag of postoperative recovery, at the end of the procedure of reinfusion.

2.7. Economic Data. In our hospital, the transfusion medicine unite has provided the following expense items: the cost of an autologous blood retransfusion system is around €68,00, while the costs of an allogenic blood transfusion, including cross-matching, delivery, and refrigerated storage, are stated to be €270.

Added costs of the postoperative drain and the ABT system are €20 and €68, respectively.

These costs were evaluated for the examined patients.

2.8. Statistic. All data are presented as mean ± SD or median (IQR) as appropriate. Groups were compared using the one-way ANOVA or *t*-test for normally distributed data and the nonparametric Kruskal-Wallis or Mann-Whitney *U* test for non-normally distributed variables.

3. Results

3.1. Preoperative Comparison of Groups Characteristics. The study group consisted of a series of sixty-four consecutive patients with mean age 73.3 ± 5.7 years, 14 male and 50 female, while the control group consisted of sixty consecutive patients with mean age 69 ± 7.2 years, 18 male and 42 female ($p < 0.05$).

The average body weight of the study group was 70.8 ± 8.8 Kg and 73.1 ± 8.0 Kg ($p = 0.43$).

3.2. Perioperative Data. In the study group, all the patients received autologous blood transfusion.

In the first six hours 400 ± 122.4 mL (min. 100; max. 600) was collected and retransfused; within 24 hours there was 198.5 ± 142.4 mL of blood drained in the drainage.

In the control group, 478.2 ± 220.3 mL (min. 250; max. 900) was drained in the first 24 hours after surgery.

Because of the intraoperative use of a tourniquet, intraoperative blood loss was negligible in both groups.

We noticed a reduction rate of allogeneic blood transfusion between the study and the control group (10.3% versus 30%; $p = 0.08$).

Six patients in the study group, four women and two men, were subjected to allogeneic transfusion, five patients received one unit of homologous blood between the second and fourth days postoperatively, and one patient received two units of homologous blood. No patient had any adverse event or febrile episodes.

In the control group, we registered 18 patients who received homologous blood transfusion; each one had received a bag of homologous whole blood.

The transfusion trigger in the ABT group ($n = 6$) was 7.5 ± 0.1 g/dL, whereas that in the control group ($n = 18$) was 7.3 ± 0.2 g/dL ($p = 0.09$).

One unit of red blood cells can be expected to result in a hemoglobin increase of 1 g/dL in a typical adult [15].

In the ABT group we recorded an increase in hemoglobin equal to 0.7 ± 0.3 (g/dL), after autologous transfusion. In this group we recorded an increase in hemoglobin equal to 1.3 ± 0.2 (g/dL) ($n = 7$ bags) versus 0.9 ± 0.1 (g/dL) ($n = 18$ bags) in the control group after homologous transfusion ($p < 0.01$).

Therefore, we noticed a greater rise in hemoglobin after homologous transfusion in the group given reinfusion (Figure 1).

The tourniquet time was 1.13 ± 0.27 hours in study group versus 1.04 ± 0.27 hours in control group ($p = 0.36$).

In the study group the mean length of stay at the hospital (LOS) was 7.88 ± 0.7 days, while it was 8.96 ± 2.47 days for the control group ($p = 0.03$).

Blood values were substantially stationary in the perioperative phase, in either group.

Really, we did not find any significant difference for hemoglobin count between groups from admission to hospital discharge (Table 1 and Figure 2); as expected, we did not find any difference between groups considering the reduction in hemoglobin for study's time points (Table 2 and Figure 3).

3.3. Complication and LOS. The results of microbiological cultures performed on blood samples taken from the postoperative blood bag at the end of the procedure of reinfusion were negative in all cases.

In our study a total knee replacement surgical procedure, along with the complementary use of a device for postoperative collection and reinfusion of shed blood resulted in an average reduction of the length of hospital stay equal to 1.08 ± 0.76 days ($p = 0.03$ versus control).

TABLE 1: Values are presented as mean ± standard deviation (Hb; g/dL).

	Study group	Control group	p value
Entry	13.7 ± 1.5	14 ± 1.2	$p = 0.12$
Postoperatively	11.8 ± 1.22	12.1 ± 1.3	$p = 0.11$
1° day	10.7 ± 1.2	10.6 ± 1.2	$p = 0.16$
2° days	10.1 ± 1.1	10.2 ± 0.9	$p = 0.28$
Discharge	9.9 ± 1.1	10.3 ± 0.9	$p = 0.14$

TABLE 2: Reduction of blood parameters; values are presented as mean ± standard deviation.

	Study group (n. 52)	Control group (n. 42)	p value
Postoperatively	1.9 ± 0.8	1.8 ± 0.5	$p = 0.22$
1° day	3 ± 1	3.2 ± 0.9	$p = 0.34$
2° days	3.6 ± 1.4	3.7 ± 1	$p = 0.21$
Discharge	3.7 ± 1.1	3.5 ± 1.1	$p = 0.21$

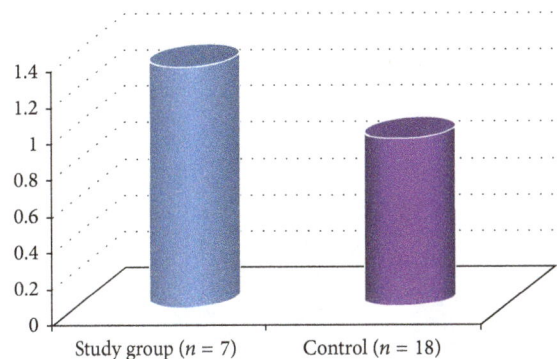

FIGURE 1: Hemoglobin increase after homologous transfusion (g/dL).

3.4. Cost Analysis. The cost of an autologous blood retransfusion system is around €68,00, while the costs of a allogeneic blood transfusion are stated to be €270, including crossmatching, delivery, and refrigerated storage.

In the present study, 18 allogeneic transfusions were given in the no-drainage group, while 7 allogeneic transfusions were given in the ABT group, at a cost of €4.860,00 and €1.890,00, respectively.

The additional costs of the postoperative drain and the ABT system were €20 and €68, respectively, in either group at a cost of €1.160,00 ($n = 58$) and €4.352,00 ($n = 64$).

The average cost per patient turned out to be lower in the group receiving reinfusion (€97.53 versus €103.79; $p < 0.01$).

4. Discussion

Primarily, autologous blood reduces the need for allogeneic blood transfusion; furthermore, it prevents the transmission of viral diseases (hepatitis C virus, hepatitis B virus, human immunodeficiency virus, and Creutzfeldt-Jacob virus), transfusion reactions, and transfusion errors [16, 17].

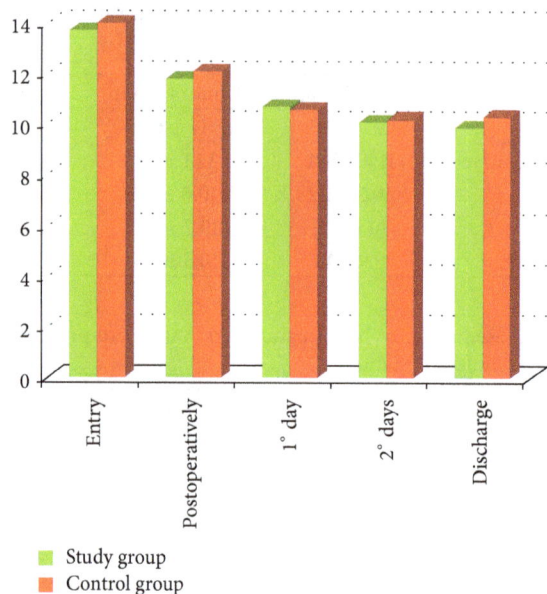

FIGURE 2: Modification of hemoglobin level in both groups during stay at the hospital period (g/dL).

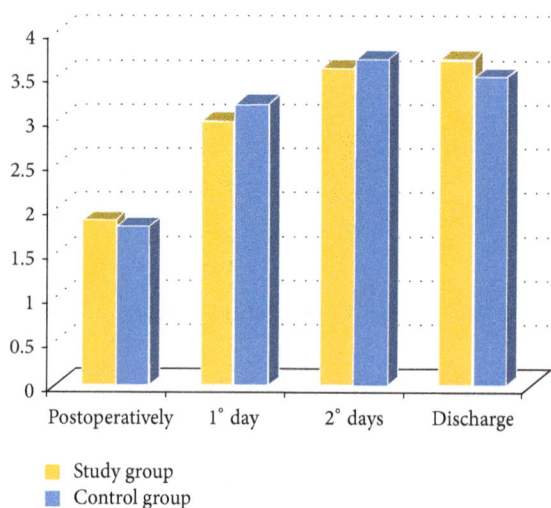

FIGURE 3: Changes in hemoglobin level in both groups during stay at the hospital period (g/dL).

The main advantage of postoperative collection and reinfusion of shed blood is this method's simplicity; hence it finds its application in traumatized patients.

However, its main disadvantage is the risk of contamination during blood collection [8, 18].

Fong et al. [19] identify some possible complications of collection of red blood cells, such as nonimmunologic haemolysis, gas embolism, nonhaemolytic transfusion reaction, coagulopathies, contamination with drugs, the intraoperative use of washing solutions in the surgical site and infectious agents, cytokines, and other microaggregates.

The risk of complications decreased due to improvement of techniques and practices as well as increased experience with autologous blood collection systems [20].

Cleveland Clinic has performed a five-year retrospective study of complications, with both homologous and collected shed blood, noting that the incidence of complications with collected blood was around 0.027% compared to 0.14% of homologous blood [21].

In our study we had no patient with adverse events or febrile illnesses.

The results of microbiological cultures performed on blood samples taken from the postoperative blood bag at the end of the reinfusion were negative in all cases.

The purpose of collection of shed blood is to reduce or eliminate the need for homologous blood transfusion and the associated risk of infectious and noninfectious complications [22].

During 2006, a meta-analysis of the recovery of red blood cells in adult elective surgery showed that recovery of blood could reduce the need for homologous blood transfusion.

The use of recovered red blood cells has reduced the exposure to allogeneic blood by 39% with an average saving of 0.67 units per patient [23].

In 2013 a meta-analysis proved that the use of a postoperative autotransfusion reinfusion system reduced significantly the demand for allogeneic blood transfusions.

It also cut the number of patients who needed allogeneic blood transfusions and the cost of hospitalization after total knee arthroplasty.

Collection of blood in orthopedic surgery results in greater safety and efficacy [24–26].

94 cases have been studied but a power analysis of the study was not performed; however, we argue that the use of a device for autologous blood collection and washing results in an average reduction of 4 units of allogeneic blood and cost savings of an average of 406.84 dollars per patient [27].

In the literature there are some authors with differing views.

These authors suggest that autologous blood transfusion drains have no effect on the proportion of transfused patients in primary total knee arthroplasty [28–34].

The postoperative hemoglobin levels, the length of hospital stay, and the adverse events are also comparable between groups [28].

In our opinion autologous blood collection and reinfusion, by the use of postoperative systems, is a procedure that allows limiting the transfusion of homologous blood to patients undergoing TKR, improving the postoperative course from a psychophysical point of view and allowing an early transfer to rehabilitation unit.

We noticed a reduction in allogenic blood transfusion between the study and the control group (10.3% versus 30%; $p = 0.08$).

Reinfusion group patients also displayed a reduction in the length of stay in hospital by 1.08 ± 0.76 days ($p = 0.03$ versus control).

Concerning costs, the question is whether savings derived from the reduction in allogeneic blood transfusion requirements outweighed the extra costs of the ABT system.

Zacharopoulos et al. [35] stated that use of the postoperative blood reinfusion systems is highly effective in reducing the demand for homologous blood transfusion for patients undergoing total knee replacement surgery, resulting in important cost savings in the management of these patients.

A previous study observing patients undergoing TKA found net savings in different cost scenarios of €5 to €106 per patient with the same ABT system as used in this study and €52 to €50 per patient with another ABT system [36].

A review of cost-effectiveness on blood-saving measures stated that cell salvage had lower costs compared with all of the alternative blood-saving strategies except acute normovolemic dilution and concluded that autotransfusion may be a cost-effective method to reduce allogeneic transfusions [37, 38].

The evidence that supports the use of red blood cell recovery in knee prosthesis is stronger and comprises randomized studies and one large retrospective review [39, 40].

The average cost per patient was found to be lower in the group receiving reinfusion (€97.53 versus €103.79; $p < 0.01$).

This work presents a lot of strengths such as the same characteristics of the sample, the surgical technique performed by the same surgeon, and the rigorous cost analysis; on the contrary we are aware of some weaknesses such as the retrospective design. So some prospective randomized studies are to be presented.

5. Conclusion

This study has confirmed the absolute safety of the device and the absence of bacteria in examined samples.

Our results emphasize the effectiveness of this procedure and have the characteristics of simplicity, low cost, easy reproducibility, and safety.

In addition, this recovery system replaces the simple postoperative surgical drainage, representing a further saving of economic resources.

Finally we conclude that the use of the shed blood recovery system Bellovac ABT constitutes a valid device, which can find wide application in orthopedics, especially in the context of total knee replacement surgery.

Conflict of Interests

The authors declare that they have no conflict of interests.

Acknowledgments

The authors would like to thank Dr. Anna Maria Morano, Dr. Marinella Zacchi, Dr. Maria Maddalena Grossi, Dr. Massimo Rugna, and Dr. Arcangela Cundari for the excellent cooperation.

References

[1] R. Y. Dodd, "The risk of transfusion-transmitted infection," *The New England Journal of Medicine*, vol. 327, no. 6, pp. 419–421, 1992.

[2] J. P. Waymack and R. W. Yurt, "The effect of blood transfusions on immune function. V. The effect on the inflammatory response to bacterial infections," *Journal of Surgical Research*, vol. 48, no. 2, pp. 147–153, 1990.

[3] M. Amin, D. Fergusson, A. Aziz, K. Wilson, D. Coyle, and P. Hébert, "The cost of allogeneic red blood cells—a systematic review," *Transfusion Medicine*, vol. 13, no. 5, pp. 275–285, 2003.

[4] D. R. Spahn and M. Casutt, "Eliminating blood transfusions: new aspects and perspectives," *Anesthesiology*, vol. 93, no. 1, pp. 242–255, 2000.

[5] A. F. C. M. Moonen, N. T. Knoors, J. J. Van Os, A. D. Verburg, and P. Pilot, "Retransfusion of filtered shed blood in primary total hip and knee arthroplasty: a prospective randomized clinical trial," *Transfusion*, vol. 47, no. 3, pp. 379–384, 2007.

[6] C.-D. Han and D.-E. Shin, "Postoperative blood salvage and reinfusion after total joint arthroplasty," *The Journal of Arthroplasty*, vol. 12, no. 5, pp. 511–516, 1997.

[7] C. M. Jensen, R. Pilegaard, K. Hviid, J. D. Nielsen, and H. J. Nielsen, "Quality of reinfused drainage blood after total knee arthroplasty," *Journal of Arthroplasty*, vol. 14, no. 3, pp. 312–318, 1999.

[8] J. W. Martin, L. A. Whiteside, M. T. Milliano, and M. E. Reedy, "Postoperative blood retrieval and transfusion in cementless total knee arthroplasty," *The Journal of Arthroplasty*, vol. 7, no. 2, pp. 205–210, 1992.

[9] M. Muñoz, D. Ariza, M. J. Garcerán, A. Gómez, and A. Campos, "Benefits of postoperative shed blood reinfusion in patients undergoing unilateral total knee replacement," *Archives of Orthopaedic and Trauma Surgery*, vol. 125, no. 6, pp. 385–389, 2005.

[10] M. B. Simpson, K. P. Murphy, H. G. Chamber, and A. L. Bucknell, "The effect of postoperative wound drainage reinfusion in reducing the need for blood transfusions in elective total joint arthroplasty: a prospective, randomized study," *Orthopedics*, vol. 17, no. 2, pp. 133–137, 1994.

[11] A. Sinha, M. Sinha, and S. Burgert, "Reinfusion of drained blood as an alternative to homologous blood transfusion after total knee replacement," *International Orthopaedics*, vol. 25, no. 4, pp. 257–259, 2001.

[12] E. L. Steinberg, P. Ben-Galim, Y. Yaniv, S. Dekel, and A. Menahem, "Comparative analysis of the benefits of autotransfusion of blood by a shed blood collector after total knee replacement," *Archives of Orthopaedic and Trauma Surgery*, vol. 124, no. 2, pp. 114–118, 2004.

[13] D. Strümper, E. W. G. Weber, S. Gielen-Wijffels et al., "Clinical efficacy of postoperative autologous transfusion of filtered shed blood in hip and knee arthroplasty," *Transfusion*, vol. 44, no. 11, pp. 1567–1571, 2004.

[14] R. L. Wixson, H. C. Kwaan, S. M. Spies, and A. M. Zimmer, "Reinfusion of platelet function wound drainage in total joint arthroplasty. Red blood cell survival and coagulopathy risk," *The Journal of Arthroplasty*, vol. 9, no. 4, pp. 351–358, 1994.

[15] J. L. Carson, B. J. Grossman, S. Kleinman et al., "Red blood cell transfusion: a clinical practice guideline from the AABB," *Annals of Internal Medicine*, vol. 157, no. 1, pp. 49–58, 2012.

[16] F. Charatan, "Organ transplants and blood transfusions may transmit West Nile virus," *British Medical Journal*, vol. 325, article 566, 2002.

[17] P. Mortimer, "Making blood safer," *British Medical Journal*, vol. 325, pp. 400–401, 2002.

[18] D. H. Clements, T. P. Sculco, S. W. Burke, K. Mayer, and D. B. Levine, "Salvage and reinfusion of postoperative sanguineous wound drainage. A preliminary report," *The Journal of Bone & Joint Surgery—American Volume*, vol. 74, no. 5, pp. 646–651, 1992.

[19] J. Fong, E. D. Gurewitsch, H.-J. Kang, L. Kump, and P. F. Mack, "An analysis of transfusion practice and the role of intraoperative red blood cell salvage during cesarean delivery," *Anesthesia and Analgesia*, vol. 104, no. 3, pp. 666–672, 2007.

[20] A. Ashworth and A. A. Klein, "Cell salvage as part of a blood conservation strategy in anaesthesia," *British Journal of Anaesthesia*, vol. 105, no. 4, pp. 401–416, 2010.

[21] R. E. Domen, "Adverse reactions associated with autologous blood transfusion: evaluation and incidence at a large academic hospital," *Transfusion*, vol. 38, no. 3, pp. 296–300, 1998.

[22] The Association of Anaesthetists of Great Britain and Ireland (AAGBI), "Safety Guideline—Blood Transfusion and the Anaesthetist: Intra-operative Cell Salvage," 2009, http://aagbi.org/publications/guidelines/docs/cell%20_salvage_2009_amended.pdf.

[23] P. A. Carless, D. A. Henry, A. J. Moxey, D. L. O'connell, T. Brown, and D. A. Fergusson, "Cell salvage for minimising perioperative allogeneic blood transfusion," *Cochrane Database of Systematic Reviews*, no. 4, Article ID CD001888, 2006.

[24] A. Shenolikar, K. Wareham, D. Newington, D. Thomas, J. Hughes, and M. Downes, "Cell salvage auto transfusion in total knee replacement surgery," *Transfusion Medicine*, vol. 7, no. 4, pp. 277–280, 1997.

[25] K. C. Sinclair, H. D. Clarke, and B. N. Noble, "Blood management in total knee arthroplasty: a comparison of techniques," *Orthopedics*, vol. 32, no. 1, article 19, 2009.

[26] D. Thomas, K. Wareham, D. Cohen, and H. Hutchings, "Autologous blood transfusion in total knee replacement surgery," *British Journal of Anaesthesia*, vol. 86, no. 5, pp. 669–673, 2001.

[27] M. M. Gómez, Y. S. Arrieta, J. J. G. Vallejo, F. J. M. de la Torre, M. D. R. R. de la Cruz, and J. M. Eloy-García, "Pre and post-operative autotransfusion. A comparative study of haematology, biochemistry and red cell metabolism in pre-donated blood an surgical drainage," *Sangre*, vol. 44, no. 6, pp. 443–450, 1999.

[28] B. J. W. Thomassen, P. H. C. den Hollander, H. H. Kaptijn, R. G. H. H. Nelissen, and P. Pilot, "Autologous wound drains have no effect on allogeneic blood transfusions in primary total hip and knee replacement: a three-arm randomised trial," *The Bone & Joint Journal*, vol. 96, no. 6, pp. 765–771, 2014.

[29] C. So-Osman, R. G. H. H. Nelissen, A. W. M. M. Koopman-van Gemert et al., "Patient blood management in elective total hip- and knee-replacement surgery (part 2): a randomized controlled trial on blood salvage as transfusion alternative using a restrictive transfusion policy in patients with a preoperative hemoglobin above 13 g/dl," *Anesthesiology*, vol. 120, no. 4, pp. 852–860, 2014.

[30] M. A. Ritter, E. M. Keating, and P. M. Faris, "Closed wound drainage in total hip or total knee replacement. A prospective, randomized study," *The Journal of Bone & Joint Surgery Series A*, vol. 76, no. 1, pp. 35–38, 1994.

[31] R. M. Marks, A. R. Vaccaro, R. A. Balderston, W. J. Hozack, R. E. Booth Jr., and R. H. Rothman, "Postoperative blood salvage in total knee arthroplasty using the Solcotrans autotransfusion system," *The Journal of Arthroplasty*, vol. 10, no. 4, pp. 433–437, 1995.

[32] G. Adalberth, S. Byström, K. Kolstad, H. Mallmin, and J. Milbrink, "Postoperative drainage of knee arthroplasty is not necessary: a randomized study of 90 patients," *Acta Orthopaedica Scandinavica*, vol. 69, no. 5, pp. 475–478, 1998.

[33] G. C. Wood, A. Kapoor, and A. Javed, "Autologous drains in arthroplasty: a randomized control trial," *Journal of Arthroplasty*, vol. 23, no. 6, pp. 808–813, 2008.

[34] A. Amin, A. Watson, J. Mangwani, D. Nawabi, R. Ahluwalia, and M. Loeffler, "A prospective randomised controlled trial of autologous retransfusion in total knee replacement," *The Journal of Bone & Joint Surgery—British Volume*, vol. 90, no. 4, pp. 451–454, 2008.

[35] A. Zacharopoulos, A. Apostolopoulos, and A. Kyriakidis, "The effectiveness of reinfusion after total knee replacement. A prospective randomised controlled study," *International Orthopaedics*, vol. 31, no. 3, pp. 303–308, 2007.

[36] M. Muñoz, D. Ariza, A. Campos, E. Martín-Montañez, and J. Pavía, "The cost of post-operative shed blood salvage after total knee arthroplasty: an analysis of 1,093 consecutive procedures," *Blood Transfusion*, vol. 11, no. 2, pp. 260–271, 2013.

[37] A. Shander, A. Hofmann, S. Ozawa, O. M. Theusinger, H. Gombotz, and D. R. Spahn, "Activity-based costs of blood transfusions in surgical patients at four hospitals," *Transfusion*, vol. 50, no. 4, pp. 753–765, 2010.

[38] L. Davies, T. J. Brown, S. Haynes, K. Payne, R. A. Elliott, and C. McCollum, "Cost-effectiveness of cell salvage and alternative methods of minimising perioperative allogeneic blood transfusion: a systematic review and economic model," *Health Technology Assessment*, vol. 10, no. 44, 2006.

[39] P. Perazzo, M. Viganò, L. de Girolamo et al., "Blood management and transfusion strategies in 600 patients undergoing total joint arthroplasty: an analysis of pre-operative autologous blood donation," *Blood Transfusion*, vol. 11, no. 3, pp. 370–376, 2013.

[40] Z. Haien, J. Yong, M. Baoan, G. Mingjun, and F. Qingyu, "Postoperative auto-transfusion in total hip or knee arthroplasty: a meta-analysis of randomized controlled trials," *PLoS ONE*, vol. 8, no. 1, Article ID e55073, 2013.

31

An Efficient Apparatus for Rapid Deoxygenation of Erythrocyte Concentrates for Alternative Banking Strategies

Lello Zolla and Angelo D'Alessandro

Department of Ecological and Biological Sciences, Tuscia University, Largo dell'Università, snc, 01100 Viterbo, Italy

Correspondence should be addressed to Lello Zolla; blood.prot@unitus.it

Academic Editor: Erwin Strasser

Erythrocyte concentrates (ECs) stored for transfusion purposes still represent a lifesaving solution in a wide series of clinically occurring circumstances, especially for traumatized and perioperative patients. However, concerns still arise and persist as to whether current criteria for collection and storage of ECs might actually represent the best case scenario or there might rather be still room for improvement. In particular, the prolonged storage of EC has been associated with the accumulation of a wide series of storage lesions, either reversible (metabolism) or irreversible (protein and morphology). Independent laboratories have contributed to propose alternative strategies, among which is the introduction of oxygen removal treatments to ECs. Convincing biochemical and preliminary clinical evidences have been produced about the benefits derived from the introduction of this practice. We, hereby, propose a rapid, efficient, and time-effective strategy for blood deoxygenation which might fit in current EC production chain. The proposed strategy resulted in the complete deoxygenation of red blood cell hemoglobin ($pO_2 < 0.0021$ mmHg). A preliminary small-scale study about the application of the present method resulted in reduced hemolysis, decreased vesiculation, and limited alterations to the red blood cell morphology, as gleaned from flow cytometry and scanning electron microscopic analyses. Further in-depth and larger-scale investigations are encouraged.

1. Introduction

Erythrocyte concentrates (ECs) are still the most widely transfused blood-derived therapeutic worldwide, as many million units of blood are collected, and million units of RBCs are administered to millions of patients every year [1, 2]. Currently, accepted European Council guidelines indicate that ECs may be stored for up to 42 days under controlled conditions before transfusion [3]. Nevertheless, recent retrospective and controversial studies have brought about concerns on the suitability of longer stored EC units for transfusion purposes [4, 5]. It has indeed been stressed that the risk of exposure to long-stored red blood cells (RBCs) is exacerbated when dealing with certain categories of recipients, such as traumatized, postoperative, and critically ill patients [5]. However, it should be worth mentioning that early results from randomized double-blind clinical prospective trials have not hitherto indicated any statistically significant disadvantage of the administration of longer stored units in comparison to fresher blood [6, 7].

While the likelihood of untoward effects related to the transfusion of older RBC units is still a matter of debate and of clinical investigations, what is now known for certain is that storage affects biochemical and biological properties of RBCs, and the extent of these accumulating changes, collectively known as "storage lesions," is proportional to the duration of the storage period [8–12]. Storage lesions include alterations to either morphology (shape changes leading from a discoid to a spherocytic phenotype) or functionality (metabolism and oxygen delivery capacity through an increase in oxygen affinity mediated by a rapid fall in 2,3-diphosphoglycerate concentrations [8–13]). Further lesions occur in stored RBCs which are reversible to some extent, such as potassium leakage to the supernatant and depletion of ATP and DPG stores, while others are not, such as the alteration of lipids and membrane proteins (membrane protein fragmentation and migration to the membrane and/or vesiculation of subsets of structural or antioxidant proteins [9]), which results in more rigid cell structures, increased osmotic fragility, higher haemolytic rates, phosphatidylserine exposure to the outer membrane leaflet, increased vesiculation rate, and reduced oxygen off-loading capacity [8–12, 14, 15].

Membrane protein fragmentation [9, 13], storage time-dependent migration of cytosolic proteins to the membrane [9, 14, 15], and increased oxidative stress-related parameters [9, 16] have been also reported to correlate with storage duration. Biochemical studies explicitly suggested that there is considerable room for improvement in the field of RBC biopreservation, especially when considering that the lifespan of RBCs *in vivo* is approximately 120 days [17]. One major phenomenon seems to lie at the root of storage lesions to RBCs: oxidative stress [9, 13, 16]. In order to cope with oxidative stress triggering phenomena, alternative RBC storage strategies have been recently proposed, such as the addition of higher loads of antioxidants (vitamin E, C, and beta-carotene) in additive solutions for storage purposes [18] or anaerobic storage [13, 19–21]. While the former strategy has been designed as to counteract oxidative stress arising over prolonged storage, the latter has been thought as to prevent overproduction of reactive oxygen species (ROS) through the elimination of the main substrate, oxygen.

The anaerobic approach (pO_2 < 4% - patent WO/1996/039026) has been reported to deliver ECs with hemolysis below 0.8% and *in vivo* survival at 24 h upon transfusion above the 75% threshold [19–21]. Independent studies from our group have evidenced that storage under helium also reduced the extent of membrane protein fragmentation or aggregation phenomena of nonleukofiltered erythrocyte concentrates [13]. However, it should be appreciated that these optimistic results are currently undergoing further clinical testing through prospective trials. The clinical milieu has so far looked at the "anaerobic perspective" with diffidence, mainly because the recently proposed protocols implied the introduction of new costly and time-consuming steps in the EC production chain. In other terms, the alternative "anaerobic perspective" appeared not to be optimized for cost/benefits or cost/effectiveness considerations.

In this view, we hereby propose a rapid strategy for cost- and time-effective deoxygenation of ECs and provide details about the likely frame of steps in which this method might be safely and efficiently introduced in clinical routine practice in the future.

2. Technical Design

2.1. Blood Collection. Whole blood (450 mL + 10%) was collected from healthy volunteer donors into citrate phosphate dextrose (CPD) anticoagulant (63 mL; pH 5.6) and leukodepleted. After the separation of plasma by centrifugation, RBCs were suspended in 100 mL of SAG-M (Saline, Adenine, Glucose, Mannitol) additive solution. We studied RBC units collected from 8 donors (male: 4, female: 4, age 45 +11.5 (mean + S.D.)). The present study was approved by the Italian National Blood Centre (Rome, Italy).

2.2. Helium Cylinders. High purity helium gas cylinders (99.999% of gas purity, $10 \, m^3$ each) were obtained from Sol S.p.A. (Pomezia, Italy).

2.3. Deoxygenation of Red Blood Cells. ECs were stored into CPD-SAGM-containing plastic bags (Fenwal Italy, Milano, Italy).

An illustration of the deoxygenation apparatus is reported in Figure 1.

Helium from gas cylinders was regulated for 1 bar output pressure through a common manometer and fluxed into the EC units through sterile connection.

A time valve (standard execution, up to 10 bar; regulation from 1 to 10 seconds) was used to regulate both influx and efflux of helium, through the opening of gas influx for 5 seconds, stabilizing the system for six minutes (in order to allow gas exchange between RBCs in the unit and the gas phase) and the opening of the second valve linked to a vacuum pump aspirating the gas from the unit.

Sterility was further guaranteed by the presence of sterility filters (AcroPak 300-Pall Life Sciences, NY, USA) in between the gas outlet from the cylinder manometer and the inlet tube into the unit and from the unit to the vacuum pump.

Each unit was conditioned with helium through 5 cycles of influx and aspiration via vacuum pump. Each cycle consisted in helium influx, six minutes gas exchange between RBCs in the unit and the gas phase and gas efflux through the opening of the vacuum pump valve.

In order to ease gas exchange, RBC units are placed on a tilting stainless steel plate for gentle agitation, as to prevent hemolysis. The stainless steel surface was thermostated at 37°C, in order to ease oxygen dissociation from hemoglobin [22–24]. Temperature stability was guaranteed by an internal resistance which was used to warm water circulating within a tunnel in the double chamber of the stainless steel plate.

The apparatus was optimized to perform deoxygenation on six units simultaneously, by means of a six-tap structure (Steroglass; Perugia, Italy) and sterility filters at the end of each tap. Depositories for six independent units were used to block the bags on the stainless steel surface for the duration of the deoxygenation process (30 minutes).

RBC units were stored under standard blood bank conditions (1–6°C) in a closed chamber conditioned with helium for up to 42 days.

2.4. Assessment of Conservation of the Deoxygenated Condition. Prior to storage, hemoglobin oxygenation levels were assayed spectrophotometrically through a double-beam spectrophotometer Cary 4 Varian and further tested with dissolved oxygen sensors by tryptophan fluorescence quenching (<0.0021 mmHg) (Steroglass, Perugia, Italy).

Since our goal was to test deoxygenation levels, albeit not hemoglobin concentration, we did not need to establish a precise path length, in agreement with the Lambert-Beer law. Conversely, we were interested in performing the assay directly on the blood unit. The internal architecture of the Cary Varian spectrophotometer allowed us to perform the analysis directly on vertically placed units, where blood was allowed to drip on the lateral surface of the plastic bag and the majority of the unit (labels included) was put below the optic path of the laser beam, in order not to disturb the reading.

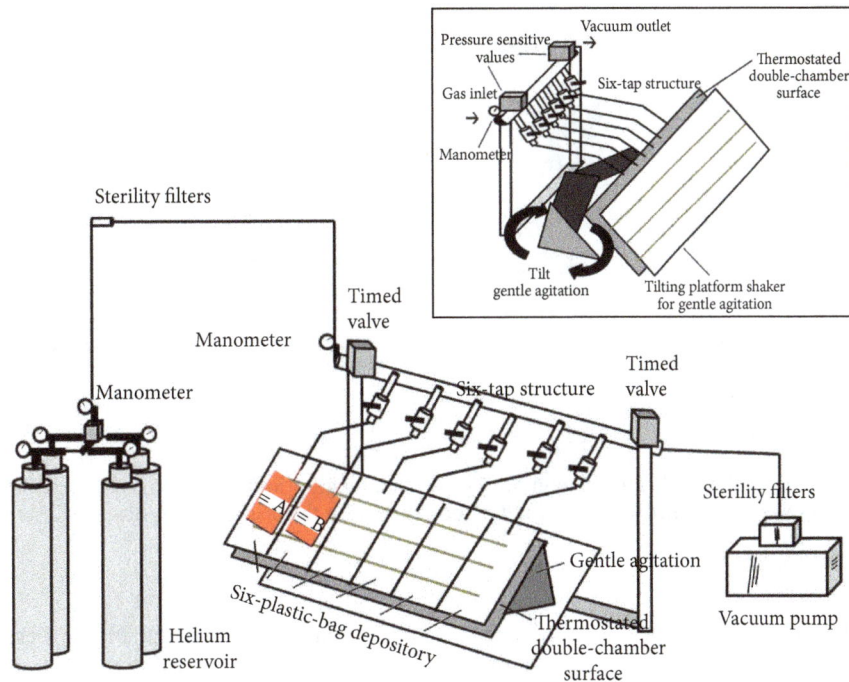

FIGURE 1: A schematization of the blood deoxygenation apparatus. Gas cylinders provide highest purity helium whose pressure is controlled through a manometer. Gas inlet is regulated in a closed system through a time valve which temporizes inlet and outlet towards a vacuum pump after 5 minutes of gas exchange within the plastic bag. Plastic bags are blocked almost horizontally as to favour gas exchange, through gentle agitation and temperature modulation. Sterility filters ensure the sterility of the whole system, either in the gas inlet or outlet tubing.

Any effect of the absorbance and scattering of the plastics was excluded in the range of $500 < \lambda < 600$ nm. When only a film of blood was visible in the lateral wall of the unit (thus excluding any scattering associated with higher volumes of packed RBCs) it was possible to measure hemoglobin absorbance without any significant scattering within a time window of 1 min. Figure 2 shows hemoglobin absorbance spectra prior to (a) and after (b) deoxygenation. The (few) inconveniences of such a home-made strategy could be easily overcome by a specifically designed plastic bag with a room of a fixed volume (0.01 cm wide, e.g.). Further testing with dissolved oxygen sensors by tryptophan fluorescence quenching indicated pO_2 below 1 ppb (<0.0021 mmHg) (Steroglass, Perugia, Italy), below the limit of detection of the instrument.

No bacterial contamination was observed at the end of the storage period in either control or deoxygenated units, as gleaned through MALDI Biotyper analyses [25].

2.5. *Hemolysis.* Hemolysis was calculated following the method by Harboe [26]. Samples were diluted in distilled water and incubated at room temperature for 30 min to lyse red blood cells. Samples from lysed RBCs were diluted 1/300 while supernatants were diluted 1/10 in distilled water. After stabilizing during 30 min and vortex mixing (Titramax 100, Heidolph Elektro, Kelheim, Germany), the absorbance of the hemoglobin was measured at 380, 415, and 450 nm (PowerWave 200 Spectrophotometer, Bio-Tek Instruments, Winooski, Vermont, USA). The mean blank was subtracted, and the corrected OD (OD*) was calculated as follows: $2 \times OD_{415} - OD_{380} - OD_{450}$.

2.6. *Flow Cytometry.* RBC supernatants of control and deoxygenated units were collected upon 42 days of storage for flow cytometry-based analyses of RBC shed microvesicles. RBC microparticles released during storage were separated from RBCs by centrifugation of RBCs transferred into 50 mL tubes for 10 minutes at 1000 ×g at room temperature. The supernatant was recentrifuged for 5 minutes at 2000 ×g at room temperature. The resulting supernatant containing RBC microparticles was collected and centrifuged for 30 minutes at 18,000 ×g at 4°C. The centrifugation speed of 18,000 ×g was selected on the basis of the method optimized by Rubin et al. [27].

The morphology of the cells and microparticles was assessed by a FACScalibur (Becton-Dickinson, USA). A standard method for approximate quantitation of RBC microparticles on the basis of their relative size and shape was applied [27, 28]. Although the method holds some pitfalls, which could be partly overcome through the use of specific antibodies against microvesicle markers (e.g., CD132 and CD235a) or annexin V (against phosphatidylserine), the presently exploited method still allows obtaining an indicative idea about the relative quantities of microparticles in a given RBC concentrate supernatant. Analyses were conducted using the instrument software by counting events in a 5-minutes time window within the gated area [27, 28]. Events were analysed on the basis of side scatter and forward scatter, as compared against a flow cytometry size calibration kit (Invitrogen, Eugene, OR) containing beads of different diameter, from ~1 μm to ~1.4 μm (RBC microparticles are smaller than those beads, as previously reported in [28]).

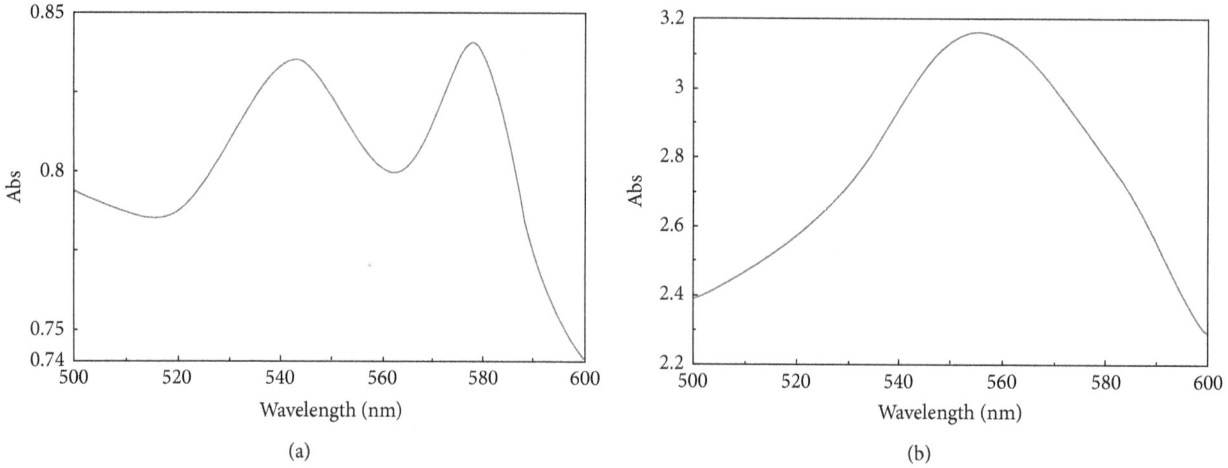

FIGURE 2: Spectrophotometric absorption of hemoglobin in the 500–600 nm range, prior to (a) or after (b) deoxygenation (30 min, 6 cycles of 5 minutes each). The assays were performed directly on red blood cells within the plastic bag, as described in the paper. No significant scattering is observed.

2.7. Scanning Electron Microscopy. Scanning electron microscopic studies of RBC were performed by means of a JEOL JSM 5200 electron microscope. Blood samples were fixed in phosphate-buffered (pH 7.2–7.4) 2.5% glutaraldehyde for 1 h, washed two times in 0.1 M phosphate buffer (pH 7.2–7.4), and mounted on poly-L-lysine-coated glass slides. The glass slides were kept in a moist atmosphere for 1 h, washed in phosphate buffer, postfixed in 1% osmium tetroxide for 1 h, rinsed in distilled water, and dehydrated in graded ethanol (50%–70%–90%–100%). After critical-point drying with liquid CO_2 in a vacuum apparatus and covering with a gold-palladium layer, the samples underwent scanning electron microscopic analysis and classification between reversible and irreversible phenotypes, as in the work of D'Alessandro et al. [9]. The percentages of discocytes, echinocytes, spheroechinocytes, stomatocytes, spherostomatocytes, and spherocytes were evaluated by counting 1000 to 1500 cells in randomly chosen fields. In detail, as reported in [9], RBCs manifesting echinocyte and stomatocyte shapes are capable of returning to the discocyte shape under certain conditions. Thus, these RBC shape changes are considered potentially reversible transformations. In contrast, RBCs assuming spheroechinocyte, spherostomatocyte, spherocyte, ovalocyte, and degenerated shapes are irreversibly changed cells.

3. Results and Discussions

Currently, whole blood withdrawn from a single donor ($\approx$450 mL) is collected in a CPD anticoagulant-containing plastic (usually bis(2-ethylhexyl)phthalate-DEHP) multiple blood-pack units. In each system, the main unit (where blood is at first collected during withdrawal) contains 63 mL of CPD solution. Three satellite units (for platelet concentrates, plasma, and erythrocyte concentrates) are also present, where cellular components are split upon centrifugation at 1500 rpm for 10 min. The satellite unit for erythrocyte concentrates contains 100 mL of SAGM as additive solution. Most commonly available centrifuges can load up to six

plastic bags for each run. Plastic bags are, then, put in a phase separator and RBCs present in the bottom of the bag are sterilely transferred through a plastic tube in the final SAGM-containing plastic bag and shipped for hypothermic storage. Before the cycle might start again with six new units, plasma and platelets require additional centrifugation steps, leaving a time frame for additional limited manipulation on EC alone. Any ideal further step to be introduced in the blood components production chain with the goal to reduce storage-induced lesions [8–12], eventually including also blood deoxygenation [13, 19–21], should be designed as to fit these preparation cycles. In our opinion, this could be best obtained by performing deoxygenation of erythrocyte concentrates in the time window ranging from the separation of blood components through centrifugation of six units to the next cycle of six units.

The aim of this technical report is to demonstrate the feasibility of a rapid and efficient deoxygenation method to be eventually introduced in clinical routine practice, whether large-scale laboratory and clinical trials will outline any significant improvement of deoxygenated RBC concentrate units over current "aerobically" stored counterparts. The deoxygenation workflow would take place in 30 minutes and does not require any transfer of erythrocytes to additional satellite units nor does it compromise safety and effectiveness of the blood therapeutic [9, 19–21]. The components of the deoxygenation apparatus (Figure 1) are relatively inexpensive (less than 2,000 €, subject to regional sales oscillations).

Helium was chosen to perform deoxygenation, since it is an inert gas, which can be easily found at the highest commercial purity. Attempts to perform deoxygenation were carried on with other gases, including Argon (expensive) and nitrogen. The latter is more difficult to be extracted from air (or commercially obtained) at the highest purity and was excluded for two main reasons: (i) even after performing multiple cycles of deoxygenation, we could still observe a 6%–10% residual oxyhaemoglobin; (ii) after twenty-eight days of storage under nitrogen, we could observe a significant haemolysis, which we interpreted as a nitrogen radical species-(RNS-) triggered phenomenon.

It could be argued that helium represents a limited resource, other than a rather expensive one. In this view, we care to stress that one single highest purity helium cylinder would theoretically suffice to perform deoxygenation of thousands of units. Although we do understand that this does not solve the issue related to the limitedness of the helium resource, this is a concern that would involve any other technology that currently adopts heliumas the working gas, such as collision-induced dissociation (CID) mass spectrometry. While these instruments have become increasingly widespread, helium based CID still represents one key approach to investigate, for example, protein, peptide, and metabolic species at the molecular level. Alternative strategies might suggest to rely upon other noble gases for deoxygenation of RBCs (such as Argon) which, however, would not make it any better in terms of availability of the raw material (in this case gas) in the long-term and on a larger scale.

As for the deoxygenation procedure, it could be argued that simple flushing with gases would easily replace the timed valve system. We could experience that after one-hour flushing we could not obtain full deoxygenation, which was instead rapidly achieved through multiple repeated cycles of gas influx/efflux through timed valves (upon manual optimization of optimal gas exchange rates). Besides, flushing resulted in the evaporation of liquid components (additive solution) altering the osmolarity of the solution and influencing RBC physiology and, inevitably, morphology. Conversely, the maintenance of temperature homeostasis through the heated stainless steel unit holder and gentle agitation, along with aspiration (without reaching vacuum as RBC would hemolyse), dramatically improved rapidity and efficiency of the deoxygenation protocol without altering RBC integrity and functionality.

It is worthwhile to note that although the Flick law would suggest to use larger plastic units for storage of ECs in order to increase the surface available for gas exchange and, thus, increase the rapidity of the deoxygenation process, in the hereby proposed method, we could obtain rapid deoxygenation with commercially available plastic bags. However, owing to plastic bag permeability to gases, in order to maintain deoxygenation of the units, we stored deoxygenated in units in helium chamber under controlled conditions.

One additional parameter that could be implemented in the process would be the acidification of pH in order to reduce haemoglobin oxygen affinity during deoxygenation. This would imply that pH should be buffered towards alkalinization later on, since an alkaline pH is known to improve RBC viability via the upmodulation of metabolism (ATP and 2,3 DPG are maintained for a longer period in alkaline solutions [29]). Though we also tried to perform deoxygenation at an acidic pH (through buffering via acidic citrate), we did not observe any significant improvement in the workflow except for the rapidity of the deoxygenation process, which was obviously faster. On the other hand, it should be also noted that deoxygenation itself promotes the alkalinization of the medium, through oxygen and bicarbonate ion removal. While it is beyond the scope of this technical note to propose

alternative additive solutions, it could be feasible enough to perform deoxygenation on RBCs collected in acidic pH CPD (or CP2D), centrifuged, and leukofiltered, prior to the transfer into a satellite unit containing a more alkaline pH commercial solutions (such as phosphate-adenine-glucose-guanosine-gluconate-mannitol (PAGGGM) [29]).

Besides, gas impermeable plastic bags would have eased storage under deoxygenated conditions, although we could achieve this goal through locating the units in a closed chamber conditioned with helium and stored at refrigerated temperatures (1–6°C). Current plastics, of which commercially available EC storage bags are made, hold some advantages as well, such as that they do not hamper spectrophotometric absorbance assays in the 500–600 nm range, as they can be adjusted vertically as to screen haemoglobin absorbance curve without any significant scattering or interference (Figure 2). Of note, we also tried to adopt oxygen sensors to monitor oxygen levels in the unit upon each deoxygenation cycle. These optic chemosensors detect the presence of oxygen through monitoring the quenched or reduced fluorescence of a specific fluorophore (polydimethylsiloxane) with a long excited-state lifetime upon collision with oxygen molecules [30]. The lower the oxygen pressures are, the lower is the likelihood of collisions between oxygen molecules and the fluorophore, which is reversely measured through fluorescence detection [30]. Unfortunately, these sensors (and the fluorophore-coated surfaces, which are meant to be inserted into the plastic bag where blood is stored) are rather expensive, and their safety in the frame of direct contact with transfusable RBCs is yet to be ascertained. Conversely, haemoglobin is totally costless and as much as informative. Within the framework of the present report, when spectrophotometric assays of haemoglobin indicated complete deoxygenation, further testing with dissolved oxygen sensors by tryptophan fluorescence quenching indicated pO_2 below 1 ppb (<0.0021 mmHg) (Steroglass, Perugia, Italy), below the limit of detection of the instrument.

3.1. A Small-Scale Study on the Effectiveness of Deoxygenation on Long-Term Storage: Preliminary Results.
While the hereby reported method is only designed as a proof of concept about the feasibility of the deoxygenation approach, we also performed a preliminary small-scale study to collect preliminary indicative (albeit not significant, since the power of the study would not allow to draw any biologically meaningful and reliable conclusion) evidences about the effects of deoxygenation on RBCs storage.

In order to determine whether the deoxygenation treatment resulted in alterations of RBC morphology and efficiency, we first tested the rapidity of the reoxygenation process. We could obtain re-oxygenated haemoglobin after less than one minute of exposure to environmental oxygen conditions. Therefore, reoxygenation of blood before its usage does not require any additional manipulation, as it would rapidly occur naturally *in vivo* during the slow process of transfusion to the recipient.

As for RBC integrity, no significant haemolysis was observed after deoxygenation treatments (0.17 ± 0.04% and 0.16 ± 0.04% in controls and deoxygenated units at day 0, resp.), while haemolysis in 42-day stored ECs under helium was significantly lower than that in controls ($0.33 \pm 0.04\%$ versus $0.64 \pm 0.08\%$, respectively, P value <0.05 ANOVA) (Figure 3).

Hereby reported preliminary results also seem to suggest that the storage of ECs under helium results in a reduced vesiculation likelihood (in Table 1, we report the counted events within the defined 5-minute time window in the gated area for side scatter and forward scatter for day 42 controls and deoxygenated counterparts). Although further more in depth investigations are mandatory, the observation about an apparent decreased vesiculation rate of deoxygenated RBCs is in agreement with previous reports by Yoshida's group [19–22].

Deoxygenation also apparently resulted in a narrower extent of the morphology alteration phenomena. We could indeed observe that while 42-day old controls displayed almost 80% of either reversibly (echinocytes and stomatocytes) and irreversibly (spheroechinocyte, spherostomatocyte, spherocyte, ovalocyte, and degenerated shapes) altered RBCs and only 20.6 ± 2.5 discocytes, the deoxygenated long stored counterparts conserved a greater percentage of unaltered discocytic phenotypes ($\approx 32.1\%$) and of reversibly modified RBCs and a lower percentage of irreversibly altered erythrocyte shapes (Table 2). It is worthwhile to stress that whether larger-scale studies will confirm these results, it would be possible to conclude that shape-based classification of deoxygenated RBCs closely resembles control RBCs stored for a shorter period (28–35 days), in relation to the values that we could previously report for untreated CPD-SAGM control erythrocytes [9, 31]. We also provide a snapshot of this phenomenon in Figure 4, which shows a scanning electron microscope-(SEM-) obtained micrograph of RBCs from EC units stored in presence (a) or in absence of oxygen (b); arrows indicate RBCs showing irreversibly altered morphologies, as previously reported [9].

An in-depth laboratory investigation is currently in progress which aims to assess the potential benefits of deoxygenated storage, including the monitoring of several parameters such as RBC morphology, vesiculation, and alterations to the membrane proteome (*paper in preparation*). On the other hand, we recently proposed a detailed study about the alterations to the metabolic fluxes upon deoxygenation and over storage duration on a weekly basis [32] and compared the results to our in-depth analyses on CPD-SAGM-stored untreated RBCs [33]. From this study, it emerged that the deoxygenation of RBCs might result in the alteration of the redox poise by upmodulating the nitric oxide (NO) metabolism, which is known to influence the production of RNS, and by blocking the oxidative stress-triggered metabolic diversion from the Emden Meyerhof classic glycolytic pathway towards the pentose phosphate pathway, which should instead provide reduced coenzymes to regenerate the antioxidant battery, such as NADPH) [31].

4. Conclusion

While the clinical improved efficiency of deoxygenated ECs it is yet to be demonstrated, preliminary laboratory evidences

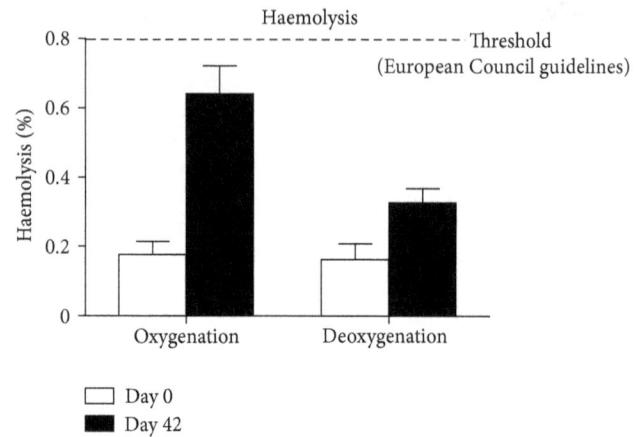

FIGURE 3: Haemolysis levels in control (left columns) red blood cells and red blood cells after deoxygenation (right columns) at day 0 (white columns) or after 42 days (black columns) of refrigerated liquid storage. At day 0, deoxygenated red blood cells do not show any significantly increased haemolysis. On the other hand, haemolysis is lower in deoxygenated red blood cells than in controls after 42 days of storage.

TABLE 1: RBC-shed microparticles.

Storage day	Microparticles (counted events in the arbitrary time window inside the gated area)
42 (control)	5234 ± 125
42 (deoxygenated)	1865 ± 78

[12, 19–21] seem to suggest that deoxygenation might soon become a critical step in the transfusion service pipelines. To this end, we hereby proposed a cheap apparatus for rapid and effective blood deoxygenation for transfusion purposes. We demonstrated its straightforward setup and functioning principles. Also, through a small-scale preliminary study, we report the effectiveness of this method in delivering deoxygenated RBCs, which do not show any substantial hemolysis after handling while they show improved morphology homeostasis maintenance and reduced vesiculation after 42 days of storage. However, since the hereby presented is but a methodology paper, it is worthwhile to stress that further more in-depth and larger-scale investigations are encouraged in order to draw any biologically meaningful conclusion.

Funding

A. D. Alessandro and L. Zolla are supported by the Italian National Blood Centre (Centro Nazionale Sangue (CNS), Istituto Superiore Sanita', Rome, Italy).

Conflict of Interests

L. Zolla and A. D. Alessandro have no direct or indirect financial relation with the trademark mentioned in this paper. L. Zolla and A. D. Alessandro disclose no conflict of interests. The proposed findings have not been patented, and the

TABLE 2: SEM erythrocyte shape classification.

Storage day	Discocyte (%)	Reversibly* changed RBC (%) (echinocyte and stomatocyte shapes)	Irreversibly* changed RBC (%) (spheroechinocyte, spherostomatocyte, spherocyte, ovalocyte, and degenerated shapes)
0	76.5 + 3.1	19.2 ± 5.7	4.3 ± 2.6
42 control	20.6 ± 2.5	43.2 ± 3.8	36.2 ± 2.9
42 deoxygenated	32.1 ± 1.9	45.4 ± 2.2	22.5 ± 3.1

*Reversible and irreversible changes were classified based on classification criteria, as previously reported by D'Alessandro et al. [9].

Control
HbO$_2$

Treated
Hb

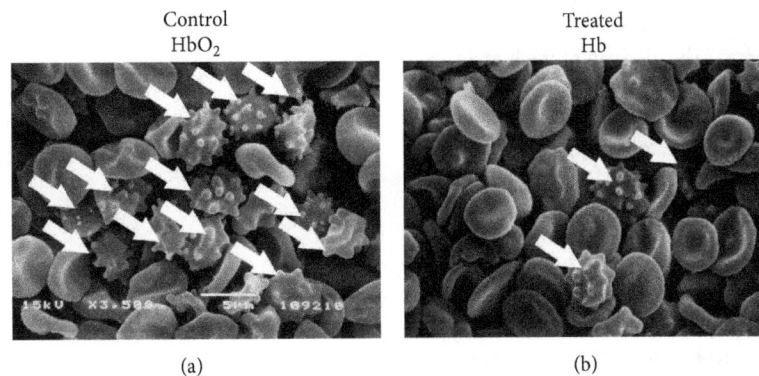

(a)   (b)

FIGURE 4: The extent of membrane shape alterations is lower in deoxygenated (b) than in control (a) red blood cells after 42 days of storage, as it emerged from preliminary scanning electron microscope (SEM) analysis.

authors claim no economic interest related to the contents of the paper at the moment of its submission.

Acknowledgments

L. Zolla and A. D'Alessandro were supported by funds from the Italian National Blood Centre (Rome, Italy). A. D'Alessandro was supported by mobility studentship funds by the Interuniversity Consortium for Biotechnologies (CIB). L. Zolla received funds from the Cofunding of Postdoctoral Research Grants "contributi per cofinanziamento assegni di ricerca-BANDO del June 14, 2012 Prot. 31/12."

References

[1] J. R. Hess, "Red cell storage," *Journal of Proteomics*, vol. 73, no. 3, pp. 368–373, 2010.

[2] A. D'Alessandro, G. Liumbruno, G. Grazzini, and L. Zolla, "Red blood cell storage: the story so far," *Blood Transfusion*, vol. 8, no. 2, pp. 82–88, 2010.

[3] European Directorate for the Quality of Medicines, "Guide to the preparation, use and quality assurance of blood components," Recommendation no. 95, 15-16th Edition. Council of Europe, 2011.

[4] C. G. Koch, L. Li, D. I. Sessler et al., "Duration of red-cell storage and complications after cardiac surgery," *The New England Journal of Medicine*, vol. 358, no. 12, pp. 1229–1239, 2008.

[5] J. L. Vincent, C. Lelubre, and M. Piagnerelli, "Association between duration of storage of transfused red blood cells and morbidity and mortality in adult patients: myth or reality?" *Transfusion*, vol. 49, no. 7, pp. 1384–1394, 2009.

[6] D. A. Fergusson, P. Hébert, D. L. Hogan et al., "Effect of fresh red blood cell transfusions on clinical outcomes in premature, very low-birth-weight infants: the ARIPI randomized trial," *JAMA*, vol. 308, no. 14, pp. 1443–1451, 2012.

[7] W. A. Flegel, "Fresh blood for transfusion: how old is too old for red blood cell units?" *Blood Transfusion*, vol. 10, no. 3, pp. 247–251, 2012.

[8] E. Bennett-Guerrero, T. H. Veldman, A. Doctor et al., "Evolution of adverse changes in stored RBCs," *Proceedings of the National Academy of Sciences of the United States of America*, vol. 104, no. 43, pp. 17063–17068, 2007.

[9] A. D'Alessandro, G. M. D'Amici, S. Vaglio, and L. Zolla, "Time-course investigation of SAGM-stored leukocyte-filtered erythrocyte concentrates: from metabolism to proteomics," *Haematologica*, vol. 97, no. 1, pp. 107–115, 2012.

[10] C. R. Valeri and N. M. Hirsch, "Restoration in vivo of erythrocyte adenosine triphosphate, 2,3-diphosphoglycerate, potassium ion, and sodium ion concentrations following the transfusion of acid-citrate-dextrose-stored human red blood cells," *The Journal of Laboratory and Clinical Medicine*, vol. 73, no. 5, pp. 722–733, 1969.

[11] O. Rubin, D. Crettaz, J. D. Tissot, and N. Lion, "Microparticles in stored red blood cells: Submicron clotting bombs?" *Blood Transfusion*, vol. 8, no. 3, pp. s31–s38, 2010.

[12] G. J. C. G. M. Bosman, E. Lasonder, M. Luten et al., "The proteome of red cell membranes and vesicles during storage in blood bank conditions," *Transfusion*, vol. 48, no. 5, pp. 827–835, 2008.

[13] G. M. D'Amici, S. Rinalducci, and L. Zolla, "Proteomic analysis of RBC membrane protein degradation during blood storage," *Journal of Proteome Research*, vol. 6, no. 8, pp. 3242–3255, 2007.

[14] S. Rinalducci, G. M. D'Amici, B. Blasi, S. Vaglio, G. Grazzini, and L. Zolla, "Peroxiredoxin-2 as a candidate biomarker to test

oxidative stress levels of stored red blood cells under blood bank conditions," *Transfusion*, vol. 51, no. 7, pp. 1439–1449, 2011.

[15] M. Antonelou, A. Kriebardis, K. Stamoulis, L. Margaritis, I. Trougakos, and I. Papassideri, "Secretory apolipoprotein J/Clusterin is an integral component of human erythrocytes and a novel biomarker of vesiculation and senescence in vivo and in stored red cells," in *Proceedings of the 31st International Congress of the International Society of Blood Transfusion (ISBT '10)*, vol. 99, p. 213, Vox Sanquinis, Berlin, Germany, 2010.

[16] R. Chaudhary and R. Katharia, "Oxidative injury as contributory factor for red cells storage lesion during twenty eight days of storage," *Blood Transfusion*, vol. 10, no. 1-4, pp. 59–62, 2011.

[17] D. Shemin and D. Rittenberg, "The life span of the human red blood cell," *The Journal of Biological Chemistry*, vol. 166, no. 2, pp. 627–636, 1946.

[18] J. Racek, R. Herynková, V. Holecek, Z. Jerábek, and V. Sláma, "Influence of antioxidants on the quality of stored blood," *Vox Sanguinis*, vol. 72, no. 1, pp. 16–19, 1997.

[19] L. J. Dumont, T. Yoshida, and J. P. AuBuchon, "Anaerobic storage of red blood cells in a novel additive solution improves in vivo recovery," *Transfusion*, vol. 49, no. 3, pp. 458–464, 2009.

[20] T. Yoshida, J. P. AuBuchon, L. J. Dumont et al., "The effects of additive solution pH and metabolic rejuvenation on anaerobic storage of red cells," *Transfusion*, vol. 48, no. 10, pp. 2096–2105, 2008.

[21] T. Yoshida and S. S. Shevkoplyas, "Anaerobic storage of red blood cells," *Blood Transfusion*, vol. 8, no. 4, pp. 220–236, 2010.

[22] W. H. Forbes and F. J. Roughton, "The equilibrium between oxygen and haemoglobin: I. The oxygen dissociation curve of dilute blood solutions," *The Journal of Physiology*, vol. 71, no. 3, pp. 229–260, 1931.

[23] S. C. Glauser and R. E. Forster 2nd, "pH dependence of the oxyhemoglobin dissociation curve at high oxygen tension," *Journal of Applied Physiology*, vol. 22, no. 1, pp. 113–116, 1967.

[24] P. Astrup, K. Engel, J. W. Severinghaus, and E. Munson, "The influence of temperature and pH on the dissociation curve of oxyhemoglobin of human blood," *Scandinavian Journal of Clinical and Laboratory Investigation*, vol. 17, no. 6, pp. 515–523, 1965.

[25] T. Elssner, M. Kostrzewa, T. Maier, and G. Kruppa, "Microorganism identification based on MALDI-TOF-MS fingerprints," *NATO Science for Peace and Security Series A*, pp. 99–113, 2011.

[26] M. Harboe, "A method for determination of hemoglobin in plasma by near-ultraviolet spectrophotometry," *Scandinavian Journal of Clinical and Laboratory Investigation*, vol. 11, no. 1, pp. 66–70, 1959.

[27] O. Rubin, J. Delobel, M. Prudent et al., "Red blood cell-derived microparticles isolated from blood units initiate and propagate thrombin generation," *Transfusion*, 2012.

[28] A. Givan, "Flow cytometry," in *Methods in Molecular Biology: Flow Cytometry Protocols*, T. S. Hawley and R. G. Hawley, Eds., Humana Press, Totowa, NJ, USA, 2011.

[29] C. F. Högman, H. Löf, and H. T. Meryman, "Storage of red blood cells with improved maintenance of 2,3-bisphosphoglycerate," *Transfusion*, vol. 46, no. 9, pp. 1543–1552, 2006.

[30] J. K. Tusa and H. He, "Critical care analyzer with fluorescent optical chemosensors for blood analytes," *Journal of Materials Chemistry*, vol. 15, no. 27-28, pp. 2640–2647, 2005.

[31] B. Blasi, A. D'Alessandro, N. Ramundo, and L. Zolla, "Red blood cell storage and cell morphology," *Transfusion Medicine*, vol. 22, no. 2, pp. 90–96, 2012.

[32] A. D'Alessandro, F. Gevi, and L. Zolla, "Red blood cell metabolism under prolonged anaerobic storage," *Molecular BioSystems*, 2013.

[33] F. Gevi, A. D'Alessandro, S. Rinalducci, and L. Zolla, "Alterations of red blood cell metabolome during cold liquid storage of erythrocyte concentrates in CPD-SAGM," *Journal of Proteomics*, vol. 76, pp. 168–180, 2012.

32

Ethical Aspects of Blood Donors and the Recipients of Their Blood

P. J. M. van den Burg[1] and K. Magnussen[2]

[1] Sanquin blood Supply, Plesmanlaan 125, 1066 CX Amsterdam, The Netherlands
[2] Centre for Donor-Haemoglobin and Iron, Blood Bank, Department of Clinical Immunology, sec. 526,
    Rigshospitalet and Hvidovre Hospital, The Capital Region, 2650 Hvidovre, Denmark

Correspondence should be addressed to P. J. M. van den Burg, p.vandenburg@sanquin.nl

Academic Editor: Jay P. Brooks

To date medical care is inextricable based on blood donors and blood products. The continuing increase and intensification of tests and guidelines also results in a change in deferral and abnormal test results. Donors and recipients of their blood are faced with this information and are confronted with a kaleidoscope of thoughts and emotions. The discussion with respect to paid versus nonpaid donation is not new, but other aspects are less often discussed. We describe these other aspects for donors and recipients of their blood and hope to open the ethical discussion; if and to what extent we should have limits?

1. Introduction

Blood transfusion has developed for about 100 years from "simple" whole blood infusion to advanced targeted therapy with specific parts of donor blood. In the same period enormous innovations were made in production techniques, laboratory techniques, and communication. The field of blood donation and transfusion nowadays plays in a rapidly growing global world with increasing needs for continuous monitoring of new threats and challenges. Simultaneously necessary ethical discussions rise on medical, financial, and political aspects. A number of ethical issues are more often discussed and published, for example, remunerated versus nonremunerated blood donation, and will not be discussed here. In this paper attention is paid towards ethical aspects of donor deferral and donor and recipient information, with focus on the donation of blood, blood products, and stem cells. These topics are less often discussed and published.

2. Donor Deferral, Good Intentions with Unwanted Adverse Effects

For optimal safety of blood donation and transfusion to recipients, guidelines for donor examination are in place. In general donors are voluntary and healthy but may, however, be confronted with deferral. This often unexpected deferral can have several unintended adverse effects as follows.

Feelings of Rejection. In general donors feel healthy, have the intention to help a patient, take their time to come to a donor centre, and may not be allowed to donate their blood. A common reason is that the haemoglobin level is just below the lower limit. The donor is informed that, although the haemoglobin level is normal, it is too low do donate. A number of these donors are frustrated and disappointed and leave the donor centre feeling that they are not good enough to help a patient [1, 2]. Most likely this has an impact since it is known that deferrals due to low hemoglobin have a strong effect on return rates of both first-time and repeat donors [3].

Confrontation with "Old" Diseases. Donors with a previous history of disorders such as cardiovascular or malignant diseases may have undergone treatment, are asymptomatic, but shall in most cases be deferred. However, these donors generally feel cured, may nearly have forgotten their disease, and are now confronted with a medical deferral. Despite the physician or nurse tries to ease the disappointed donor, a number of donors relive their disease.

Confrontation with Unrealised Risks. A number of donor guidelines have a preventive character and are based on enhanced risks of diseases. The risk may be almost negligible while the disease is very serious. In case of deferral with respect to increased risks of v-CJD, for example, cornea transplant or hepatitis B risks in case of endoscopy, the donors are confronted with risks they mostly are not aware of.

Feelings of Discrimination. Blood donors belonging to minority groups are prone to feel discriminated upon, when deferred. All who come to donate wants to help, and, when deferred on top of the feeling of rejection, they may also feel discriminated upon. Groups where the incidence of blood-borne infectious disease is higher than that in the background population are deferred to reduce the number of infected blood components from donors who, at the time of donation, were in the window period. Examples of such groups are men who have sex with men (MSM) and couples where one of them come from countries that cause deferral due to risk of contagious and blood-borne infections. Especially the MSM discussion, already started in 1977, is still a matter of debate with many social and ethical aspects [4, 5]. Donors may feel that they, or their partner, are discriminated upon just because of sexual preference or race. In line with this discussion, donors appeal on a supposed right to donate blood that does not exist [6]. It could also be that this reaction to the deferral is actually a result of becoming aware of risks that the donor perhaps repressed or did not realise before! In some countries there have been lawsuits because of this point that interferes with very personal aspects.

3. The Problem of Different or Absence of Guidelines

Guidelines can differ, mostly on minor points, between blood establishments and other institutions that collect blood and blood products. Donors can be faced with these differences when different institutions are visited or consulted. We can explain how these differences can exist; however, this may not give a professional impression to donor who asks himself how substantiated our guidelines are. Another point of discussion is not the differences, but the absence of a guideline in specific situations, for example, the Ehlers-Danlos syndrome. The physician should make a decision regarding both donor and recipient safety. The problem occurs when two physicians make different decisions in the same case. We should be aware that this situation degrades the professional position we have.

The reasons for deferral are usually sound, but are not always easy to explain to the blood donors. Mostly the donor is rationally agreeing with the deferral; the personal and emotional experience of this deferral could, however, be rather different. In those situations the donor leaves the blood bank less happy than he came and maybe also worried. The donor may ask "is my intention to donate blood worth the inconvenience." It is important to be aware of the adverse

effects of our rules of deferral already when making the guidelines. Knowing the psychological and practical effects will help us to deal with the problems and enable better assessment regarding the deferrals. Every deferral reduces the probability for retaining the donor [7, 8]. Possible ways of reducing this effect are donor information, education of the staff in deferral rules and donor communication, and to contact the donor after the deferral.

4. Information to Donors and Recipients

Confrontation of Donors with (Unexpected) Information. Despite donors fill in elaborate questionnaires and test negative in obligatory tests, the recipients of their blood may experience transfusion complications. In certain situations, for example, posttransfusion infections or TRALI, it is warranted to reexamine the donor. The donor is confronted with the knowledge that a recipient could have complaints or disease because of his blood and feels guilty. On the other hand, the donor could have, for example, an infection that was not known and was not discovered during screening of the donor's blood.

Confrontation of Recipients with (Unexpected) Information. The recipients are entitled to receive information about the risk of adverse effects to blood transfusion. But after discharge from hospital, adverse effects are hopefully not what the recipient is thinking about. Still, in case of look back due to the risk of a "window donation," the recipient is, perhaps years after transfusion, confronted with the risk of carrying an infection. Also, before informing the recipient, the physician is troubled with the consideration whether informing the recipient is the best way to go, for example, is case of a short life expectancy. Another striking example is the awareness of risks of transmitting the Creutzfeldt-Jakob disease and later its variant type in relation to Bovine Spongiform Encephalopathy, which resulted in many ethical discussions whether or not to inform recipients [9, 10].

Influences of Nonanonymous Transfusions. Donors and recipients, whenever possible, should be anonymous. In case of "related stem cell donation" or patients with very rare blood groups and antibodies against common antigens, this is not always possible. The same is the case in countries where family replacement donations are used. This could have positive effects, but they are by far outbalanced by the negative effects. The donor experiences an emotional pressure that his donation is necessary for the treatment of the patient. As a possible result, the donor could be embarrassed to disclose risk behaviour or medication, both of which could influence the answers in the donor questionnaire. The recipient may not want to be indebted towards a particular donor or the donor may feel that the recipient is now in debt to him. Also the donor will be aware of the patient's condition and could feel guilty if the condition is aggravated.

Confrontation with (Unforeseen) Information. These issues with respect to test results or risks for diseases are applicable to the field of, mainly unrelated, stem cell transplantations. After transplantation the donor can develop a disease that could also have been "transmitted" by the stem cells. Also the recipients can develop a disease that is likely or could have originated form the transplanted cells. In what case should we inform the donor or the recipient? Do therapeutic options play a role or is it relevant for genetic counselling of relatives?

The Scope of Informed Consents. All the possible risks of blood, blood products, or stem cell donation can be included in the information to donors and recipients as part of the informed consent [10, 11]. However, do we serve the needs of donors and recipients when we strive to give all information? Do we want to face donors and recipients of their blood to all conceivable results and adverse effects? Do the donors and the recipients of their blood want to be informed about all the information that physicians, or lawyers, want to give? Independent of these questions we should also realise that donors and recipients do not read or understand all information and also are selective for the information provided [10–12].

Confrontation with Test Results. An increasing number of tests are developed to improve the safety and efficacy of blood transfusion. And information to the donor, about the tests that are done, is mandatory. In these informed consents attention should be paid to the kind of tests and information about, possible unexpected, test results [13]. Whenever a test is positive, the donor is retested and informed when confirmed positive. Clearly, confirmed positive test results for infectious diseases have great influence. However, (temporary) deferral because of seemingly unimportant false-positive test results is often misunderstood and has negative psychosocial effects [14–16]. Beside results from infectious disease tests, donors can also be confronted with other tests that interfere with donorship such as positive DAT results or cold agglutinins that hinders leucofiltration. How specific and reliable must a test result be to inform donors about them? To what extent must donors be protected for results that have no consequences at that moment in time, and shall mainly be an emotional burden?

5. Information and Advices

Information and advice about risks and adverse effects are important, also, because in some cases knowledge may reduce the risk. In the case of needle injury, correct phlebotomy technique together with compression and only light use of the donation arm after the donation will reduce the risk of needle injury [17].

Iron deficiency is common among the general population and even more common among blood donors. Iron deficiency may result in overt anemia or a lower haemoglobin than what would have been the normal haemoglobin level for a particular person. Iron deficiency in itself also have effects, like muscle fatigue, reduced endurance, and perhaps also impaired cognitive skills, and also means low iron stores in case of pregnancy or blood loss [18–20].

There are striking differences with respect to the fact if we advise, treat, or only wait longer for the next donation. Some blood centres do not test for iron deficiency or only do so when the haemoglobin level is below the limit for donation, but still more develop protocols to avoid the blood donors from developing iron deficiency and to diagnose the iron deficiency before the donor develops anaemia. In some institutions it is common to give dietary advices; other institutions advise or subscribe iron supplementation; other increase the interval between donations or permanently defer the donor. To what extent do we want to interfere with life style or treat donors who are healthy? Do we accept adverse effects of ironsupplementation in healthy asymptomatic donors to increase with these efforts their haemoglobin, which is subsequently donated in the following donation? Should we accept the adverse effects of iron deficiency that is caused by donations, without acting on the current knowledge?

6. Conclusion

In this paper we describe a number of ethical issues that could play a role in donors and recipients of blood, blood products, and stem cells. We try to focus on these issues to get attention and awareness that these items are of influence. In counselling donors it is important that we not only send the message we want to give but also receive the verbal and nonverbal information of donors. Only by receiving that information of the donor, we are able to give adequate information. Most likely, we shall be confronted with other ethical aspects in the future. Medical and ethical aspects are like a snapshot and will need renewal regularly.

References

[1] K. Magnussen, N. Bork, and L. Asmussen, "The effect of a standardized protocol for iron supplementation to blood donors low in hemoglobin concentration," *Transfusion*, vol. 48, no. 4, pp. 749–754, 2008.

[2] B. H. Newman, D. T. Newman, R. Ahmad, and A. J. Roth, "The effect of whole-blood donor adverse events on blood donor return rates," *Transfusion*, vol. 46, no. 8, pp. 1374–1379, 2006.

[3] T. Hillgrove, V. Moore, K. Doherty, and P. Ryan, "The impact of temporary deferral due to low hemoglobin: future return, time to return, and frequency of subsequent donation," *Transfusion*, vol. 51, no. 3, pp. 539–547, 2011.

[4] M. Goldman, Q. L. Yi, X. Ye, L. Tessier, and S. F. O'Brien, "Donor understanding and attitudes about current and potential deferral criteria for high-risk sexual behavior," *Transfusion*, vol. 51, no. 8, pp. 1829–1834, 2011.

[5] D. Fox, "The expressive dimension of donor deferral," *American Journal of Bioethics*, vol. 10, no. 2, pp. 42–43, 2010.

[6] I. M. Franklin, "Is there a right to donate blood? Patient rights; donor responsibilities," *Transfusion Medicine*, vol. 17, no. 3, pp. 161–168, 2007.

[7] B. Custer, A. Chinn, N. V. Hirschler, M. P. Busch, and E. L. Murphy, "The consequences of temporary deferral on future whole blood donation," *Transfusion*, vol. 47, no. 8, pp. 1514–1523, 2007.

[8] B. Custer, K. S. Schlumpf, D. Wright, T. L. Simon, S. Wilkinson, and P. M. Ness, "Donor return after temporary deferral," *Transfusion*, vol. 51, no. 6, pp. 1188–1196, 2011.

[9] D. Steinberg, "Informing a recipient of blood from a donor who developed Creutzfeldt-Jakob disease: the characteristics of information that warrant its disclosure," *Journal of Clinical Ethics*, vol. 12, no. 2, pp. 134–140, 2001.

[10] J. Hart, B. Leier, and S. Nahirniak, "Informed consent for blood transfusion: should the possibility of prion risk be included?" *Transfusion Medicine Reviews*, vol. 19, no. 3, pp. 177–183, 2004.

[11] L. A. Alaishuski, R. D. Grim, and R. E. Domen, "The informed consent process in whole blood donation," *Archives of Pathology and Laboratory Medicine*, vol. 132, no. 6, pp. 947–951, 2008.

[12] L. A. Sherman, "Legal issues in blood banking: elements of informed consent," *Clinics in Laboratory Medicine*, vol. 16, no. 4, pp. 931–946, 1996.

[13] M. F. Verweij and B. C. J. Hamel, "Unexpected findings in identifiable stored blood samples after analysis without consent: moral arguments for and against disclosure," *Genetic Counseling*, vol. 13, no. 2, pp. 115–121, 2002.

[14] M. Hanson, "Blood donor screening: factors influencing decision making," *Archives of Pathology and Laboratory Medicine*, vol. 118, no. 4, pp. 457–461, 1994.

[15] H. Kamel and P. Tomasulo, "A healthy donor or unsuspecting patient," *Transfusion*, vol. 49, no. 5, pp. 818–820, 2009.

[16] S. Kleinman, B. Wang, Y. Wu et al., "Retrovirus epidemiology donor study," *Transfusion*, vol. 44, no. 5, pp. 658–666, 2004.

[17] B. H. Newman, "Donor reactions and injuries from whole blood donation," *Transfusion Medicine Reviews*, vol. 11, no. 1, pp. 64–75, 1997.

[18] T. Brownlie, V. Utermohlen, P. S. Hinton, and J. D. Haas, "Tissue iron deficiency without anemia impairs adaptation in endurance capacity after aerobic training in previously untrained women," *American Journal of Clinical Nutrition*, vol. 79, no. 3, pp. 437–443, 2004.

[19] T. D. Brutsaert, S. Hernandez-Cordero, J. Rivera, T. Viola, G. Hughes, and J. D. Haas, "Iron supplementation improves progressive fatigue resistance during dynamic knee extensor exercise in iron-depleted, nonanemic women," *American Journal of Clinical Nutrition*, vol. 77, no. 2, pp. 441–448, 2003.

[20] L. E. Murray-Kolb and J. L. Beard, "Iron treatment normalizes cognitive functioning in young women," *American Journal of Clinical Nutrition*, vol. 85, no. 3, pp. 778–787, 2007.

33

Low Dose Perioperative Intravenous Tranexamic Acid in Patients Undergoing Total Knee Arthroplasty: A Double-Blind Randomized Placebo Controlled Clinical Trial

Mahdi Motififard,[1] Mohammad Ali Tahririan,[1] Mehdi Saneie,[1] Sajad Badiei,[1,2] and Amin Nemati[1,2]

[1]Orthopedic Department, Kashani Teaching Hospital, Isfahan University of Medical Sciences, Isfahan, Iran
[2]Students Research Center, Isfahan University of Medical Sciences, Isfahan, Iran

Correspondence should be addressed to Mehdi Saneie; saneie.mehdi@yahoo.com

Academic Editor: Pär Johansson

Background and Objectives. The null hypothesis of this study was that TA has no effect on postsurgical bleeding in patients undergoing TKA. *Methods*. This study was a double-blind randomized trial. In the first group (T) patients received 500 mg of intravenous Tranexamic acid (TA) twice (once preoperatively and once 3 hours postoperatively) and in the second group (P) they received slow infusion of normal saline as placebo. The primary outcome of the study was the level of Hb 48 hours after surgery. *Results*. Hb levels 48 hours after surgery as the primary outcome were 10.92 ± 0.97 and 10.23 ± 0.98 (g/dL) in groups T and P, respectively, and the difference was statistically significant ($P = 0.001$). Statistically significant differences were also observed in Hb levels 6 and 24 hours after surgery, the drain output 48 hours after surgery, and the number of units of packed cells transfused between study groups ($P < 0.05$). There was no significant difference in duration of hospitalization between the study groups ($P =$ n.s.). *Conclusions*. The low dose perioperative intravenous TA significantly reduces blood loss, requirement for blood transfusion, and drain output in patients undergoing TKA. However, duration of hospitalization did not change significantly.

1. Introduction

Nowadays, total knee arthroplasty (TKA) is one of the most common procedures in orthopedic surgery and about half of the patients need blood transfusion [1, 2]. Allogeneic blood transfusion is the standard approach to increase hemoglobin (Hb) level. However, it can cause some complications such as hemolytic and nonhemolytic transfusion reactions and transmission of infectious diseases and can also increase morbidity and mortality [3, 4]. Thus, reducing the need for blood transfusion becomes a major concern for orthopedic surgeons. Several strategies have been suggested to reduce intraoperative and perioperative blood loss and as a result reduce blood transfusion [5–8]. One of them is the use of pharmacologic agents such as Tranexamic acid (TA). Pneumatic tourniquets are usually used to reduce intraoperative bleeding during TKA surgery. However, this will result in

more bleeding after surgery [9]. Previous studies showed that there is a transitional activation of the fibrinolytic system after surgery which can be indices by the use of tourniquets [10]. Hence, antifibrinolytic agents could theoretically be effective in reducing bleeding.

TA is a synthetic derivative of Lysin that competitively blocks the lysine-binding sites in the plasmin and plasminogen activator molecules and its usage has become more popular in recent years [11]. Several application methods such as oral, local, and intravenous methods have been described and each one has its own advantages and disadvantages. Intravenous administration is a conventional method. There are previous studies that have focused on the administration of intravenous TA with different protocols. However, in all of these studies there were deficiencies such as lack of outcome measure, study design, or sample size. There is no consensus on its use protocol and the question still remains about the dosage, timing, and the administration method. Therefore, this study was designed. The null hypothesis of this study was that TA does not have an impaction on blood loss after TKA. This hypothesis was evaluated by measuring the decrease in Hb, the drain output volume, and the volume of blood needed to be transfused.

2. Materials and Methods

2.1. Participants and Setting. This study was a double-blind randomized clinical trial which was performed at Kashani teaching hospital, a tertiary referral center in Isfahan, Iran. During the period of study (January 2012 to March 2013) a total number of 95 patients were enrolled in the study. Eligible patients were individuals with osteoarthritis who were indicated for primary TKA. Patients with previous history of cerebrovascular disease, thromboembolism, myocardial infarction, and those who were candidates for bilateral TKA were excluded.

2.2. Surgical Technique and Intervention. All surgeries were performed under spinal anesthesia which was done by the anesthesiologist colleague. Two grams of intravenous Cephazolin (EXIR, Borujerd, Iran) was administered thirty minutes before the surgery.

All operations were performed in the morning between 8 am and 12 pm by a single skilled surgeon (MM) using posterior cruciate substituting cemented total knee prosthetics (Zimmer, Warsaw, IN). Surgeries were performed through an anterior skin incision from 8 centimeters above the patella to 2 centimeters distal to the tibial tubercle. A pneumatic tourniquet was used which inflated before the skin incision and deflated just before the soft tissue repair at the end of surgery. During the surgery sterilized gauzes were used for blood absorption while electrical coater and suction were established to control bleeding. At the end of surgery during soft tissue repair in extension position a low vacuum intra-articular drain was used for postoperative wound drainage which was removed 48 hours after surgery.

Eligible patients were randomly assigned to one of two groups: in the first group (Group T) they received intravenous (IV) Tranexamic acid (Caspian Tamin pharmaceutical Co., Rasht, Iran) 500 mg diluted in 100 mL of 0.9% saline chloride twice; the first dose was infused in over 10 minutes about 30 minutes before inflation of tourniquet and the second dose after staying in the recovery room for three hours. In the second group (Group P), patients received IV slow infusion of 100 mL of 0.9% sodium chloride twice. The timing was the same as that of Group T.

All patients were mobilized on the first day after surgery. DVT prophylaxis was performed by Low Molecular Weight Heparin (Clexane, Sanofi, UK) 40 mg/day postoperatively which continued for 14 days. Postoperative transfusion was done in patients with hemoglobin level less than 8 g/dL and less than 10 g/dL in patients with comorbidities and untolerated anemic symptoms. Postoperative complications including hyper coagulable states such as DVT, PTE, myocardial infarction, and cerebrovascular events were evaluated by

means of clinical signs and symptoms. Further evaluations were performed when needed. Patients were discharged if they had been mobilized and the wound was dry without any discharge.

2.3. Measurements and Outcomes. The primary outcome of this study was the Hb level 48 hours after surgery which was evaluated by one of the study investigators (MS). The secondary outcomes were Hb levels, 6 and 24 hours after surgery, drain output during the first 48 hours after surgery, and blood product administration after surgery and duration of hospitalization. Hb levels were checked every day at 7 am. Drain output was measured during the first 48 hours after surgery. The total volume of blood drained in this period was considered as the output. Drains were replaced if filled before 48 hours.

2.4. Blindness and Randomization. Eligible patients were allocated to one of the two groups using "Random allocation software," which has been used for this purpose in several previous studies [12]. This study was a double-blind one. Neither the patient nor the physician who evaluated the study outcomes knew whether a patient was in group T or P.

2.5. Sample Size and Statistical Analyses. Sample size was calculated using a statistical formula considering $\alpha = 0.05$ and $\beta = 0.2$ expecting at least 0.5 gr/dL difference in Hb levels between the two study groups. With these inputs the sample size was calculated to be 45 in each group. Statistical analyses were performed using SPSS (SPSS, Inc., Chicago, IL, version 20). Qualitative variables were compared using the Chi-square test and presented as number (%). Quantitative variables had normal distribution and were compared using the paired t-test and presented as mean ± standard deviation. Written informed consent was obtained from all patients at the beginning of the study. The protocol of this study was approved in the review board of Isfahan University of Medical Sciences (number: 392114).

3. Results

Ninety-five patients were assessed for eligibility criteria. Among them four patients did not consent to participate in the research project and one patient was a candidate for bilateral TKA and, thus, the mentioned 5 patients were excluded from the study. The participant flow diagram is shown in Figure 1. There was no significant difference in the demographic variables age and sex between the study groups (Table 1).

Hb levels 48 hours after surgery were 10.92 ± 0.97 (gr/dL) and 10.23 ± 0.98 (gr/dL) for groups T and P, respectively, and the difference was statistically significant ($P = 0.001$). The differences in Hb levels between groups, 6 and 24 hours after surgery, were also found to be statistically significant ($P = 0.04$ and 0.001, resp.). Detailed data are shown in Table 2.

Drain outputs were 268.66±116.68 milliliters and 478.11± 254.19 milliliters for groups T and P, respectively, and the difference was statistically significant ($P = 0.001$). In other

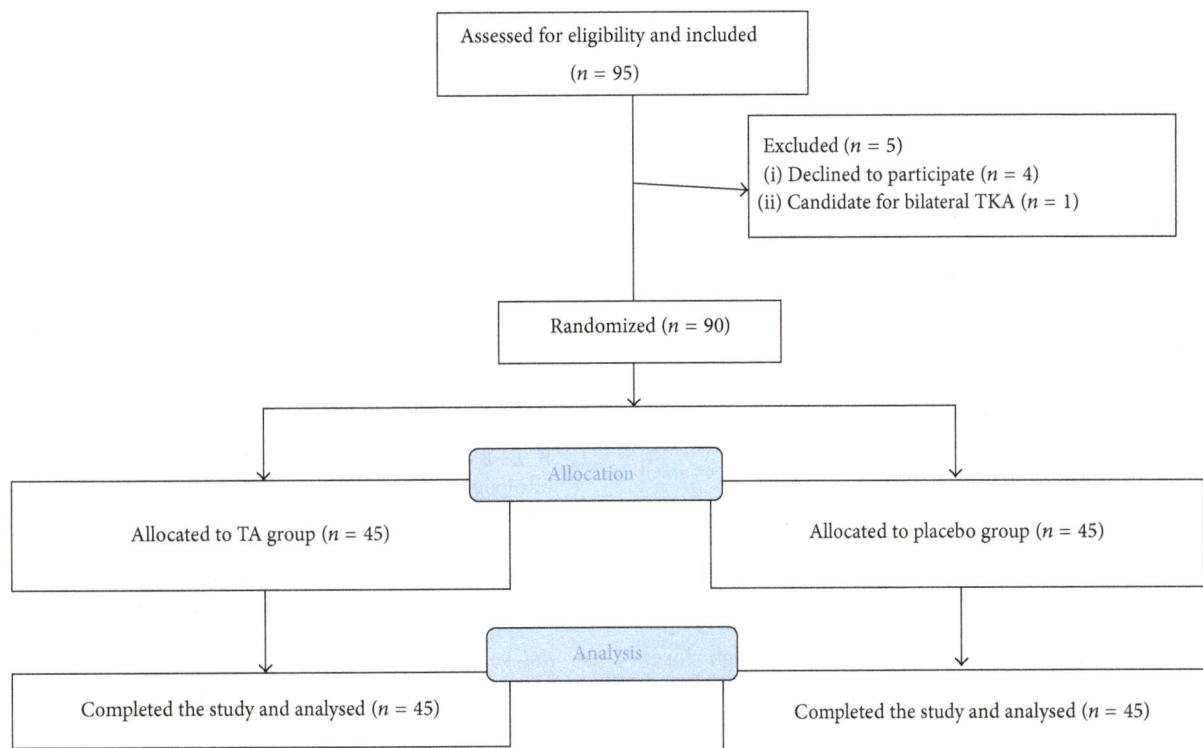

FIGURE 1: Participants' flow diagram.

TABLE 1: Demographic variables between study groups.

Variable	Group T ($n = 45$)	Group P ($n = 45$)	P value
Age (year)	67.04 ± 8.01	65.66 ± 4.97	n.s.
Sex			
Women	35 (77.78%)	32 (71.12%)	n.s.
Men	10 (22.22%)	13 (28.88%)	

Data are presented as mean ± standard deviation and number (%). n.s.: nonsignificant. $P < 0.05$ is considered statistically significant.

TABLE 2: Hb level before and during the study period between study groups.

Hb level (g/dL)	Group T	Group P	P value
Before surgery	12.90 ± 1.11	12.63 ± 1.24	n.s.
6 hours after surgery	11.77 ± 1.26	11.21 ± 1.31	0.04*
24 hours after surgery	11.01 ± 1.17	9.96 ± 1.15	0.001*
48 hours after surgery	10.92 ± 0.97	10.23 ± 0.98	0.001*

Data are presented as mean ± standard deviation. n.s.: nonsignificant. *$P < 0.05$ is considered statistically significant.

words, the mean drain output of patients in group T was approximately 43% less than that of patients in group P. Patients in group P received 1.28 ± 0.75 units of packed cells while patients in group T received 0.26 ± 0.49 units ($P = 0.001$) which shows that blood transfusion in group T occurred nearly 79% less than in group P. Duration of hospitalization was 6.02 ± 2.97 days in group T and 6.93 ± 2.71 days in group P. The difference was not statistically significant

(P = n.s.). There were no instances of DVT or any other adverse reactions for blood transfusion in study patients.

4. Discussion

Our findings reject the null hypothesis of the study and showed that usage of low dose perioperative TA reduces blood loss and the need for blood transfusion in patients undergoing primary unilateral TKA. In this study we evaluated the effect of the reception of 500 mg intravenous TA once before and once after surgery on postoperative blood loss by means of measuring the Hb levels which was done several times after surgery. Another method was measuring the drain output in the first 48 hours after surgery. It was found that twice receiving 500 mg of TA, once 30 minutes before surgery, and once three hours after surgery significantly reduces the loss of Hb, drain volume, and need for blood transfusion. However, it does not reduce the hospitalization period of patients.

There are some previous studies that have evaluated the impact of intravenous TA on blood loss after TKA with different doses and regimens. These studies can be divided into three groups. In the first group there are studies that have evaluated the effectiveness of low dose regimens of TA. The administration dose in this group of studies was 10–15 mg/Kg (1 gram or lower). Hiippala et al. administered 15 mg/Kg of TA and found a significant decrease in drain volume and transfusion rate but did not find a significant decrease in the drop of Hb levels [13].

Sarzaeem et al. conducted a well-designed double-blind randomized clinical trial which showed that administration of a single 500 mg dose of TA significantly reduces the need for blood transfusion and reduces Hb drop and drain output after surgery [14]. In another randomized trial, Maniar et al. compared four methods of TA administration and showed that a single dose of intravenous TA did not give effective results [15]. In other studies Orpen et al. [16] and McConnell et al. [17] did not find significant reduction in Hb drop, transfusion rate, and drain output while Lin et al. [18] administered 10 mg/Kg of TA and showed significant reduction in total blood loss and transfusion rate. As can be seen, there is no consensus among different studies. However, it is the authors' belief that the reason in some studies no significant changes were seen in the outcome was because of their low sample sizes and that studies with larger sample sizes showed the effectiveness of TA.

In the second group there are studies that evaluated the intermediate dose regimens (1-2 grams). Most of these studies administered 10–15 mg/kg for the first dose and another 10–15 mg/kg during the first 12 hours after surgery [10, 19–27].

In the last group there are studies in which high doses of TA (more than 2 grams) were administered [28–30]. They administered TA with different protocols in doses larger than those of the second group. Jansen et al. used 15 mg/kg of TA before the surgery and the same dose every 8 hours for 3 days after surgery and found a significant reduction in Hb level drop [30]. In another study Dahuja et al. [28] used the same regimen for 2 days and reached results similar to those achieved by Jansen el al. Most studies in the second and third group revealed that TA is effective in reducing blood loss and Hb drop after surgery, a result studies in the first group did not reach.

Another important variable that was evaluated in this study was the hospitalization period of study patients. Few of the previous studies have considered this item and most of them concluded that TA may reduce the duration of hospital stay [31, 32]. In this study it was found that although TA reduces Hb drop and the need for transfusion, it does not have a significant impact on the period of hospitalization. This issue should be considered in further cost effectiveness studies for the routine use of TA in TKA.

One of the strengths of this study is that all surgeries were performed by a single expert surgeon and a single prosthetic brand was used which excludes the possible role of technical effects on our results.

This study also had some downsides. First of all, intraoperative bleeding was not evaluated. Other downsides are that the diagnosis of TA complications such as DVT or PTE was based on clinical signs and symptoms, not the gold standard diagnostic tests, and that other nonthrombotic adverse events of TA were not evaluated.

In conclusion it is deduced that perioperative intravenous administration of TA in two 500 mg doses, first dose before and second dose three hours after surgery, reduces Hb drop and drain output volume and the need for blood transfusion after TKA. The failure of previous studies to show this effect is due to their low sample size and study design. On the other hand this study showed that low dose perioperative intravenous TA does not influence the hospitalization period.

Disclosure

The level of evidence of this study is Level I.

Conflict of Interests

The authors declare that there is no conflict of interests regarding the publication of this paper.

References

[1] B. E. Bierbaum, C. Hill, J. J. Callaghan et al., "An analysis of blood management in patients having a total hip or knee arthroplasty," *The Journal of Bone & Joint Surgery—American Volume*, vol. 81, no. 1, pp. 2–10, 1999.

[2] M. S. Noticewala, J. D. Nyce, W. Wang, J. A. Geller, and W. Macaulay, "Predicting need for allogeneic transfusion after total knee arthroplasty," *The Journal of Arthroplasty*, vol. 27, no. 6, pp. 961–967, 2012.

[3] M. E. Stokes, X. Ye, M. Shah et al., "Impact of bleeding-related complications and/or blood product transfusions on hospital costs in inpatient surgical patients," *BMC Health Services Research*, vol. 11, article 135, 2011.

[4] J. R. Tuttle, S. A. Ritterman, D. B. Cassidy, W. A. Anazonwu, J. A. Froehlich, and L. E. Rubin, "Cost benefit analysis of topical tranexamic acid in primary total hip and knee arthroplasty," *The Journal of Arthroplasty*, vol. 29, no. 8, pp. 1512–1515, 2014.

[5] C. E. R. Gibbons, M. C. Solan, D. M. Ricketts, and M. Patterson, "Cryotherapy compared with Robert Jones bandage after total knee replacement: a prospective randomized trial," *International Orthopaedics*, vol. 25, no. 4, pp. 250–252, 2001.

[6] K. Ishida, N. Tsumura, A. Kitagawa et al., "Intra-articular injection of tranexamic acid reduces not only blood loss but also knee joint swelling after total knee arthroplasty," *International Orthopaedics*, vol. 35, no. 11, pp. 1639–1645, 2011.

[7] T. Onodera, T. Majima, N. Sawaguchi, Y. Kasahara, T. Ishigaki, and A. Minami, "Risk of deep venous thrombosis in drain clamping with tranexamic acid and carbazochrome sodium sulfonate hydrate in total knee arthroplasty," *The Journal of Arthroplasty*, vol. 27, no. 1, pp. 105–108, 2012.

[8] J. Parvizi, S. Chaudhry, M. R. Rasouli et al., "Who needs autologous blood donation in joint replacement?" *The Journal of Knee Surgery*, vol. 24, no. 1, pp. 25–31, 2011.

[9] M. Alipour, M. Tabari, M. Keramati, A. M. Zarmehri, and H. Makhmalbaf, "Effectiveness of oral Tranexamic acid administration on blood loss after knee artroplasty: a randomized clinical trial," *Transfusion and Apheresis Science*, vol. 49, no. 3, pp. 574–577, 2013.

[10] G. Benoni and H. Fredin, "Fibrinolytic inhibition with tranexamic acid reduces blood loss and blood transfusion after knee arthroplasty: a prospective, randomised, double-blind study of 86 patients," *The Journal of Bone & Joint Surgery—British Volume*, vol. 78, no. 3, pp. 434–440, 1996.

[11] J. Tan, H. Chen, Q. Liu, C. Chen, and W. Huang, "A meta-analysis of the effectiveness and safety of using tranexamic acid in primary unilateral total knee arthroplasty," *The Journal of Surgical Research*, vol. 184, no. 2, pp. 880–887, 2013.

[12] M. Saghaei, "Random allocation software for parallel group randomized trials," *BMC Medical Research Methodology*, vol. 4, article 26, 2004.

[13] S. Hiippala, L. Strid, M. Wennerstrand et al., "Tranexamic acid (Cyklokapron) reduces perioperative blood loss associated with total knee arthroplasty," *British Journal of Anaesthesia*, vol. 74, no. 5, pp. 534–537, 1995.

[14] M. M. Sarzaeem, M. Razi, G. Kazemian, M. E. Moghaddam, A. M. Rasi, and M. Karimi, "Comparing efficacy of three methods of tranexamic acid administration in reducing hemoglobin drop following total knee arthroplasty," *The Journal of Arthroplasty*, vol. 29, no. 8, pp. 1521–1524, 2014.

[15] R. N. Maniar, G. Kumar, T. Singhi, R. M. Nayak, and P. R. Maniar, "Most effective regimen of tranexamic acid in knee arthroplasty: a prospective randomized controlled study in 240 patients," *Clinical Orthopaedics and Related Research*, vol. 470, no. 9, pp. 2605–2612, 2012.

[16] N. M. Orpen, C. Little, G. Walker, and E. J. P. Crawfurd, "Tranexamic acid reduces early post-operative blood loss after total knee arthroplasty: a prospective randomised controlled trial of 29 patients," *The Knee*, vol. 13, no. 2, pp. 106–110, 2006.

[17] J. S. McConnell, S. Shewale, N. A. Munro, K. Shah, A. H. Deakin, and A. W. G. Kinninmonth, "Reduction of blood loss in primary hip arthroplasty with tranexamic acid or fibrin spray," *Acta Orthopaedica*, vol. 82, no. 6, pp. 660–663, 2011.

[18] P.-C. Lin, C.-H. Hsu, W.-S. Chen, and J.-W. Wang, "Does tranexamic acid save blood in minimally invasive total knee arthroplasty?" *Clinical Orthopaedics and Related Research*, vol. 469, no. 7, pp. 1995–2002, 2011.

[19] J. C. Álvarez, F. X. Santiveri, I. Ramos, E. Vela, L. Puig, and F. Escolano, "Tranexamic acid reduces blood transfusion in total knee arthroplasty even when a blood conservation program is applied," *Transfusion*, vol. 48, no. 3, pp. 519–525, 2008.

[20] M. A. Camarasa, G. Ollé, M. Serra-Prat et al., "Efficacy of aminocaproic, tranexamic acids in the control of bleeding during total knee replacement: a randomized clinical trial," *British Journal of Anaesthesia*, vol. 96, no. 5, pp. 576–582, 2006.

[21] M. H. Ellis, B. Fredman, E. Zohar, N. Ifrach, and R. Jedeikin, "The effect of tourniquet application, tranexamic acid, and desmopressin on the procoagulant and fibrinolytic systems during total knee replacement," *Journal of Clinical Anesthesia*, vol. 13, no. 7, pp. 509–513, 2001.

[22] J. M. Engel, T. Hohaus, R. Ruwoldt, T. Menges, I. Jürgensen, and G. Hempelmann, "Regional hemostatic status and blood requirements after total knee arthroplasty with and without tranexamic acid or aprotinin," *Anesthesia and Analgesia*, vol. 92, no. 3, pp. 775–780, 2001.

[23] K. Ido, M. Neo, Y. Asada et al., "Reduction of blood loss using tranexamic acid in total knee and hip arthroplasties," *Archives of Orthopaedic and Trauma Surgery*, vol. 120, no. 9, pp. 518–520, 2000.

[24] P. N. Kakar, N. Gupta, P. Govil, and V. Shah, "Efficacy and safety of tranexamic acid in control of bleeding following TKR: a randomized clinical trial," *Indian Journal of Anaesthesia*, vol. 53, no. 6, pp. 667–671, 2009.

[25] N. Tanaka, H. Sakahashi, E. Sato, K. Hirose, T. Ishima, and S. Ishii, "Timing of the administration of tranexamic acid for maximum reduction in blood loss in arthroplasty of the knee," *The Journal of Bone & Joint Surgery—British Volume*, vol. 83, no. 5, pp. 702–705, 2001.

[26] M. Veien, J. V. Sørensen, F. Madsen, and P. Juelsgaard, "Tranexamic acid given intraoperatively reduces blood loss after total

knee replacement: a randomized, controlled study," *Acta Anaesthesiologica Scandinavica*, vol. 46, no. 10, pp. 1206–1211, 2002.

[27] E. Zohar, B. Fredman, M. Ellis, I. Luban, A. Stern, and R. Jedeikin, "A comparative study of the postoperative allogeneic blood-sparing effect of tranexamic acid versus acute normovolemic hemodilution after total knee replacement," *Anesthesia and Analgesia*, vol. 89, no. 6, pp. 1382–1387, 1999.

[28] A. Dahuja, G. Dahuja, V. Jaswal, and K. Sandhu, "A prospective study on role of tranexamic acid in reducing postoperative blood loss in total knee arthroplasty and its effect on coagulation profile," *The Journal of Arthroplasty*, vol. 29, no. 4, pp. 733–735, 2014.

[29] S. T. Hiippala, L. J. Strid, M. I. Wennerstrand et al., "Tranexamic acid radically decreases blood loss and transfusions associated with total knee arthroplasty," *Anesthesia and Analgesia*, vol. 84, no. 4, pp. 839–844, 1997.

[30] A. J. Jansen, S. Andreica, M. Claeys, J. D'Haese, F. Camu, and K. Jochmans, "Use of tranexamic acid for an effective blood conservation strategy after total knee arthroplasty," *British Journal of Anaesthesia*, vol. 83, no. 4, pp. 596–601, 1999.

[31] P. T. Diamond, M. R. Conaway, S. H. Mody, and K. Bhirangi, "Influence of hemoglobin levels on inpatient rehabilitation outcomes after total knee arthroplasty," *The Journal of Arthroplasty*, vol. 21, no. 5, pp. 636–641, 2006.

[32] L. M. Napolitano, "Perioperative anemia," *The Surgical Clinics of North America*, vol. 85, no. 6, pp. 1215–1227, 2005.

34

An Audit on Near-Miss Events in Transfusion Medicine: The Experience of the Teaching Hospital in Northeastern Malaysia

M. N. Noor Haslina, M. Y. Shafini, B. Rosnah, R. Marini, S. Salamah, and M. A. Mohd Fakhri

Transfusion Medicine Unit, Hospital Universiti Sains Malaysia, 16150 Kubang Kerian, Kelantan, Malaysia

Correspondence should be addressed to M. N. Noor Haslina, drhaslina@kb.usm.my

Academic Editor: Silvano Wendel

The rate of near misses in transfusion is important as it indicates situations with the potential of adverse outcome. The aim of this study was to assess the frequency of mislabeled and miscollected samples received by our transfusion medicine unit. This study was conducted from January to December 2009 in Transfusion Medicine Unit, Hospital Universiti Sains Malaysia. The total number of near-miss events reported and analysed over the 1-year period was 178 (0.40%). All mislabeled and miscollected samples and its location cases were identified. Mislabeled and miscollected (WBIT) samples were 66.3% and 33.7%, respectively. The highest number of mislabeled and miscollected samples was from accident and emergency unit and medical ward, respectively. Continuous monitoring and analysis of near misses data should be mandatory in order to improve the safety of transfusion.

1. Introduction

Hospital Universiti Sains Malaysia is a teaching hospital in northeastern Malaysia with a total of 800 beds. The services that are offered by the transfusion medicine laboratory range from routine immunohematology, that is, ABO and Rh grouping, group screen and hold, group cross match, antibody titre and direct Coombs test, to special tests that is, red cell antibody identification, platelet antibody screening, cold agglutinin test, Donath Leinsteiner test, and so forth. We also provide peripheral stem cell collection and preparation for the haemato-oncology unit in the hospital. The laboratory is run by 6 medical technologists, 3 senior medical technologists, 1 scientific officer, and 2 haematologists.

Most errors result from human actions. Hence, the errors may be preventable, and hospital-wide efforts at prevention are required [1]. Safety and reliability in blood transfusion are not static are dynamic nonevents. Collection of the patient's sample for pretransfusion testing initiates a complex chain of events in the transfusion process [2].

Half of the reported serious adverse events from transfusion are consequences of medical errors. The greatest risk in transfusion medicine is actually human error, resulting in the use of the incorrect blood component [3].

Mislabeled sample is defined as that not meeting local standards for sample acceptance. Miscollected sample is defined as sample in which the ABO or D type of the blood in the tube is different from the result already in the record for the patient's name on the tube with the exception of change in blood type due to bone marrow transplantation [4].

A major cause of ABO-incompatible transfusion is the "wrong blood in tube" (WBIT) phenomenon, that is, the sample is not from the recipient identified on the label [5]. An audit of mislabeled and miscollected samples should be carried out to identify the causes of errors, and the conclusions should be reported to the institution staffs for the prevention of similar errors [3].

This study was done to identify the rate of near-misses in our laboratory as an effective mean of highlighting human and system failure associated with transfusion.

2. Materials and Methods

This prospective study was conducted from January to December 2009 in Transfusion Medicine Unit, Hospital

Universiti Sains Malaysia. All the blood samples were taken by the medical officer or house officer at the respective wards as we did not have specific phlebotomy staff. The samples should be labeled clearly and should include patient's full name, registration number or identity card number, date and time of collection, and the initial/signature of the person who was taking the blood. Failure to comply with the above requirements resulted in sample rejection. The sample would also be rejected if the request form was inadequately filled up or there were discrepancies between the information on the sample label and the request form.

Mislabeled sample was defined as the sample that did not fulfill the above criteria for acceptance by the laboratory. Miscollected sample was also called wrong blood in tube (WBIT) or defined as samples in which the blood group result was different from the result on the file from the prior testing. All mislabeled and miscollected cases were included as near-miss events.

Samples which were properly labeled but were not acceptable to the laboratory for other reasons (i.e., insufficient volume of blood in the tube or presence of haemolysis) were not included.

All staffs in our immunohaematology laboratory could report events that were considered near-miss errors.

Locations with a high proportion of mislabeled and miscollected samples were identified every month.

3. Results

The number of samples submitted to the transfusion laboratory in 2009 was 44194.

The total number of near-miss events reported and analysed over the 1-year period was 178 (0.4%). Mislabeled samples were 66.3% (118/178) (wrong registration number, wrong name, and others, that is, incomplete form/discrepancies between sample labels and forms were 39, 52 and 29 cases resp.) and miscollected (WBIT) samples were 33.7% (60/178) cases (Table 1). The mean reporting rate was 15 events per month. During the same period, 33958 blood components were issued by our transfusion medicine unit, corresponding to a reporting rate of five near-miss events per 1000 units issued. Frequency of events and samples received was shown in Table 2.

The highest number of mislabeled samples was from accident and emergency unit whereas the highest number of miscollected samples was from medical ward. All the mislabeled and miscollected samples were detected by the laboratory staffs during the pretransfusion testings.

4. Discussion

Errors in the collection and labeling of patient sample for pretransfusion testing are known to be an important source of transfusion-related patient morbidity and mortality [4]. Near-miss events are five times more frequent than actual transfusion errors, and the majority of errors are detected before the blood was issued [5]. A study by Ibojie and Urbaniak showed that 75% of transfusion errors were detected as near-misses [6].

We reported that total near-miss cases encountered by our transfusion medicine laboratory for the year of 2009 was 178 cases (0.4%). It was observed that the frequency of mislabeled samples was higher than miscollected samples which were 6.3% and 33.7%, respectively. These findings were supported by Gonzalez-Porras et al. who reported that the frequency of inappropriately labeled samples was higher than those of miscollected samples and wrong blood in tube (WBIT) which were 6.45% and 0.06%, respectively [3].

We observed that the rate for mislabeled samples was 1 in every 374 samples, and 1 in 736 samples for the miscollected samples which was higher than reported by Dzik et al. A study on the performance of sample collection in 71 hospitals from 10 different nations showed that the median hospital performance resulted in a rate for mislabeling of 1 in every 165 samples. There was a very low rate of miscollected samples in Sweden and Finland. However, outside these nations, miscollected samples occurred at a median rate of 1 in every 1986 samples [7].

We observed that the emergency department and medical wards contributed to the high rate of near-miss events that were mislabeled and miscollected samples. These results were supported by Lundy et al. who reported that other than the general ward areas where the majority of transfusion activity took place, the accident and emergency (A & E) department and the transfusion laboratory were the two departments where significant numbers of near-miss events occurred [8].

Sample collection is the step in the work process where the majority of events first occurred. Prescription/request is also highlighted as a potentially high-risk step in the work process which contributes to the near-miss events [8]. In our hospital, mislabeled and miscollected samples were discovered during crosschecking of sample information on the request forms and sample tubes before the pretransfusion testings. We found that all the mislabeled occurred in the ward during the labeling process where blood was taken from the intended patients but was wrongly labeled either in the name or registration number. We observed that all of the miscollected samples were associated with phlebotomy where blood was taken from other patients and labeled for the intended patients. Our findings were supported by Ibojie and Urbaniak who observed that almost half of the near-misses were due to problems with patient identification at phlebotomy [6]. The majority of events were reported to occur outside the blood bank and effort of prevention is required [1].

Near-miss events were discovered at the sample-handling step in the laboratory during crosschecking of the details on the request forms and sample tubes and after the product were issued, which were 53% and 24%, respectively. In 33% of these events, the discovery was made by chance [8].

Near-miss events also occurred at some point after issue from the laboratory but before administration; these included events in which the wrong unit was collected from the site of storage [8].

Way of labeling also contributes to near-miss events where it is reported that preprinted label gives higher rate of

TABLE 1: Reported events: breakdown of reporting types and rates per units transfused.

Near-miss events reported over 12 months	Mislabeled	Miscollected	Units transfused over 12 months	Near-miss events per 1000 units transfused
178	118	60	33958	5.2

TABLE 2: Frequency of events and samples received.

Total samples received	Frequency of mislabeled	Frequency of miscollected
44194	1 in every 374 samples	1 in every 736 samples

error in transfusion medicine compared to handwritten label [3].

Failing to check patient identification at the bedside and remote labeling of samples in areas such as the nurse's station have demonstrated a clear correlation with high risk events [8].

Medical staffs are most frequently involved in error. Errors involving doctors are related to errors associated with sample collection. Nursing staff, laboratory staff, phlebotomy staff, clerical staff, and "other" grades of staff are also observed to involve in the near-miss events [8].

Clinical staffs were reported to give a higher rate of inappropriate labeled compared to that of blood bank staff which was 8.8% and 2.1%, respectively [3]. Most errors observed result from human actions and should be preventable [1].

Ongoing monitoring and analysis of labeling and collection should be mandatory in order to improve the safety of transfusion [3]. Baseline performance data may be useful in formulating national standards of performance for sample collection from patients [7]. Hospitals can monitor the performance of the sample collection process by doing periodic analysis of mislabeled and miscollected samples [7]. Statistical process control (SPC) techniques are formal methods for monitoring process over time. It is used to document a critical process that is in control and to alert responsible parties when a process wanders out of control. It is a useful tool to assess the effect of new interventions intended to improve blood transfusion therapy [4]

It is reported that difficulty in gaining access to medical staff for transfusion or haemovigilance training is one of the major obstacles in establishing best practice and compliance [8]. Phlebotomy training for nurses working in the A & E department is important to improve the phlebotomy service [8]. It is observed that the percentage of inappropriately labeled samples has decreased with educational intervention, and hand-written labels represent the best method of labeling compared to preprinted labels [3].

The use of barcode patient identification has shown significant improvement in the procedure for the administration of blood. Previous study has evaluated a barcode patient identification system involving hand-held computers for blood sample collection for compatibility testing and administration of blood. The study found that it was easy to operate and prevented staff from becoming distracted and interrupted during the process of transfusion therapy [9]. This was supported by another study that barcodes identification technology was being implemented in order to improve performance sample labeling and the bedside check [10].

The rate of mislabeled and miscollected samples (WBIT) can be used to track the performance of sample collection [7].

5. Conclusions

Most near-miss events result from human actions and thus may be preventable. The majority of events occur outside the blood bank, and the bedside of the patient is the main location. Education of the staff responsible for transfusion to comply with the existing guidelines is a key step towards improving performance.

References

[1] J. V. Linden, K. Wagner, A. E. Voytovich, and J. Sheehan, "Transfusion errors in New York State: an analysis of 10 years' experience," *Transfusion*, vol. 40, no. 10, pp. 1207–1213, 2000.

[2] M. F. Murphy, B. E. Stearn, and W. H. Dzik, "Current performance of patient sample collection in the UK," *Transfusion Medicine*, vol. 14, no. 2, pp. 113–121, 2004.

[3] J. R. Gonzalez-Porras, I. F. Graciani, M. Alvarez et al., "Tubes for pretransfusion testing should be collected by blood bank staff and hand labelled until the implementation of new technology for improved sample labelling. Results of a prospective study," *Vox Sanguinis*, vol. 95, no. 1, pp. 52–56, 2008.

[4] W. S. Dzik, N. Beckman, K. Selleng et al., "Errors in patient specimen collection: application of statistical process control," *Transfusion*, vol. 48, no. 10, pp. 2143–2151, 2008.

[5] D. MacIvor, D. J. Triulzi, and M. H. Yazer, "Enhanced detection of blood bank sample collection errors with a centralized patient database," *Transfusion*, vol. 49, no. 1, pp. 40–43, 2009.

[6] J. Ibojie and S. J. Urbaniak, "Comparing near misses with actual mistransfusion events: a more accurate reflection of transfusion errors," *British Journal of Haematology*, vol. 108, no. 2, pp. 458–460, 2000.

[7] W. H. Dzik, M. F. Murphy, G. Andreu et al., "An international study of the performance of sample collection from patients," *Vox Sanguinis*, vol. 85, no. 1, pp. 40–47, 2003.

[8] D. Lundy, S. Laspina, H. Kaplan, B. Rabin Fastman, and E. Lawlor, "Seven hundred and fifty-nine (759) chances to learn: a 3-year pilot project to analyse transfusion-related near-miss events in the Republic of Ireland," *Vox Sanguinis*, vol. 92, no. 3, pp. 233–241, 2007.

[9] M. F. Murphy and J. D. S. Kay, "Barcode identification for transfusion safety," *Current Opinion in Hematology*, vol. 11, no. 5, pp. 334–338, 2004.

[10] W. H. Dzik, "New technology for transfusion safety," *British Journal of Haematology*, vol. 136, no. 2, pp. 181–190, 2007.

35

Comprehensive Look at Blood Transfusion Utilization in Total Joint Arthroplasty at a Single Academic Medical Center under a Single Surgeon

Sean Robinson, Owen McGonigle, Sam Volin, Yung-Chi Sung, Matthew Moore, Charles Cassidy, and Eric Smith

Department of Orthopaedic Surgery, Tufts Medical Center, Boston, MA 02111, USA

Correspondence should be addressed to Sean Robinson; sean.robinson@tufts.edu

Academic Editor: Rajendra Chaudhary

The utilization of autologous and allogeneic transfusions in total joint arthroplasties was to characterize patients who may benefit from giving preoperative blood donations. We conducted a retrospective chart review of 525 patients to document preoperative hematocrit, estimated blood loss, length of stay, transfusions, and medical comorbidities. Results of our review showed that total hip arthroplasty revision (THA-R) had the highest prevalence of transfusions (60%) followed by total hip arthroplasty (THA, 53%), total knee arthroplasty-revision (TKA-R, 33%), and total knee arthroplasty (TKA, 23%). There was significant waste of autologous donations: 92% of TKA patients, 64% of THA, and 33% of THA-R patients wasted on average 1.527, 1.321, and 1.5 autologous units, respectively. Pre-operative hematocrit was the strongest predictor of future transfusion need across all procedures, and primary THA had additional predictors in age and gender.

1. Introduction

Anemia is a significant and frequent complication of total joint replacements. Anemia after total joint replacement has been shown to increase length of stay, decrease immediate postoperative physical function, and increase the likelihood of requiring a blood transfusion [1]. Allogeneic blood transfusion, while important in treating anemia, are not without risks and have been shown to lead to immunosuppression, blood-borne disease transmission, immunologic reactions, allergic reactions, and increased mortality [1–3].

Developing strategies to treat or prevent postoperative anemia while limiting the exposure of patients to allogeneic blood has become an important focus. Multiple studies have found that low preoperative hemoglobin is a major risk factor for perioperative and postoperative transfusion after total joint arthroplasty [4–7]. Attempts to improve preoperative hematocrit, including iron therapy and erythropoietin stimulating agents, have been inconsistent in demonstrating a significant effect on preoperative hematocrit [8]. Additional strategies have included perioperative blood salvage (i.e., cell saver), hemodilution, and preoperative donation of blood for autologous transfusion [9–12].

Using autologous donations for transfusion avoids many of the adverse events associated with allogeneic transfusion as noted above [2, 13]. Autologous donations, if utilized effectively, decrease the cost of obtaining, storing, and using allogeneic blood [14–16]. In practice, however, obtaining preoperative autologous donations is often time consuming, expensive, and inefficient. Additionally, many patients who donate will not require a transfusion [4, 9, 11]. In their study of 9,482 patients, Bierbaum et al. concluded that the utilization of autologous blood is inefficient and the process of determining those who may need transfusion is underdeveloped [4]. Understanding which patients are most at risk of developing anemia after total joint replacement is important for optimal preoperative, intra-operative, and postoperative care, as well as maximal utilization of blood resources.

The purpose of this study was to review the blood transfusion utilization of patients undergoing total knee arthroplasty (TKA), total knee arthroplasty revision (TKA-R), total hip arthroplasty (THA), and total hip arthroplasty revision (THA-R) at a single academic institution under a single surgeon. We evaluated this cohort for potential risk factors that may predispose one to a transfusion and documented the usage and waste of preoperative autologous blood donations. To our knowledge, no studies have evaluated data from a single surgeon and institution with a uniform protocol from preoperative evaluation through postoperative followup. This study may provide a unique perspective that eliminates confounding factors that may arise in studies that include multiple surgeons with many different protocols.

2. Materials and Methods

A retrospective chart review was conducted of all TKA, TKA-R, THA, and THA-R preformed from March 2009 to March 2011 at a single academic medical center with the senior author performing all procedures. Approval was granted from the Institutional Review Board. In total, 526 patients were enrolled in the study: 246 total knee arthroplasties, 155 total hip arthroplasties, 67 total knee revisions, and 58 total hip revisions.

The senior author's protocol for patients in this study started with a preoperative clinic visit where the decision was made to proceed with surgery. Preoperative evaluation for all patients included an anesthesia consult, EKG, chest X-ray, and standard preoperative labs including a complete blood count, chemistry profile, type and screen, prothrombin time and INR. Additional labs or studies were ordered on selected patients if deemed appropriate based on history or physical exam.

Autologous donations were collected two weeks prior to the operation for patients who were thought to be at increased risk for blood transfusions. Determination of risk was individualized and included factors such as preoperative hematocrit, medical comorbidities, age, gender, general health, and patient's desire to donate. See Table 3 for details regarding the average number of units of autologous packed red blood cells donated for each procedure. Each unit collected was 220 cc.

On the day of surgery, all primary and revision total knee arthroplasties had a thigh tourniquet placed and inflated (tourniquet pressures varied from 275 to 325 mmHg based on thigh size) prior to skin incision. At the time of closure, a hemovac drain was placed in all primary and revision total knee arthroplasties. There were no drains used in any primary or revision total hip arthroplasties. Upon admission to the post anesthesia care unit (PACU), all patients had a hematocrit drawn. Patients were transferred to the surgical ward as per PACU protocol. Hematocrit (HCT) values were measured daily during the patient's hospital stay. Hemovac drains were removed on postoperative day 1 regardless of drain output. Patients were discharged to home or rehab based on evaluation by the arthroplasty service in coordination with physical and occupational therapy. The decision to transfuse during the hospital stay was based on a global evaluation by the arthroplasty service which included patient symptoms,

hematocrit value, vital signs, urine output, and estimated blood loss in surgery. There was no cut-off hematocrit below which a transfusion was required, or value above which no transfusion could be given; however, a hematocrit of 25.5% or less was used as a cut-off guide for most patients.

Data for evaluation in this study was obtained by reviewing clinical charts, anesthesia records, and patients' hospital records. Information recorded from the clinical chart included the procedure, preoperative hematocrit value and patient co-morbidities. Comorbidites were grouped into general categories which included cardiovascular, gastrointestinal, hematology/oncology, pulmonary, renal, musculoskeletal, endocrine—other than diabetes mellitus (DM), diabetes mellitus, psychiatric illnesses, neurologic disease (including seizures, history of stroke), liver disease, gynecologic disorders, dyslipidemias, and autoimmune disorders. The patients hospital record and anesthesia record were evaluated for hematocrit values, hematocrit value at which the patient was transfused, number of units transfused, number of allogeneic transfusions, number of autologous transfusions, number of wasted autologous units, and additional breakthrough transfused units beyond the autologous donation. Complications occurring both intraoperatively and postoperatively were also recorded.

2.1. Statistical Methods/Analysis of Data. General demographics were first determined with an average and standard deviations (Table 1). The total transfusion data was determined and further stratified by allogeneic transfusions, autologous transfusions, and breakthrough transfusion requirement (Tables 2 and 3). Two comparative groups were created: transfused patients versus nontransfused patients (Table 4) and patients who gave an autologous donation versus patients who did not (Table 5). Age, length of stay (LOS), preoperative HCT, estimated blood loss (EBL), 14 comorbidities were compared, and a P value was assigned to each comparative group. Logistic regressions were conducted to predict patient transfusion using age, gender, and pre-op HCT as predictors. A test of the full model against a constant only model was conducted for each of the four groups (THA, TKA, THA-R, and TKA-R) to determine the predictors of transfusion. Additionally, coefficient of determination (R^2), Wald's criteria, and EXP(B) were used to determine the chance of future events (transfusion) for each variable: preoperative hematocrit, age, gender, and comorbidities.

3. Results

3.1. TKA. A logistic regression analysis was conducted to predict patient transfusion for 246 patients. A test of the full model against a constant only model indicated that preoperative hematocrit was a significant predictor of transfusion (chi square = 27.866, $P < 0.0001$ with df = 1). Age, gender, and comorbidities were not found to significantly predict transfusion ($P > 0.05$).

Nagelkerke's R^2 of 0.173 indicated a small positive relationship between Preoperative hematocrit and transfusion. Prediction success overall was 81.1%. The Wald criterion

TABLE 1: General demographics.

			Gender			Age Mean (range)		
			Men	Women	Total	Men	Women	Range
TKA	Total patients	246	92	154	62.7	61.5	63.5	21–88
	Unilateral	241						
	Bilateral	5						
TKA-R	Total patients	67	22	45	63.8	69.7	61	30–85
	Unilateral	65						
	Bilateral	2						
THA	Total patients	155	70	85	59.1	56.6	61.3	19–86
	Unilateral	152						
	Bilateral	3						
THA-R	Total patients	58	33	25	56.7	55.3	58.5	26–91
	Unilateral	57						
	Bilateral	1						
	Total	526	217	309	61.1	59.8	62.1	19–91

TABLE 2: General transfusion data.

	Pre-op HCT	HCT on day of transfusion	Number of patients (%) requiring transfusion			Total units			Units transfused
			Total	Women	Men	Total	Allogeneic	Autologous	Avg. units per patient
TKA	35.8	24.8	54 (22%)	41	13	79	62	17	1.4
TKA-R	37.2	24.9	22 (33%)	12	10	60	60	0	2.7
THA	38.8	24.0	82 (53%)	56	26	154	111	43	1.9
THA-R	38	24.5	35 (60%)	15	20	124	119	5	3.5

TABLE 3: Autologous blood donation and utilization.

	Total donators (%)	Units donated	Donators who required transfusion	Patients who wasted total donation	Avg. donated units wasted	Patients with breakthrough transfusions	Avg. breakthrough units
TKA	62 (25%)	1.65	13	80%	1.3	7%	2
TKA-R	0	0	0	0%	0	0	0
THA	45 (29%)	1.5	22	51%	1.4	32%	1.6
THA-R	6 (11%)	1.3	4	33%	1.5	0	0

TABLE 4: Transfused versus Nontransfused patients.

		TKA	P value	TKA-R	P value	THA	P value	THA-R	P value
Age	*Not transfused*	62.0	0.007	61.3	0.004	56.1	0.07	52.8	0.06
	Transfused	65.1		69.0		61.8		59.2	
LOS	*Not transfused*	3.4	0.03	3.8	0.09	3.5	0.04	4.0	0.43
	Transfused	3.8		4.6		4.1		5.7	
Pre-op HCT	*Not transfused*	40.5	0.001	38.7	0.001	40.4	0.001	40.5	0.008
	Transfused	37.3		34.3		37.4		36.5	
EBL	*Not transfused*	57	0.05	96	0.008	279	0.03	736	0.003
	Transfused	75		285		349		1326	
Comorbidities	*Not transfused*	2.92	0.2	2.08	0.07	2.52	0.07	2.29	0.002
	Transfused	3.07		3.27		2.74		3.03	

TABLE 5: Autologous donation patient versus Nondonation patients.

		TKA	P value	THA	P value	THA-R	P value
Age	Auto donation	57.4	0.001	54.1	0.001	49	0.1
	No auto donation	64.5		61.1		57.6	
Pre-op HCT	Auto donation	39.0	0.01	37.8	0.03	39.7	0.2
	No auto donation	40.1		39.2		37.9	
EBL (mL)	Auto donation	64.2	0.2	331.3	0.3	845	0.2
	No auto donation	59.8		310.0		1120.4	
Comorbidities	Auto donation	2.7	0.1	2.4	0.09	3.3	0.2
	No auto donation	3.0		2.7		2.8	

demonstrated that preoperative HCT made significant contributions to prediction ($P < 0.0001$). EXP(B) value indicates that when preoperative HCT is decreased by 1% the odds ratio is 1.258, and therefore patients are 1.258 more likely to need transfusion.

3.2. TKA-R. A logistic regression analysis was conducted to predict transfusion for 67 patients. A test of the full model against a constant only model indicated that preoperative hematocrit was a significant predictor of transfusion (chi square = 11.264, $P < 0.005$ with df = 1). Age, gender, and comorbidities were not found to significantly predict transfusion ($P > 0.05$).

Nagelkerke's R^2 of 0.216 indicated a small positive relationship between preoperative HCT and transfusion. Prediction success overall was 70.1%. The Wald criterion demonstrated that pre-op HCT made significant contributions to prediction ($P < 0.005$). EXP(B) value indicates that when pre-op HCT is decreased by 1%, the odds ratio is 1.203, and therefore patients are 1.203, more likely to need transfusion.

3.3. THA. A logistic regression analysis was conducted to predict patient transfusion for 155 patients. A test of the full model against a constant-only model indicated that age, gender, and preoperative hematocrit significantly predicted transfusion (chi square = 35.141, $P < 0.0001$ with df = 3). Comorbidities were not found to significantly predict transfusion ($P > 0.05$).

Nagelkerke's R^2 of 0.279 indicated a small positive relationship between the predictors (age, gender, and preoperative HCT) and prediction (transfusion or not). Prediction success overall was 70.7%. The Wald criterion demonstrated that age, gender, and preoperative HCT made significant contributions to prediction ($P < 0.05$). EXP(B) value indicates when age is raised by one unit (one year), the odds ratio is 1.029, and therefore patients are 1.029 more times likely to need transfusion. In addition, EXP(B) value indicates that for female patients the odds ratio is 2.326, and therefore female patients are 2.326 more times likely to need transfusion. Finally, EXP(B) value indicates that when preoperative HCT is decreased by 1%, the odds ratio is 1.236 and therefore patients are 1.236, more likely to need transfusion.

3.4. THA-R. A logistic regression analysis was conducted to predict patient transfusion for 58 patients. A test of the full model against a constant only model indicated that preoperative hematocrit significantly predicted transfusion (chi square = 5.896, $P < 0.05$ with df = 1). Age, gender, and comorbidities were not found to significantly predict transfusion ($P > 0.05$).

Nagelkerke's R^2 of 0.133 indicated a small positive relationship between the preoperative HCT and transfusion. Prediction success overall was 64.9%. The Wald criterion demonstrated that preoperative HCT made a significant contribution to prediction ($P < 0.05$). EXP(B) value indicates that when preoperative HCT is decreased by 1%, the odds ratio is 1.206, and therefore patients are 1.206 more likely to need transfusion.

4. Discussion

This study reviewed the utilization of blood transfusion after total joint arthroplasty at a single academic medical center performed by a single orthopaedic surgeon. Data collected was analyzed for preoperative risk factors that are predictive of transfusion as well as how preoperative autologous blood donations were utilized. In a previous study, Bierbaum et al. analyzed similar blood usage but among a cohort of 330 orthopaedic surgeons spread over various geographic locations throughout the United States. They determined that preoperative hemoglobin and lack of pre-donated units were the most consistent predictors of allogeneic transfusion need [4]. They also concluded that autologous blood donation and utilization was grossly inefficient. Bierbaum et al. noted a limitation in the lack of a uniformed protocol among surgeons participating whereas the present study has the advantage of a consistent protocol from preoperative visit to postoperative followup.

Logistic regression analysis of our collected data demonstrated preoperative hematocrit as a consistent predictor of future transfusion—similar to several other studies [4, 9, 11, 12]. For each one-point decrease in preoperative hematocrit, the odd ratio demonstrated an increased possibility for transfusion for all procedures (OR 1.203–1.258). These odds ratios are additive, and, therefore, those patients with a hematocrit several points lower than normal had a much higher risk of transfusion. In addition to preoperative hematocrit, predictors of transfusion for total hip arthroplasty (THA) included age and gender. For each year increase in age, the chance of transfusion increased by 1.029. Additionally, female patients were more likely to receive transfusion with an odds ratio of 2.326. This relationship, to our knowledge, has not been demonstrated in previous studies.

Preoperative hematocrit was equally shown to be a predictor of future transfusion in total knee arthroplasty (TKA), total knee arthroplasty revision (TKA-R), and total hip arthroplasty-revision (THA-R) groups; however, no other variables (age, gender, and comorbidities) were found to be significant predictors for transfusion. It is unclear why age and gender were found to be significant only in THA patients.

A review of our overall blood usage (both allogeneic and autologous) shows that we were frequently unsuccessful in predicting those who will require a transfusion. In all, THA-R had the greatest proportion of patients receiving transfusions followed closely by THA, TKA-R, and TKA. While TKA had the fewest patient requiring transfusion in all, this group had 62 patients (25%) providing an autologous donation. In addition, only 13 (21%) of those patients providing donation actually required transfusion; therefore, the vast majority of donators wasted their entire donation. This waste accounts for a large fee in blood draw, storage, and retrieval [14–16]. On the other hand, zero patients provided a donation in the TKA-R arm of the study, but 33% of patients required allogeneic blood (average of 2.7 units). As for THA and THA-R, these groups had the highest percentage of patients requiring a transfusion (53% and 60%, resp.) and required the most units of blood (154 units and 124 units, resp.), but only 29% and 11% provided an autologous donation, respectively. Inconsistency in choosing appropriate patients for pre-donation is not limited to our study; similar difficulty has been documented in other studies [4, 9, 12].

Ultimately better models are needed to predict the patients who are most and least likely at risk for needing a transfusion in the perioperative period. Improved patient selection will help reduce risks to the patient, decrease wasted blood, and lower expenses.

Shortcomings of this study include its nonrandomized nature. We did not perform a power analysis to determine the number of charts to review, so it is unclear if collecting more data might allow trends we found to become significant. While we attempted to extract information from our chart review believed to be important preoperative risk factors, additional information could always be considered for analysis. Future reviews could include BMI, race, or history of previous transfusion requirements. In addition, comorbidities were grouped into broad categories rather than evaluating specific conditions. This may have hidden the role that certain disease processes play in predisposing patients to anemia after surgery, particularly in less commonly seen diseases. Future evaluation looking at the effect of specific diseases would be beneficial. To do this, however, we would likely need a much larger patient database for proper power.

Finally, there was no specific protocol for transfusion of patients. While the same generalized principles were applied to all the patients in the decision to transfuse, results may have been affected because there was no uniform outline for when patient should or should not be transfused. While theoretically possible to implement, this may be difficult based on the number of factors to consider when deciding to transfuse.

Despite these flaws, we have provided the first comprehensive summary of blood transfusion utilization at a single academic institution under a single surgeon. Our results confirmed previous findings that that preoperative hematocrit is the most significant factor that determines need for postoperative blood transfusion. In addition, our data suggests that age and gender, particularly in THA, may play an important role. The inefficiencies of autologous blood collection and utilization were again demonstrated. Continued analysis of additional variables (BMI, race, and more specific comorbidity data with a scoring system such as the Charlson comorbidity score [17]) may better stratify and identify those patients most at risk for transfusion.

References

[1] D. R. Spahn, "Anemia and patient blood management in hip and knee surgery: a systematic review of the literature," *Anesthesiology*, vol. 113, no. 2, pp. 482–495, 2010.

[2] M. C. Fernandez, M. Gottlieb, and J. E. Menitove, "Blood transfusion and postoperative infection in orthopedic patients," *Transfusion*, vol. 32, no. 4, pp. 318–322, 1992.

[3] C. E. Stevens, R. D. Aach, and F. B. Hollinger, "Hepatitis B virus antibody in blood donors and the occurrence of non-A, non-B hepatitis in transfusion recipients. An analysis of the transfusion-transmitted viruses study," *Annals of Internal Medicine*, vol. 101, no. 6, pp. 733–738, 1984.

[4] B. E. Bierbaum, C. Hill, J. J. Callaghan et al., "An analysis of blood management in patients having a total hip or knee arthroplasty," *Journal of Bone and Joint Surgery*, vol. 81, no. 1, pp. 2–10, 1999.

[5] J. R. Gonzalez-Porras, E. Colado, M. P. Conde, T. Lopez, M. J. Nieto, and M. Corral, "An individualized pre-operative blood saving protocol can increase pre-operative haemoglobin levels and reduce the need for transfusion in elective total hip or knee arthroplasty," *Transfusion Medicine*, vol. 19, no. 1, pp. 35–42, 2009.

[6] S. Guerin, C. Collins, H. Kapoor, I. McClean, and D. Collins, "Blood transfusion requirement prediction in patients undergoing primary total hip and knee arthroplasty," *Transfusion Medicine*, vol. 17, no. 1, pp. 37–43, 2007.

[7] R. Yomtovian, "Autologous transfusion complications," in *Transfusion Reactions*, M. Popovsky, Ed., pp. 237–280, AABB Press, Bethesda, Md, USA, 1996.

[8] A. Kumar, "Perioperative management of anemia: limits of blood transfusion and alternatives to it," *Cleveland Clinic Journal of Medicine*, vol. 76, supplement 4, pp. S112–S118, 2009.

[9] A. M. Hatzidakis, R. M. Mendlick, T. McKillip, R. L. Reddy, and K. L. Garvin, "Preoperative autologous donation for total joint arthroplasty: an analysis of risk factors for allogenic transfusion," *Journal of Bone and Joint Surgery*, vol. 82, no. 1, pp. 89–100, 2000.

[10] D. C. Ayers, D. G. Murray, and D. M. Duerr, "Blood salvage after total hip arthroplasty," *Journal of Bone and Joint Surgery*, vol. 77, no. 9, pp. 1347–1351, 1995.

[11] J. L. Knight, D. Sherer, and J. Guo, "Blood transfusion strategies for total knee arthroplasty: minimizing autologous blood

wastage, risk of homologous blood transfusion, and transfusion cost," *Journal of Arthroplasty*, vol. 13, no. 1, pp. 70–76, 1998.

[12] G. A. Nuttall, P. J. Santrach, W. C. Oliver Jr. et al., "The predictors of red cell transfusions in total hip arthroplasties," *Transfusion*, vol. 36, no. 2, pp. 144–149, 1996.

[13] G. E. Hill, W. H. Frawley, K. E. Griffith, J. E. Forestner, and J. P. Minei, "Allogeneic aiiogeneic blood transfusion increases the risk of postoperative bacterial infection: a meta-analysis," *Journal of Trauma*, vol. 54, no. 5, pp. 908–914, 2003.

[14] J. D. Birkmeyer, L. T. Goodnough, J. P. AuBuchon, P. G. Noord-sij, and B. Littenberg, "The cost-effectiveness of preoperative autologous blood donation for total hip and knee replacement," *Transfusion*, vol. 33, no. 7, pp. 544–551, 1993.

[15] N. Blumberg, S. A. Kirkley, and J. M. Heal, "A cost analysis of autologous and allogeneic transfusions in hip-replacement surgery," *American Journal of Surgery*, vol. 171, no. 3, pp. 324–330, 1996.

[16] J. Etchason, L. Petz, E. Keeler et al., "The cost effectiveness of preoperative autologous blood donations," *New England Journal of Medicine*, vol. 332, no. 11, pp. 719–724, 1995.

[17] M. E. Charlson, P. Pompei, K. A. Ales, and C. R. MacKenzie, "A new method of classifying prognostic comorbidity in longitudinal studies: development and validation," *Journal of Chronic Diseases*, vol. 40, no. 5, pp. 373–383, 1987.

36

Comparison of Epidemiological Methods for Estimation of Hepatitis B Incidence and Residual Risk for Blood Donors in Southern Brazil

Emil Kupek[1] and Andrea Petry[2]

[1] Departamento de Saúde Pública/CCS, Universidade Federal de Santa Catarina, 88040-900 Florianopolis, SC, Brazil
[2] Hematology and Hemotherapy Center of Santa Catarina (HEMOSC), Florianopolis, SC, Brazil

Correspondence should be addressed to Emil Kupek, kupek@ccs.ufsc.br

Academic Editor: M. Popovsky

Background and Objective. The objective of this work was to compare three methods for estimating hepatitis B virus (HBV) incidence and residual risk. *Methods*. Computerized blood donor records in southern Brazil were examined for the period 2004–2006. The methods for estimating HBV incidence included stand-alone HBsAg, HBsAg yield method, and an extension of the latter which added recent anti-HBc seroconversions as incident HBV cases. *Results*. HBV incidences for the above methods were 9.91, 20.09, and 22.93 per 100000 repeat donors, respectively. In the same order, corresponding residual risks were 1 : 62482, 1 : 30821, and 1 : 47559, respectively. First-time donors had 52 higher HBV incidence compared to repeat donors. *Conclusion*. Although the three methods compared produced overlapping 95% confidence intervals, their variation was considerably lower for the method which included recent anti-HBc seroconversions. First-time donors are primary cause for concern regarding HBV transmission via blood transfusion in southern Brazil.

1. Introduction

There is a consensus that infection caused by hepatitis B virus (HBV) is a worldwide public health concern of high priority, given over 2 billion people who have already been infected and about 350 million of them living with a chronic infection [1]. About a million deaths per year are attributed to this infection and its complications, primarily liver cancer and cirrhosis [1, 2].

Three quarters of the world population live in high-prevalence areas for HBV [2]. In developing countries with endemic regions for this infection, such as the Southeast of Asia, China, Africa, many Middle East countries, Pacific islands, and the Amazon region, serologic surveys show that majority of the population has been infected and that 8–15% are chronic HBV carriers. Because 5–12% of the women of childbearing age have been infected with HBV, the risk of perinatal transmission reaches the level of 70–90%, resulting in many newborns infected at birth. In addition,

many children are infected during childhood through direct contact with infected blood, ulcerative wounds, or saliva. Approximately one quarter of the children infected with HBV until five years of age become chronic carriers of the virus. On the other hand, adolescent and adult populations acquire HBV through sexual contacts and have between 1% and 5% risk of becoming chronic carriers [3].

Such a high disease burden is even more absurd in the light of the fact that HBV infection is preventable by affordable vaccine (about U$10 per person for the standard vaccine schedule). Among developing countries, Brazil has recently started its own production of a DNA-recombinant hepatitis B vaccine whose effectiveness has been confirmed in various studies [4–6]. Other important measures to prevent HBV transmission include screening the blood donors and pregnant women.

In Brazil, at least 15% of the population has been infected with HBV, and about 1% of them remain as chronic carriers [7]. As a consequence, the residual risk for not detecting the virus through serological tests for blood donor screening is also high compared to the developed countries. Routine blood screening for HBV in Brazil includes HBsAg (HBV surface antigen) and anti-HBc (antigen to HBV core antibody). The residual risk is the product of the infectious window period and the virus incidence in blood donor population [8, 9]. The latter depends primarily on the effectiveness of predonation interview in eliminating donor candidates with risky sexual behavior. However, other important factors for HBV prevalence in the general population such as the risk of perinatal transmission and vaccine coverage are not within the scope of blood donor selection procedures.

Despite a significant reduction in residual risk for HBV in southern Brazil in the past two decades [10–13], it is still much higher than in the developed countries. In addition, the risk reduction was not linear in time, showing temporary peaks whose significance has not yet been elucidated [11]. Although nucleid acid testing (NAT) for human immunodeficiency virus (HIV) and hepatitis C has recently started as a pilot scheme in some Brazilian blood banks, it seems unlikely that it is going to be extended to HBV. Therefore, a significant reduction in infectious window period due to the NAT is not a viable option for reducing the residual risk for HBV in Brazil in near future. It is thus necessary to implement alternative methods to estimate the virus incidence in blood donors.

The most frequently used method to estimate HBV incidence in blood donors is based on the serologic marker HbsAg alone, with adjustment for approximately one quarter of the population with primary antibody response [8, 9]. Although widely applied in various countries [14], including in Brazil1 [1, 15], this method is restricted to repeat donors and depends on the duration of interdonation interval which is pretty variable between the blood banks. In addition, this method requires a large number of repeat donors to obtain reasonably accurate estimates [16].

Another way to estimate HBV incidence in blood donors is by testing for both immunoglobulin G (IgG) and M (IgM) for anti-HBc to distinguish between an old and a recent infection. Thus a recent (<6 moths) infection is diagnosed if either IgM anti-HBc or HBsAg is positive. However, these are not serological tests used for routine screening as only total anti-HBc is used for this purpose worldwide. The same restriction is applied to yet another method to estimate HBV incidence in blood donors based on anti-HBc positive test result and any of the following: a positive test result for anti-HBe (antigen to HBV antibody "e"), anti-HBc IgM, DNA for HBV on current or previous donation, anti-HBs (antigen to HBV antibody "s") without vaccination against hepatitis B [17].

Yet another method for estimating HBV incidence with routine serologic markers in blood donor screening (HBsAg and anti-HBc), known as "HBsAg yield approach," has been proposed and tested by various authors during the 2010 decade [16, 18–20]. A recent comparison of the most popular method based on stand-alone HBsAg [8, 9] and the HBsAg yield approach showed very close agreement of the HBV incidence estimates in the United States blood donor population [20].

A major advantage of the HBsAg yield approach over the stand-alone HBsAg method is to provide HBV incidence estimate for the first-time donors as well. It also makes use of both serologic markers routinely used for HBV screening in blood donor candidates. This paper extends this idea to include anti-HBc seroconverting repeat donors when the time between the last seronegative and the first seropositive test result for this marker was less than a year. Such a short period makes the assumption of a recent HBV infection more plausible. As anti-HBc marker is much more prevalent than the HBsAg marker, the precision of the estimates based on Poisson distribution of the incident cases using both markers also tends to improve.

2. Material and Methods

The main objective of this paper was to compare three methods to obtain hepatitis B incidence estimate and residual risk for blood donors in southern Brazil: the stand-alone HbsAg method [8, 9], the HBsAg yield approach, and an extension to the latter which includes anti-HBc seroconverting repeat donors. In addition, deferral rate for HBV serological markers was also calculated for both repeat and first-time donors.

Computerized data from four blood banks in the state of Santa Catarina, southern Brazil, were gathered for the period 2003–2006. The blood banks were located in the cities of Florianopolis, Joinville, Criciúma, and Lages. Over 95000 blood donor candidates with complete serological test results were included in the analysis. Among these, 36350 were repeat donors during the 2003–2006 period and their total follow-up time summed to 103819 person-years.

Serological tests in blood banks in Lages, Criciuma, and Joinville included enzyme-linked immunosorbent assays (ELISA) for HBsAg (produced by "Organon Teknika BV") and anti-HBc (produced by "Ortho Diagnostic Systems"). In the blood bank in Florianopolis, the serological tests included microparticle enzyme immunoassay (MEIA) for HBsAg and anti-HBc (produced by "ABBOTT Laboratories"). Mean infectious window periods were 59 and 82 days for HBsAg and for the second-generation anti-HBc, respectively [15].

Other screening tests included EIA for HIV-1 and HIV-2, hepatitis C antibody, human T-cell lymphotropic virus type 1 and 2, antibody for *Treponema pallidum* (using Veneral Disease Research Laboratory test) and antibody for *Trypanosoma cruzi*. For the purpose of blood donation screening, positive test results for any blood screening test eliminate the possibility of transfusing the blood to a recipient. As this paper focuses on HBV transmission, the outcome of interest here is having a positive test result for either HBsAg or anti-HBc or both.

Next section briefly describes the three methods for hepatitis B incidence estimation. For all methods, corresponding residual risk was calculated by multiplying the HBV incidence estimate by the duration of infectious window period.

2.1. The Stand-Alone HBsAg Method. Residual risk for HBV is the probability of seroconversion during infectious window period [8, 9]. It is calculated as the product of HBV incidence and duration of the window period. For repeat donors, un unbiased estimate of the date of seroconversion is the the midpoint of the interval between the last seronegative and subsequent seropositive test result for HBsAg. The incidence numerator is the number of HBsAg seroconverting donors, and its denominator is the time at risk for HBV infection for all blood donors tested except those who would be eliminated for some other reason (e.g., tested positive for some other serologic marker, inadequate weight, risky sexual behavior).

However, some seroconverting donors show transient antigenemia and do not reach the level of HBsAg high enough to be detected by the test [9]. Therefore, the following adjustment is made. The probability of transient antigenaemia, denoted by S, is estimated by dividing its average duration of 63 days with the median interdonation period among HBsAg seroconverting donors [8]. The overall probability of detecting a new case of HBV infection, denoted by P, is based on the study that showed 70% prevalence of donors with transient antigenaemia and 5% prevalence of long-term HBV carriers, leading to the formula $P = 0.7S + 0.05$. The reciprocal value of P gives the adjustment factor to be multiplied by HBsAg incidence, providing corrected HBV incidence.

2.2. HBsAg Yield Method. The central idea of this approach is to determine the fraction of blood donors who tested positive for HBsAg and negative for anti-HBc, separately for repeat donors and first-time donors, as well as the ratio of the two [16, 18–20]. Repeat blood donors also provide the information on the interval between the last seronegative and the first seropositive test result which can be used to estimate their exposure time and thus density-type incidence by dividing the number of seroconverting donors with corresponding person-time at risk for being an HBsAg yield case. Multiplying this estimate by the above ratio extrapolates the incidence estimate to the first-time donors as well.

In this study, the donors with positive test results on HBV screening were verified by follow-up test results and S/O values for HBsAg. Only the donors whose S/O values equaled or exceeded the cutoff of 6 on screening and whose anti-HBC negative test results on screening was followed by subsequent anti-HBC positive test result were considered HBsAg yield cases [20].

2.3. HBsAg Yield Method with Inclusion of Anti-HBc Seroconverting Repeat Donors. Although a large multicenter study showed the lack of specificity of anti-HBc EIA tests in diagnosing acute HBV infection [21], this is less problematic in the case of repeat donors with the interdonation interval between the last two donations being less than a year. The most plausible cause of such seroconversion is an acute HBV infection. The time at risk for HBV infection and incidence are calculated in the same way as for HBsAg yield approach, only now it is extended to anti-HBc seroconverting repeat donors. In other words, this approach counts both HBsAg

and anti-HBc seroconverting repeat donors in the incidence numerator. The seroconverting anti-HBc repeat donors were repeatedly tested in the followup of the screening test, and only those who repeated a positive anti-HBc test result were considered confirmed incident cases of HBV infection.

2.4. Statistical Methods. Descriptive statistics provide some basic information of blood donor characteristics (age, sex, number of previous donations) and HBV screening test results (HBV surface antigen and core antibody) with 95% confidence intervals based on binomial distribution.

A recent HBV infection was considered confirmed when donor tested positive on two consecutive tests for HBsAg and suspected if the second test has not been made. The fraction of confirmed cases was multiplied by the confirmation rate among those with two consecutive tests for HBsAg to estimate the likely number of incident HBV cases in blood donors who were invited for the second HBsAg test after the first one showed a positive result but failed to do so. This number was added to the number of confirmed cases to produce the estimate of the number of seroconverting repeat blood donors with 95% confidence intervals based on Poisson distribution.

The 95% confidence interval (CI) for the residual risk was estimated using the 95% CI for incidence, which in turn was based on the exact 95% Poisson CI for its numerator. In addition, the HBsAg yield method has the duration of the so-called yield window period (the time between HbsAg and anti-HBc positive test results) as another source of variation. As present study found only one HBsAg yield case and therefore observed no yield window variation, this information was based on simulation of a Poisson distribution ($n = 1000$) with the mean equal to the observed yield window of 45 days. Thus the 95% CI for incidence was the span between the percentiles of 2.5 and 97.5 of the simulated Poisson distribution. Stata statistical software was used for the simulation [22].

For the stand-alone HBsAg method and its extension to anti-HBC seroconverting donors, residual risk was calculated by multiplying the estimated HBV incidence by the duration of infectious window period of 59 days (0.1615 years) for the HBsAg test. In addition, a refined infectious window period of 30 and 38 days was used to make the results comparable to the seminal US study for the HBsAg yield method [20]. The span between 30 and 38 days corresponds to the time range necessary to produce 1 to 20 copies of HBV DNA per 20 mL, respectively, as a minimal infectious dose for a transfused component [23]. Both extremes of the time range were used and the results averaged to obtain the residual risk estimate for this method.

3. Results

Some basic characteristics of the blood donors analyzed are presented in Table 1.

Age distribution was similar for first-time and repeat donors, although the former had somewhat higher percentage of male donors and almost 20% lower percentage of

TABLE 1: Demographic characteristics of blood donor candidates, collection site, and intended recipient in southern Brazil, 2004–2006.

Donor profile	Categories	First-time donors		Repeat donors		All donors	
		n	%	n	%	n	%
Sex	Male	20001	33.90	10250	28.12	30251	31.70
	Female	38997	66.10	26195	71.88	65192	68.30
Age (years)	18-19	5805	9.84	1712	4.70	7517	7.88
	20–29	24859	42.14	15423	42.32	40282	42.21
	30–39	15322	25.97	10042	27.55	25364	26.58
	40–49	9382	15.90	6471	17.76	15853	16.61
	50–65	3630	6.15	2797	7.67	6427	6.73
Blood collection site	Blood bank	53600	90.85	34355	94.27	87955	92.15
	Mobile unit	5398	9.15	2090	5.73	7488	7.85
Donation directed to	Any recipient	33591	56.94	27731	76.09	61322	64.25
	Specific recipient	25164	42.65	8679	23.81	33843	35.46
	Self	24	0.04	14	0.04	38	0.04

donations not directed to any specific recipient such as a member of family or a friend.

Median interdonation period for repeat donors was 507 days with interquartile range between 277 and 811 days.

Deferral rate due to the HBV serological markers was 70 times higher in the first-time donors compared to the repeat donors (Table 2). The difference between male and female deferral rate was statistically significant for the first-time donors but not for the repeat donors.

Based on stand-alone HBsAg, the HBV incidence in the repeat blood donors was estimated at 9.91 per 100.000 per year. The corresponding residual risk was 1 : 62482 blood donations with 95% confidence interval between 1 : 11213 and 1 : 2476780 donations (Tables 2 and 3).

By adding ten anti-HBc seroconverting donors to the one HBsAg seroconverting donors the estimate of recent HBV seroconversions increased to 11, producing HBV incidence of 20.09 per 100.000 per year and associated residual risk of 1 : 30821 donations with 95% CI between 1 : 17229 and 1 : 61734 donations (Table 4).

Among the 116 first-time donors who tested HBsAg positive and anti-HBC negative on screening, 86 was considered confirmed positive by S/O values greater than 6 and subsequent anti-HBC positive results. Only one of three repeat donors who tested HBsAg positive and anti-HBC negative on screening were confirmed by the same criteria, as the other two donors tested subsequently negative on anti-HBC on two occasions (3 and 6 months after the screening). All ten anti-HBc soroconverting repeat donors within 12 months of their last donation tested repeatedly positive for this serological marker but none tested positive for HBsAg. None of the donors who tested positive on either HBsAg or anti-HBc on screening was found positive on anti-HBs test in the followup.

In order to make the above results comparable to a recent US study [20], the residual risk and corresponding 95% CI for the HBsAg yield rate method were also calculated using 30 and 38 days for the infectious window period [23] and taking the average. For the repeat donors, the estimates were 1 : 41934 and 1 : 53184, with the mean of 1 : 47559 and

95% CI between 1 : 12280 and 1 : 2100046. For the first-time donors, the corresponding values were 1 : 807 and 1 : 1023 with the mean value of 1 : 915 and 95% CI between 1 : 552 and 1 : 1435.

The ratio of the first-time to repeat donor yield rate was 51.97 (Table 5), thus indicating almost 52 times higher HBV incidence in the former. Weighted mean HBV incidence per 100000 for all donors was 751.67 with corresponding residual risk of 1 : 824.

4. Discussion

HBV incidence estimates per 100000 for repeat donors were pretty close between the HBsAg yield method (20.09) and the method that included recent anti-HBc seroconverting donors (22.93) but more than twice the value obtained by the stand-alone HBsAg method (9.91). However, the difference among the estimates should be interpreted with caution as only one case of HBsAg seroconversion and relatively small sample size for this type of study may considerably reduce their precision.

Although the confidence intervals for corresponding residual risk estimates overlapped considerably for all methods, they were extremely wide for both the HBsAg yield method and the stand-alone HBsAg method. Only the method including recent anti-HBc seroconverting donors produced reasonable confidence intervals that may be useful for comparison purposes. Smaller variance of the latter method was due to the increase in the total number of seroconverting donors by adding the anti-HBc seroconversions within the last 12 months to the HBsAg seroconversions in repeat donors. Anti-HBc seroconversion within such a short period is most likely a recent case of HBV infection as it was confirmed by repeatedly positive anti-HBc test results for all cases in the followup to the positive screening test result. It should be noticed that the stand-alone HBsAg method does not account for the variation in the adjustment factor due to the variation of the median of the interdonation period among repeat donors, neither does the HBsAg yield method account for the HBsAg yield rate variation in the population,

Table 2: Deferral for either anti-HBc or HBsAg positive test result among candidates for blood donation in southern Brazil, 2004–2006.

	First-time blood donors			Repeat blood donors		
Sex	Tested	Confirmed	Prevalence (%) and CI[1]	Tested	Confirmed	Prevalence (%) and CI[1]
Female	19894	375	1.88 1.70–2.08	10215	2	0.020 0.002–0.071
Male	38881	875	2.25 2.11–2.40	26135	9	0.034 0.016–0.065
All	58775	1250	2.13 2.01–2.25	36350	11	0.0303 0.015–0.054

[1] 95% exact binomial confidence interval.

Table 3: HBV incidence and residual risk for stand-alone HBsAg in repeat blood donors in southern Brazil, 2004–2006.

Parameter	Value
Number of HBsAg seroconverting donors	1
Median of interdonation intervals (days)	329
Probability of transient antigenaemia[1]	0.1915
Probability of detecting HBV seroconversion by stand-alone HBsAg test[2]	0.1840
Time at risk (person-years) for HBsAg seroconverting donors	0.45
Time at risk (person-years) for all repeat donors	54788.73
Incidence per 100.000 per year (95% CI)[3]	1.825 (0.00, 6.73)
Adjustment factor[4]	5.43
Adjusted incidence per 100.000 per year (95% CI)	9.91 (0.00, 36.54)
Residual risk (95% CI)[5]	1 : 62482 (1 : 16946, 1 : ∞)

[1] Assuming 63 days of average duration for transient antigenaemia [8], that is, 63/329.
[2] Assuming 75% of blood donors with ELISA detectable HBsAg8.
[3] Confidence interval.
[4] Reciprocal value of the probability of detecting HBV seroconversion by stand-alone HBsAg test, that is, 1/0.184 = 5.43.
[5] Assuming Poisson distribution for one HBsAg seroconverting case.

Table 4: HBV incidence and residual risk for stand-alone HBsAg and anti-HBc seroconverting repeat blood donors in southern Brazil, 2004–2006.

Parameter	Value
Number of HBsAg or anti-HBc seroconverting donors[1]	11
Time at risk (person-years) for HBsAg or anti-HBc seroconverting donors	24.93
Time at risk (person-years) for all repeat donors	54788.73
Incidence per 100.000 per year (95% CI)[2]	20.09 (10.03, 35.94)
Residual risk (95% CI)[3]	1 : 3082 (1 : 17229, 1 : 61734)

[1] One HBsAg positive and anti-HBc negative, and ten HBsAg negative and anti-HBc positive donors.
[2] Confidence interval.
[3] Assuming Poisson distribution for 11 seroconverting cases.

thus underestimating the confidence intervals for residual risk. Nevertheless, in smaller settings such as regional or even smaller national blood banks, the confidence intervals can still be prohibitively high for comparison purposes. The key reason for this is the rarity of confirmed HBsAg seroconversion even in a high HBV prevalence area analyzed in the present study. The transient nature of this marker and its relatively high false positive rate when compared to anti-HBc underline the limitations of the HBV incidence methods based solely on the HBsAg test result.

The above finding is different from that of the US study that found a close agreement between the stand-alone HBsAg and HBsAg yield rate method [20]. However, the US study also found the HBV incidence ratio of first-time to repeat donors to be 2.42 compared to almost 52 found with the data in hand.

The importance of anti-HBc for HBV screening has been demonstrated in numerous studies. In the United

States, HBV DNA testing of HBsAg negative blood showed that anti-HBc detected HBV in 1 per 49000 transfusion units that would be eligible for transfusion, which is a rate comparable to the estimated residual risk for HBV infectious window period [24]. In Asia, there is a great concern with preventing the transmission of occult HBV infection given high HBV prevalence in this part of the world. HBsAg negative blood can still contain HBV during chronic stages of infection, and anti-HBc testing can greatly increase the chance of its detection, especially in low endemic areas [25]. However, in areas with anti-HBc prevalence of 10% or higher, this strategy may not be sufficient to meet the increasing demands for blood safety, thus calling for nucleic acid amplification tests (NAT) [25].

Many commercially available kits for anti-HBc have demonstrated high sensitivity and reasonable specificity for high values of cut-off but only one of them has shown high specificity for moderate cut-off values among first-time donors in Germany [26]. This means that false positive test results are likely in low endemic areas such as Germany, with anti-HBc seroprevalence of 1.8% in first-time donors. However, this problem is bound to be considerably diminished for repeat donors whose anti-HBc seroconversion was registered within the last 12 months and who tested repeatedly positive, as in the present study with Brazilian blood donors. A more

TABLE 5: HBsAg yield rate method for first-time and repeat blood donors in southern Brazil, 2004–2006.

Parameter	First-time (n = 58679)	Repeat (n = 35432)
HBsAg− & anti-HBc−[1]	57435	35404
HBsAg− & anti-HBc+[1]	1122	10
HBsAg+ & anti-HBc−[1]	86	1
HBsAg+ & anti-HBc+[1]	6	0
Yield rate (per 100000)	146.56	2.82
Incidence[2] per 100000 (95% CI)[3]	1191.71 (848.80, 1741.28)	22.93 (0.58, 78.30)
Residual risk (95% CI)[4]	1 : 520 (1 : 730, 1 : 356)	1 : 27003 (1 : 7908, 1 : 1067578)

[1] Number of blood donors for each HBV markers combination ("−" and "+" after the markers stand for negative and positive test results, resp.).

[2] For the repeat donors, the incidence was calculated by dividing the yield rate by the 45 days (0.123 years) of time between the anti-HBc negative test result on screening and subsequent anti-HBC positive for the one HBsAg yield case. For the first time donors, the incidence was estimated by multiplying the repeat donors incidence with the ratio of the first-time to the repeat donors yield rate.

[3] Confidence interval.

[4] Using 59 days for the infectious window period.

recent German study confirmed adequate sensitivity of most anti-HBc tests used for routine blood screening but also reported their improved specificity [27].

Although occult HBV infection is a great concern in Asia [25, 28, 29], it seems rare among blood recipients in low endemic areas, including in Brazil [30]. HBV is likely to be more prevalent in immunocompromised patients such as those with HIV but it is highly unlikely that both HIV and HBV would be missed on blood donor screening [31]. In addition, clinical observation indicated low transmission rate of occult HBV compared to the window period, especially in the presence of anti-HBs [32]. On the other hand, anti-HBc-positive and HBsAg negative blood donors without detectable anti-HBs are at least moderately infectious and may be highly infectious in immunocompromised blood recipients [30].

The magnitude of HBV incidence in southern Brazil is striking when compared to the developed countries. For example, in the United States the incidence per 100000 during the 2006–2008 period was estimated at 2.47 and 6.97 for repeat and first-time donors, respectively [20]. This compares to the present study data on the same scale in the range of 9.91 to 22.93 for repeat donors. However, it is among the first-time donors where the incidence of 1191 per 100000 in southern Brazil is more than 170 times that of the US estimate. Unlike the US study where the HBV incidence ratio from first-time to repeat donors was 2.42, in the present study it almost reached the value of 52. The deferral rate due to HBV screening serological markers of 2.13% among Brazilian first-time donors is also higher than in the Unites States.

Other studies from the same region also found very high HBV incidence but also showed the data pointing out to

considerable variability in the ratio of the first-time to repeat donor yield rate [10–12, 33]. The most recent one found this ratio close to 26 for the whole state of Santa Catarina and a considerable regional variation [33]. Such a large variation is certainly a limiting factor for precision and interpretation of HBV incidence and associated residual risk.

The main reason for such a large difference in HBV incidence between Brazil and the United States is the late start of universal vaccination of children in Brazil, so that the prevention of HBV infection is restricted to the population of less than 20 years of age, which is only a small part of the total blood donor population. Although HBV vaccination campaigns in Brazil started in the beginning of the 1990 decade, adequate vaccine supplies for universal vaccination in children were available only after 1998 [34]. In southern Brazil, the vaccine coverage currently exceeds 90% in the first year of life but less than 20% of the newborn are vaccinated within 48 hours after birth, thus missing the opportunity to reduce vertical transmission. Under the circumstances, HBV vaccination directed specifically to blood donors seems the most efficient way to bridge the gap between older unvaccinated donors and younger HBV-vaccinated generation which is yet to become eligible for blood donation.

There are several limitations of the study presented here that should be borne in mind. First, despite the population of almost 100000 donors analyzed in our study, it is still of limited size for rare outcomes such as HBsAg seroconversion in repeat donors, thus leading to a large variation of the HBV incidence and residual risk estimates. Second, HBV DNA testing was not available to obtain a more precise estimate of the HBV incidence against with which the three methods used in this work could be compared. Third, the incidence of occult HBV infection was beyond the scope of this work but is certainly an important topic to be addressed in future studies of this type.

Despite the above limitations, this is to our knowledge the first study to apply HBsAg yield method to Brazilian blood donors and compare its results with other methods, including a novel approach of counting recently seroconverted anti-HBC donors as incident cases of HBV infection. Larger population studies are needed to overcome the shortcomings of the present data. An opportunity of this kind is envisaged with the participation of some Brazilian blood banks in the REDS-II project.

5. Conclusions

Although all three methods for estimating HBV incidence and residual risk compared in this study (stand-alone HBsAg, HBsAg yield method, and HBsAg yield method enhanced by anti-HBc seroconversion within the last 12 months) produced overlapping 95% confidence intervals, the last two methods produced incidence estimates about twice as high as the first one. Adding recently seroconverting anti-HBc donors to the HBsAg positive ones considerably reduced the variance of the HBV incidence and residual risk estimates. The first-time donors had about 52 times higher HBV incidence as estimated by the HBsAg yield method.

As the benefits of universal child vaccination against HBV have not yet reached the blood donor population in Brazil, enhancing the HBV vaccination of blood donors remains a valuable policy.

Acknowledgments

The authors would like to thank the HEMOSC board of directors and Ana Paula Duarte from the HEMOSC computerized records office for their collaboration in assembling the data records, as well as the HEMOSC blood donors who made this work possible.

References

[1] "CDC-Centers for disease control and prevention," Hepatitis B virus, 2005, http://www.cdc/ncidod/diseases/hepatitis/b/education.htm.

[2] "WHO-World Health Organization," Hepatitis B, 2002, http://www.who/cds/csr/lyo/2002.2:Hepatitis B.

[3] O. D. White and F. J. Fenner, *Medical Virology*, Academic Press, New York, NY, USA, 1994.

[4] R. M. Martins, G. Bensabeth, L. C. Arraes, G. G. Barbosa, M. L. Oliveira, and L. A. B. Camacho, "Estudo multicêntrico de imunogenicidade e reatogenicidade de vacinas contra hepatite B: informe preliminar," *Epidemiologia e Serviços de Saúde*, vol. 12, no. 3, pp. 165–166, 2003.

[5] A. Petry and E. J. Kupek, "Effectiveness of recombinant DNA vaccines against hepatitis B in blood donors in an endemic region of South Brazil," *Revista da Sociedade Brasileira de Medicina Tropical*, vol. 39, no. 5, pp. 462–466, 2006.

[6] M. D. D. S. Oliveira, R. M. B. Martins, M. A. Matos et al., "Seroepidemiology of hepatitis B virus infection and high rate of response to hepatitis B virus Butang vaccine in adolescents from low income families in Central Brazil," *Memorias do Instituto Oswaldo Cruz*, vol. 101, no. 3, pp. 251–256, 2006.

[7] "Ministério da Saúde. Portaria 121 (Brasília, 24/09/1995)," in *Coletânea de Legislação em Hemoterapia e Hematologia*, A. R. Carneiro and M. E. D. Lopes, Eds., Sociedade Brasileira de Hematologia e Hemoterapia, Rio de Janeiro, Brazil, 2002.

[8] G. B. Schreiber, M. P. Busch, S. H. Kleinman, and J. J. Korelitz, "The risk of transfusion-transmitted viral infections. The retrovirus epidemiology donor study," *New England Journal of Medicine*, vol. 334, no. 26, pp. 1685–1690, 1996.

[9] J. J. Korelitz, M. P. Busch, S. H. Kleinman et al., "A method for estimating hepatitis B virus incidence rates in volunteer blood donors," *Transfusion*, vol. 37, no. 6, pp. 634–640, 1997.

[10] E. J. Kupek, "Residual transfusion risk for hepatitis B and C in southern Brazil, 1991–1999," *Journal of Viral Hepatitis*, vol. 8, no. 1, pp. 78–82, 2001.

[11] E. Kupek, "Transfusion risk for hepatitis B, hepatitis C and HIV in the state of Santa Catarina, Brazil, 1991–2001," *The Brazilian Journal of Infectious Diseases*, vol. 8, no. 3, pp. 236–240, 2004.

[12] N. Rosini, D. Mousse, C. Spada, and A. Treitinger, "Seroprevalence of HbsAg, Anti-HBc and anti-HCV in Southern Brazil, 1999–2001," *The Brazilian Journal of Infectious Diseases*, vol. 7, no. 4, pp. 262–267, 2003.

[13] A. F. B. Andrade, M. Oliveira-Silva, S. G. C. Silva, I. J. F. Motta, and C. R. Bonvicino, "Seroprevalence of hepatitis B and C virus markers among blood donors in Rio de Janeiro, Brazil,
1998–2005," *Memorias do Instituto Oswaldo Cruz*, vol. 101, no. 6, pp. 673–676, 2006.

[14] S. A. Glynn, S. H. Kleinman, D. J. Wright, and M. P. Busch, "NHLBI retrovirus epidemiology donor study. International application of the incidence rate/window period model," *Transfusion*, vol. 42, no. 8, pp. 966–972, 2002.

[15] V. Canutti Jr., "Risco transfusional: metodologia e estudo," in *Atualização em Hemoterapia*, D. T. Covas and M. A. Zago, Eds., vol. 5 of *Série de Monografias da Escola Brasileira de Hematologia*, pp. 90–99, Fundação Hemocentro de Ribeirão Preto, Ribeirão Preto, SP, Brazil, 1998.

[16] M. P. Busch, S. A. Glynn, S. L. Stramer et al., "A new strategy for estimating risks of transfusion-transmitted viral infections based on rates of detection of recently infected donors," *Transfusion*, vol. 45, no. 2, pp. 254–264, 2005.

[17] S. Laperche, M. Maniez, V. Barlet et al., "A revised method for estimating hepatitis B virus transfusion residual risk based on antibody to hepatitis B core antigen incident cases," *Transfusion*, vol. 48, no. 11, pp. 2308–2314, 2008.

[18] R. Y. Dodd, E. P. Notari IV, and S. L. Stramer, "Current prevalence and incidence of infectious disease markers and estimated window-period risk in the American Red Cross blood donor population," *Transfusion*, vol. 42, no. 8, pp. 975–979, 2002.

[19] S. Zou, S. L. Stramer, E. P. Notari, F. Musavi, C. T. Fang, and R. Y. Dodd, "Estimating current incidence and residual risk of hepatitis B viral infection among blood donors in the United States through a novel approach," *Vox Sanguinis*, vol. 95, supplement 1, pp. 22–23, 2008.

[20] S. Zou, S. L. Stramer, E. P. Notari et al., "Current incidence and residual risk of hepatitis B infection among blood donors in the United States," *Transfusion*, vol. 49, no. 8, pp. 1609–1620, 2009.

[21] W. Hughes, A. Barr, B. C. Dow, E. A. Follett, and J. A. Barbara, "A multicentre assessment of the specificity of ten anti-HBc screening tests," *Transfusion Medicine*, vol. 5, no. 3, pp. 225–230, 1995.

[22] StataCorp, *Stata Statistical Software: Release 9*, StataCorp LP, College Station, Tex, USA, 2005.

[23] S. H. Kleinman and M. P. Busch, "Assessing the impact of HBV NAT on window period reduction and residual risk," *Journal of Clinical Virology*, vol. 36, no. 1, pp. S23–S29, 2006.

[24] S. H. Kleinman, M. C. Kuhns, D. S. Todd et al., "Retrovirus Epidemiology Donor Study. Frequency of HBV DNA detection in US blood donors testing positive for the presence of anti-HBc: implications for transfusion transmission and donor screening," *Transfusion*, vol. 43, no. 6, pp. 696–704, 2003.

[25] C. J. Liu, S. C. Lo, J. H. Kao et al., "Transmission of occult hepatitis B virus by transfusion to adult and pediatric recipients in Taiwan," *Journal of Hepatology*, vol. 44, no. 1, pp. 39–46, 2006.

[26] M. Schmidt, C. M. Nübling, H. Scheiblauer et al., "Anti-HBc screening of blood donors: a comparison of nine anti-HBc tests," *Vox Sanguinis*, vol. 91, no. 3, pp. 237–243, 2006.

[27] M. K. Hourfar, L. A. Walch, G. Geusendam et al., "Sensitivity and specificity of anti-HBc screening assays - Which assay is best for blood donor screening?" *International Journal of Laboratory Hematology*, vol. 31, no. 6, pp. 649–656, 2009.

[28] Z.-L. Fang, H. Zhuang, X.-Y. Wang, X.-M. Ge, and T. J. Harrison, "Hepatitis B virus genotypes, phylogeny and occult infection in a region with a high incidence of hepatocellular carcinoma in China," *World Journal of Gastroenterology*, vol. 10, no. 22, pp. 3264–3268, 2004.

[29] S. Datta, A. Banerjee, P. K. Chandra, A. Chowdhury, and R. Chakravarty, "Genotype, phylogenetic analysis, and transmission pattern of occult hepatitis B virus (HBV) infection in families of asymptomatic HBsAg carriers," *Journal of Medical Virology*, vol. 78, no. 1, pp. 53–59, 2006.

[30] C. M. D. Silva, C. Costi, C. Costa et al., "Low rate of occult hepatitis B virus infection among anti-HBc positive blood donors living in a low prevalence region in Brazil," *Journal of Infection*, vol. 51, no. 1, pp. 24–29, 2005.

[31] M. V. F. Sucupira, F. C. A. Mello, E. A. Santos et al., "Patterns of hepatitis B virus infection in Brazilian human immunodeficiency virus infected patients: high prevalence of occult infection and low frequency of lamivudine resistant mutations," *Memorias do Instituto Oswaldo Cruz*, vol. 101, no. 6, pp. 655–660, 2006.

[32] D. Candotti and J. P. Allain, "Transfusion-transmitted hepatitis B virus infection," *Journal of Hepatology*, vol. 51, no. 4, pp. 798–809, 2009.

[33] C. Maresch, P. J. Schluter, A. D. Wilson, and A. Sleigh, "Residual infectious disease risk in screened blood transfusion from a high-prevalence population: Santa Catarina, Brazil," *Transfusion*, vol. 48, no. 2, pp. 273–281, 2008.

[34] E. J. A. Luna, M. A. S. M. Veras, B. Flannery, and J. C. de Moraes, "Household survey of hepatitis B vaccine coverage among Brazilian children," *Vaccine*, vol. 27, no. 39, pp. 5326–5331, 2009.

Permissions

The contributors of this book come from diverse backgrounds, making this book a truly international effort. This book will bring forth new frontiers with its revolutionizing research information and detailed analysis of the nascent developments around the world.

We would like to thank all the contributing authors for lending their expertise to make the book truly unique. They have played a crucial role in the development of this book. Without their invaluable contributions this book wouldn't have been possible. They have made vital efforts to compile up to date information on the varied aspects of this subject to make this book a valuable addition to the collection of many professionals and students.

This book was conceptualized with the vision of imparting up-to-date information and advanced data in this field. To ensure the same, a matchless editorial board was set up. Every individual on the board went through rigorous rounds of assessment to prove their worth. After which they invested a large part of their time researching and compiling the most relevant data for our readers.

The editorial board has been involved in producing this book since its inception. They have spent rigorous hours researching and exploring the diverse topics which have resulted in the successful publishing of this book. They have passed on their knowledge of decades through this book. To expedite this challenging task, the publisher supported the team at every step. A small team of assistant editors was also appointed to further simplify the editing procedure and attain best results for the readers.

Apart from the editorial board, the designing team has also invested a significant amount of their time in understanding the subject and creating the most relevant covers. They scrutinized every image to scout for the most suitable representation of the subject and create an appropriate cover for the book.

The publishing team has been an ardent support to the editorial, designing and production team. Their endless efforts to recruit the best for this project, has resulted in the accomplishment of this book. They are a veteran in the field of academics and their pool of knowledge is as vast as their experience in printing. Their expertise and guidance has proved useful at every step. Their uncompromising quality standards have made this book an exceptional effort. Their encouragement from time to time has been an inspiration for everyone.

The publisher and the editorial board hope that this book will prove to be a valuable piece of knowledge for researchers, students, practitioners and scholars across the globe.

List of Contributors

Mariia Zhurova
Department of Laboratory Medicine and Pathology, University of Alberta, 8249-114 Street, Edmonton, AB, Canada T6G 2R8

John Akabutu
Alberta Cord Blood Bank, Suite 408 College Plaza, 8215-112 Street, Edmonton, AB, Canada T6G 2C8

Jason Acker
Research and Development, Canadian Blood Services, 8249-114 Street, Edmonton, AB, Canada T6G 2R8

Z. Kabiri and M. Benajiba
Centre National de Transfusion Sanguine, rue Lamfadel Cherkaoui, Madinat Al Irfane, P.O. Box 180, 10000 Rabat, Morocco

N. Dakka, H. Bellaoui and Z. Kabiri
Departement de Biologie, Faculte des Sciences, University MDV Rabat Agdal, 1014 Rabat, Morocco

K. Hajjout
Centre Regional de Transfusion Sanguine, rue Lamfadel Cherkaoui, Madinat Al Irfane, P.O. Box 180, 10000 Rabat, Morocco

M. B. Kagu and Waheed K.Moshood
North-East Zonal Centre, National Blood Transfusion Service, Maiduguri, Nigeria

M. B. Kagu, Sagir G. Ahmed, Mohammed B.Malah and Jimoh M. Kehinde
Department of Haematology & Blood Transfusion, University of Maiduguri Teaching Hospital, P.M.B.1414 Maiduguri, Borno State, Nigeria

Aisha A.Mohammed
Department of Haematology & Blood Transfusion, Aminu Kano Teaching Hospital, P. M. Bc 3452 Kano, Nigeria

Cherie Mastronardi, Qi-Long Yi, Craig Jenkins and Wanda Lefresne
Canadian Blood Services, 1800 Alta Vista Drive, Ottawa, ON, K1G 4J5, Canada K1G4J5

Peter Schubert and Elena Levin
Canadian Blood Services, Centre for Blood Research, 2350 Health Sciences Mall, University of British Columbia, Vancouver, BC, Canada V6T 1Z3

William Sheffield and Varsha Bhakta
Canadian Blood Services Research and Development, McMaster University, HSC 4N66, 1200 Main Street West, Hamilton, ON, Canada L8N 3Z5

Adele Hansen
Canadian Blood Services Research and Development, 8249 114th Street, Edmonton, AB, Canada T6G 2R8

Tamiko Stewart and Jason P. Acker
Canadian Blood Services, Network Centre for Applied Development, Suite 207, 2150Western Parkway, Vancouver, BC, Canada V6T 1V6

Richard Dillon, Yvonne Francis, Laura Cameron, Claire N. Harrison and Deepti Radia
Department of Haematology, Guy's and St Thomas' NHS Foundation Trust, London SE1 9RT, UK

IbrahimMomoh
Department of Haematology, Kings College Hospital, London SE5 9RS, UK

Rahul Chaurasia, Shamsuz Zaman, Bankim Das and Kabita Chatterjee
Department of Transfusion Medicine, All India Institute of Medical Sciences, New Delhi 110029, India

Lauren M. McDaniel
University of Pittsburgh School of Medicine, Pittsburgh, PA 15261, USA

Darrell J. Triulzi
Department of Pathology, University of Pittsburgh, Pittsburgh, PA 15213, USA

Darrell J. Triulzi and James Cramer
The Institute for Transfusion Medicine, Pittsburgh, PA 15213, USA

Brian S. Zuckerbraun, Jason L. Sperry, Andrew B. Peitzman and Matthew D. Neal
Division of Trauma and General Surgery, Department of Surgery, University of Pittsburgh, Pittsburgh, PA 15213, USA

Jay S. Raval
Department of Pathology and Laboratory Medicine, University of North Carolina, Chapel Hill, NC 27599, USA

L. Siransy Bogui, B. Dembele, Y. Sekongo, S. Abisse and S. Konaté
National Blood Transfusion Center, 52 boulevard de Marseille, BP 15 Abidjan, Cote d'Ivoire

L. Siransy Bogui, Y. Sekongo, S. Abisse and M. Sombo
Laboratory of Immunology, UFR of Medical Sciences, BP 34 Abidjan 01, Cote d'Ivoire

B. Dembele
Laboratory of Immunology, UFR of Pharmaceutical and Biological Sciences, BP 34 Abidjan 01, Cote d'Ivoire

M. Sombo
Hospital and University Centre of Cocody, BP 1843 Abidjan 08, Cote d'Ivoire

ShichunWang, Tiantian Wang, Yahan Fan, Shan Huang, Zhongmei Yi, Ruiqing Li and Shuming Zhao
Department of Blood Transfusion, Southwest Hospital, TheThird Military Medical University, No. 30 Street Gaotanyan, Chongqing 400038, China

Florent Fouelifack Ymele and Jeanne Hortense Fouedjio
Yaounde Central Hospital, P.O. Box 31186, Yaounde, Cameroon

Florent Fouelifack Ymele and Basile Keugoung
Research, Education and Health Development Associates Group (REHDAG), Dschang, Cameroon

Basile Keugoung
Ministry of Public Health, Yaounde, Cameroon

Sandrine Mendibi and Jeanne Hortense Fouedjio
Faculty of Medicine and Biomedical Sciences, University of Yaounde I, P.O. Box 1364, Yaounde, Cameroon

Nadege Kouam
Institute for Training and Demographic Research, P.O. Box 5644, Yaounde, Cameroon

Jacqueline Dongtsa Mabou
Yaounde Central Hospital, Blood Bank Unit, P.O. Box 31186, Yaounde, Cameroon

Babatunde O. Akinbami
Department of Oral and Maxillofacial Surgery, University of Port Harcourt Teaching Hospital, Choba, PMB 6173 Port Harcourt, 500004 Rivers State, Nigeria

Bisola Onajin-Obembe
Department of Anaesthesia, University of Port Harcourt Teaching Hospital, PMB 6173 Port Harcourt, 500004 Rivers State, Nigeria

Johanne Charbonneau, Marie-Soleil Cloutier and Élianne Carrier
Research Chair of Social Aspect of Blood Donation, INRS-Centre Urbanisation Culture Société, 385 Sherbrooke Street East, Montreal, QC, Canada H2X 1E3

Alani Sulaimon Akanmu, Olufemi Abiola Oyedeji, Titilope Adenike Adeyemo, and Ann Abiola Ogbenna
Department of Hematology & Blood Transfusion, Faculty of Clinical Sciences, College of Medicine, University of Lagos, PMB 12003, Lagos, Nigeria

Dietmar Enko, FranzWallner and Gabriele Halwachs-Baumann
Department of Laboratory Medicine, Central Hospital Steyr, Sierningerstraße 170, 4400 Steyr, Austria

Barbara Mayr and Claudia Habres
University of Applied Sciences for Health Professions Upper Austria, Bachelor Program Biomedical Science, Central Hospital Steyr, Sierningerstraße 170, 4400 Steyr, Austria

Sana Saleem, Anum Wasim, Sidra Sabih, Ayisha Farooq Khan, Madiha Hasan Rizvi, Umaima Ayesha Jillani, Mujtaba Jamal Syed, Madiha Mumtaz, Abdul Moid Shehzad, Om Dawani, Saima Khan, Sheheryar Munir, Nava Asad and Abdul Nafey Kazi
Dow Medical College, Dow University of Health Sciences, Karachi 74200, Pakistan

Yasmeen Mumtaz
Department of Community Medicine, Dow Medical College, Dow University of Health Sciences, Karachi 74200, Pakistan

Leibovici Vera
Department of Dermatology, Hadassah-Hebrew University Hospital, P.O. Box 12018, Jersalem, Israel

Donchin Milka
Brown School of Public Health, Hadassah University Hospital, Jersalem, Israel

Strauss-Liviatan Nurith
Private Practice, P.O. Box 84027, 90805 Mevaseret Zion, Israel

Shinar Eilat
Magen David Adom National Blood Services, 52621 Ramat Gan, Israel

Pule Ishmael Pule, Boitshwarelo Rachaba, Mgaywa Gilbert Mjungu Damas Magafu and Dereje Habte
Faculty of Medicine, University of Botswana, Private Bag 00713, Gaborone, Botswana

A. Benahadi, S. Boulahdid, B. Adouani, A. Laouina, K. Hajjout, M. Benajiba and R. Alami
Centre National de Transfusion Sanguine, Rue Lamfadal Charkaoui, Madinat Al Irfane, BP 180, Rabat, Morocco

A. Benahadi, S. Boulahdid, B. Adouani, A. Laouina, A. Mokhtari and A. Soulaymani
Laboratoire de Génétique et de Biométrie, Faculté des Sciences, University Ibn Tofaïl, Kenitra, Morocco

Leonard Kouegnigan Rerambiah, Rose Marlène Mouguiama, Phanie Brunelle Issanga, Axel Sydney Biyoghe, Sylvestre Akone Assembe and Joel Fleury Djoba Siawaya
Centre National de Transfusion Sanguine (CNTS), Libreville, Gabon

Laurence Essola Rerambiah
Service d'Anesthésie-Réanimation du Centre Hospitalier Universitaire de Libreville, Libreville, Gabon

Armel Mbourou Etomba
Centre National d'Hémodialyse de Libreville, Libreville, Gabon

Batchelili Batchilili
Centre Hospitalier Universitaire d'Angondjé, Libreville, Gabon

Joel Fleury Djoba Siawaya
Unité de Recherche et deDiagnostic Spécialisé/Laboratoire National de Santé Publique (URDS/LNSP), Libreville, Gabon

Nada Hosny, Fikry Goubran, Basma BadrEldin Hasan and Noha Kamel
Clinical Pathology Department, Faculty of Medicine, Suez Canal University, Ismailia 41522, Egypt

Håkon Reikvam
Department of Haematology, Institute of Internal Medicine, University of Bergen, 5021 Bergen, Norway

Kjersti Svendheim, Anne S. Røsvik and Tor Hervig
Department of Immunology and Transfusion Medicine, Haukeland University Hospital, 5021 Bergen, Norway

Anne S. Røsvik and Tor Hervig
Gades Institute, University of Bergen, 5021 Bergen, Norway

Benedict Nwogoh and Usimenahon Aigberadion
Department of Haematology and Blood Transfusion, University of Benin Teaching Hospital, P.M.B 1111, Benin City 300283, Nigeria

Alexander Ikenna Nwannadi
Department of Haematology, Benue State University, Makurdi 102119, Nigeria

Tadesse Belayneh and Zewditu Abdissa
Department of Medical Anesthesiology, College of Medicine and Health Sciences, University of Gondar, Kebele 16, P.O. Box 196, Gondar, Ethiopia

Gashaw Messele
Department of Surgery, College of Medicine and Health Sciences, University of Gondar, Kebele 16, P.O. Box 196, Gondar, Ethiopia

Birehanemeskel Tegene
Department of Medical Microbiology, College of Medicine and Health Sciences, University of Gondar, Kebele 16, P.O. Box 196, Gondar, Ethiopia

Gaston Godin
Research Group on Behavior and Health, Laval University, FSI-Vandry, Room3493, Quebec City, QC, Canada G1V 0A6ss

Marc Germain
Medical Affairs, Héma-Québec, 1070, avenue des Sciences-de-la-Vie, Québec City, QC, Canada G1V 5C3

Adelbert B. James, Cassandra D. Josephson, Marta I. Castillejo and John D. Roback
Department of Pathology and Laboratory Medicine, Center for Transfusion and Cellular Therapies, Emory University School of Medicine, Atlanta, GA 30322, USA

George B. Schreiber
Independent Consultant, Bethesda, MD 20814, USA

Narcisse Elenga
Pediatric Unit, Cayenne Hospital, rue des Flamboyants, BP 6006, 97306 Cayenne Cedex, French Guiana

Loic Niel
French Guianese Blood Agency, Cayenne Hospital, rue des Flamboyants, BP 6006, 97306 Cayenne Cedex, French Guiana

Wilhellmuss I. Mauka, Sia E. Msuya and Rune N. Philemon
Institute of Public Health, Department of Community Medicine, Kilimanjaro Christian Medical University College, P.O. Box 2240, Moshi, Tanzania

Wilhellmuss I. Mauka
Northern Zone Blood Transfusion Centre, P.O. Box 823, Moshi, Tanzania

Michael J. Mahande and Sia E. Msuya
Institute of Public Health, Department of Epidemiology and Biostatistics, Kilimanjaro Christian Medical University College, Moshi, Tanzania

Sia E. Msuya
Department of Community Medicine, Kilimanjaro Christian Medical Centre, Moshi, Tanzania

Rune N. Philemon
Department of Pediatrics, Kilimanjaro Christian Centre, Moshi, Tanzania

Antonio Crescibene
Orthopedics and Traumatology Unit, San Francesco di Paola Hospital, Via Promintesta, 87027 Paola, Italy

Marcello Napolitano
Immunohaematology and Transfusion Medicine Unit, Cosenza Hospital, Via Migliori, 87100 Cosenza, Italy

Raffaella Sbano
Radiology Unit, San Francesco di Paola Hospital, Via Promintesta, 87027 Paola, Italy

Enrico Costabile
Orthopedics and Traumatology Unit, Cosenza Hospital, Via Migliori, 87100 Cosenza, Italy

Hesham Almolla
Radiology Unit, Cosenza Hospital, Via Migliori, 87100 Cosenza, Italy

I.Majid, S. Alshryda, B. Somanchi, E. Morakis and A. Foster
Royal Manchester Children Hospital, Central Manchester University Hospitals, Oxford Road, Manchester M13 9WL, UK

A. Crescibene, F. Martire and M. Candela
Orthopedics and Traumatology Unit, San Francesco di Paola Hospital, Azienda Sanitaria Provinciale di Cosenza, Via Promintesta, 87027 Paola, Italy

P. Gigliotti
Kidney and Transplantation Research Center, Azienda Ospedaliera di Cosenza, Via Felice Migliori, 87100 Cosenza, Italy

A. Rende
Transfusion Medicine Unit, San Francesco di Paola Hospital, Azienda Sanitaria Provinciale di Cosenza, Via Promintesta, 87027 Paola, Italy

Lello Zolla and Angelo D'Alessandro
Department of Ecological and Biological Sciences, Tuscia University, Largo dell'Universitá, snc, 01100 Viterbo, Italy

P. J. M. van den Burg
Sanquin blood Supply, Plesmanlaan 125, 1066 CX Amsterdam, The Netherlands

K.Magnussen
Centre for Donor-Haemoglobin and Iron, Blood Bank, Department of Clinical Immunology, sec. 526, Rigshospitalet and Hvidovre Hospital, The Capital Region, 2650 Hvidovre, Denmark

Mahdi Motififard, Mohammad Ali Tahririan, Mehdi Saneie, Sajad Badiei and Amin Nemati
Orthopedic Department, Kashani Teaching Hospital, Isfahan University of Medical Sciences, Isfahan, Iran

Sajad Badiei and Amin Nemati
Students Research Center, Isfahan University of Medical Sciences, Isfahan, Iran

M. N. Noor Haslina, M. Y. Shafini, B. Rosnah, R. Marini, S. Salamah and M. A. Mohd Fakhri
Transfusion Medicine Unit, Hospital Universiti Sains Malaysia, 16150 Kubang Kerian, Kelantan, Malaysia

Sean Robinson, Owen McGonigle, Sam Volin, Yung-Chi Sung, Matthew Moore, Charles Cassidy and Eric Smith
Department of Orthopaedic Surgery, Tufts Medical Center, Boston, MA 02111, USA

Emil Kupek
Departamento de Saúde Pública/CCS, Universidade Federal de Santa Catarina, 88040-900 Florianopolis, SC, Brazil

Andrea Petry
Hematology and Hemotherapy Center of Santa Catarina (HEMOSC), Florianopolis, SC, Brazil

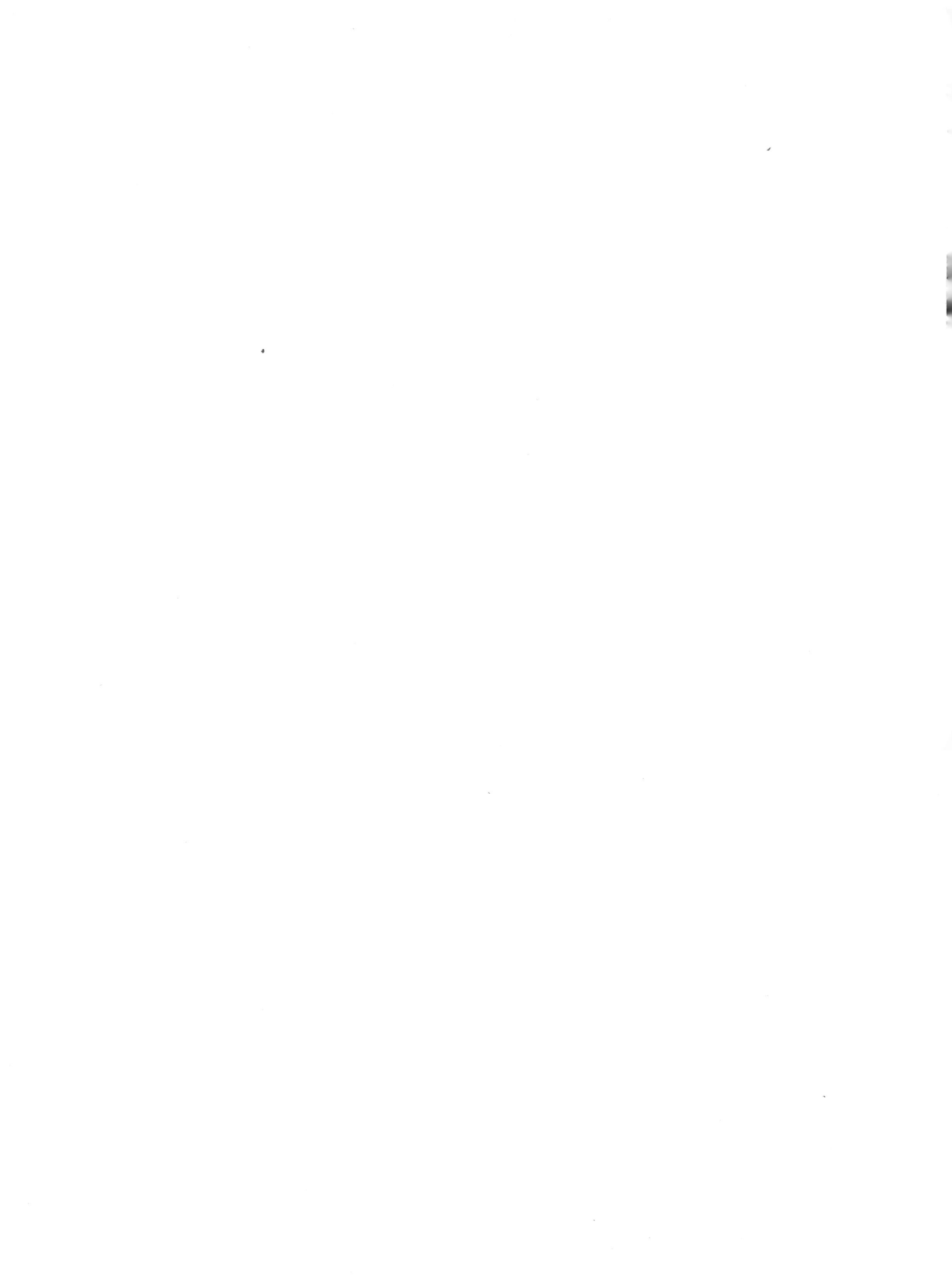